Monoclonal Antibodies and T Cell Products

Editor

David H. Katz, M. D.

President and Director
Medical Biology Institute
La Jolla, California

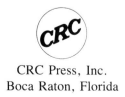

CRC Press, Inc.
Boca Raton, Florida

Library of Congress Cataloging in Publication Data

Main entry under title:

Monoclonal antibodies and T cell products.

   Includes bibliographies and index.
   1. Antibodies, Monoclonal. 2. T cells.
I. Katz, David H. [DNLM: 1. Antibodies.
2. Hybrid cells—Immunology. 3. T-Lymphocytes
—Immunology. QW 575 M749]
QR186.85.M658   616.07′9   81-21604
ISBN 0-8493-6580-5   AACR2

Direct all inquiries to CRC Press, Inc., 2000 Corporate Blvd., N.W., Boca Raton, Florida 33431.

©1982 by CRC Press, Inc.

International Standard Book Number 0-8493-6580-5

Library of Congress Card Number 81-21604
Printed in the United States

PREFACE

This monograph is comprised of a selective collection of review chapters on the topical subject of hybridomas. This relatively new technology, developed by Cesar Milstein and Georges Köhler in 1975, promises to revolutionize certain aspects of biomedical research and the application of research findings into the public domain. Not only has the hybridoma technology been utilized for construction of cell lines producing monoclonal antibodies, but more recently T cell hybridomas secreting biological products of potential usefulness have been constructed in several different laboratories around the world. This monograph thus focuses on both types of lymphoid hybridomas. Although much has been written about hybridoma technology and its applications in recent years, this is a rapidly evolving field of basic research that, thereby, deserves frequent updating to keep both active and interested investigators abreast of the progress being made in the area. It is the authors' hope that this volume serves such a useful purpose.

THE EDITOR

David H. Katz, M.D., received his Bachelor of Arts degree in Biology at the University of Virginia, Charlottesville, in 1963. He obtained his M.D. degree at Duke University Medical School in 1968, following which he obtained postdoctoral house-staff clinical training in internal medicine on the Osler Medical Service at Johns Hopkins Hospital. After completion of his internship and fellowship in Medicine at Hopkins, Dr. Katz spent two years as Staff Associate in the Laboratory of Immunology at the National Institute of Allergy and Infectious Diseases of the NIH in Bethesda, Maryland. His first faculty appointment came in 1971 in the Department of Pathology at Harvard Medical School in Boston, Massachusetts. While on the Faculty of Medicine at Harvard from 1971 to 1976, Dr. Katz rose to the rank of Associate Professor. In 1976, Dr. Katz left Harvard to found a new Department of Cellular and Developmental Immunology at Scripps Clinic and Research Foundation, La Jolla, California. In early 1982, Dr. Katz left Scripps Clinic to undertake new responsibilities as President and Director of the newly created Medical Biology Institute, also located in La Jolla.

Dr. Katz has a wide range of interests in basic immunological research including mechanisms of cell–cell interactions and communication, genetic control of cell differentiation and function, and the regulation of IgE responses in animals and man. He is the author of over 200 publications, including one textbook entitled *Lymphocyte Differentiation, Recognition and Regulation,* published by Academic Press. In addition to serving on the editorial boards of eight journals, Dr. Katz is a Member of the National Board of Trustees and Medical Scientific Advisory Board of the Leukemia Society of America and is a member of the National Cancer Institute's Cancer Special Program Advisory Council.

ACKNOWLEDGMENTS

The Editor wishes to acknowledge the splendid assistance of Beverly Burgess, Lucy Gunnill, and Rebecca Mead in organizing this monograph.

CONTRIBUTORS

Amnon Altman, Ph.D.
Associate Member
Department of Immunology
Medical Biology Institute
La Jolla, California

John H. Elder, Ph.D.
Assistant Member II
Department of Immunopathology
Scripps Clinic and Research Foundation
La Jolla, California

Zelig Eshhar, Ph.D.
Senior Scientist
Department of Chemical Immunology
The Weizmann Institute of Science
Rehovot, Israel

Gideon Goldstein, M.D., Ph.D.
Vice President
Immunobiology Division
Ortho Pharmaceutical Corporation
Raritan, New Jersey

Perrie Hausman, Ph.D.
Cornell University Medical College
New York, New York

David H. Katz, M.D.
President and Director
Medical Biology Institute
La Jolla, California

John Lifter, Ph.D.
Immunobiology Division
Ortho Pharmaceutical Corporation
Raritan, New Jersey

Fu-Tong Liu, Ph.D.
Associate Member
Department of Immunology
Medical Biology Institute
La Jolla, California

Robert Mittler, Ph.D.
Immunobiology Division
Ortho Pharmaceutical Corporation
Raritan, New Jersey

Henry L. Niman, Ph.D.
Assistant Member
Department of Immunopathology
Scripps Clinic and Research Foundation
La Jolla, California

Howard Raff, Ph.D.
Department of Microbiology/
Immunology
University of Washington
Seattle, Washington

Joyce Rauch, Ph.D.
Research Associate
Montreal General Hospital Research
Institute
Montreal, Quebec, Canada

Bruce Richardson, M.D., Ph.D.
University of California
Research Associate
Howard Hughes Medical Institute
San Francisco, California

Robert D. Schreiber
Department of Molecular Immunology
Scripps Clinic and Research Foundation
La Jolla, California

Robert S. Schwartz, M.D.
Director
Cancer Research Center
Professor of Medicine
Tufts University School of Medicine
Director, Hematology/Oncology
Tufts-New England Medical Center
Boston, Massachusetts

John D. Stobo, M.D.
Associate Professor of Medicine
University of California
Head,
Section of Rheumatology/Clinical
Immunology
Moffitt Hospital
San Francisco, California

B. David Stollar, M.D.
Professor
Department of Biochemistry and
Pharmacology
Tufts University School of Medicine
Boston, Massachusetts

TABLE OF CONTENTS

Chapter 1
Monoclonal Antibodies (mAbs) as Useful Research and Diagnostic Probes 1
Fu-Tong Liu and David H. Katz

Chapter 2
mAbs as Probes of Protein Structure: Molecular Diversity Among the
Envelope Glycoproteins (gp70s) of the Murine Retroviruses 23
Henry L. Niman and John H. Elder

Chapter 3
Use of mAbs to Probe the Function and Specificity of Cells Participating
in the Autologous Mixed Lymphocyte Reaction (AMLR) 53
Bruce Richardson, Perrie Hausman, Howard Raff, and John Stobo

Chapter 4
mAbs to Human Lymphocyte Surface Antigens 71
Gideon Goldstein, John Lifter, and Robert Mittler

Chapter 5
Applications of Hybridoma Technology to Autoimmunity 91
Joyce Rauch, Robert S. Schwartz, and B. David Stollar

Chapter 6
Functional T Cell Hybridomas Producing Nonspecific Immunoregulatory Factors 113
Amnon Altman, Robert D. Schreiber, and David H. Katz

Chapter 7
Functional T Cell Hybridomas Producing Antigen–Specific
Immunoregulatory Factors 133
Zelig Eshhar

Index 171

Chapter 1

MONOCLONAL ANTIBODIES (mAbs) AS USEFUL RESEARCH AND DIAGNOSTIC PROBES

Fu-Tong Liu and David H. Katz

TABLE OF CONTENTS

I.   Introduction 2

II.   mAbs of Defined Immunoglobulin (Ig) Classes and Subclasses 2
     A.   Murine IgE 2
     B.   Other Ig Classes 5

III.   mAbs Specific for Receptors and Soluble Proteins 5
     A.   mAbs as Useful Reagents for Purification of Proteins 6
     B.   mAbs as Probes to Study Structure-Function Relationship of
          Soluble Proteins 7
          1.   β-Galactosidase 7
          2.   Complement Components 8
     C.   mAbs as Probes to Study the Structure–Function Relationship
          of Biological Receptors 8
          1.   Acetylcholine Receptor 8
          2.   Ig FcR 9
          3.   Other Systems 10
     D.   mAbs as Probes to Study Multiprotein Complexes 11

IV.   Identification of Cell Surface Markers by mAbs 11

V.   mAbs as Diagnostic Probes 12
     A.   Detection of Human Peptides and Proteins 13
     B.   Detection of Membrane Proteins 13
     C.   Immunodiagnosis of Tumors 14
     D.   Immunodiagnosis of Viral, Bacterial, and Parasitic Infections 14
          1.   Immunodiagnosis of Hepatitis B (HBs) 14
          2.   Immunoassay for Streptococcal Antigen 15
          3.   Immunodiagnosis of Parasitic Infections 15

VI.   Conclusion 16

Acknowledgments 17

References 17

I. INTRODUCTION

The hybridoma technique for obtaining a monoclonal antibody of defined specificity, as first reported by Köhler and Milstein,[1] has an enormous impact on many areas of biological and medical research. Table 1 is a summary of various research areas where mAb has been applied. The number of publications pertaining to hybridomas is amazingly large and a thorough review of the use of mAb in research is almost impossible. There are already a few review books and many review papers on various applications of the hybridoma technology. Some of these references are included in Table 1.[2–10] In this chapter, we would like to make a general review of the use of mAb as research and diagnostic probes using a few examples in each area.

II. mAbs OF DEFINED IMMUNOGLOBULIN (Ig) CLASSES AND SUBCLASSES

In the next two sections, many advantages of mAb over conventional polyclonal antibodies will be pointed out. Although it is obvious that mAb is by far the superior reagent for various purposes, many of these problems can still be tackled to a certain extent with conventional antibodies. However, if one needs to have homogeneous Ig of certain classes or subclasses, the hybridoma technique (or any other technique) providing mAb may be the only resort. This is especially true if one deals with an Ig class present only in minute quantities, such as IgE.

A. Murine IgE

The discovery of IgE has contributed significantly to the understanding of human immediate hypersensitivity reactions. Unlike most Ig classes, IgE is normally present in very low concentrations in serum. Our current knowledge of the physicochemical properties and biological function of IgE has substantially benefited from the discovery of rare IgE-producing myelomas of the human and rat. However, none of the available human or rat IgE myeloma proteins has a known antigenic specificity. Although the mouse has been a good model system for the study of mechanisms and regulation of IgE synthesis, such studies have been hampered due to the lack of any known IgE-producing murine myelomas.

Bottcher et al.[11] reported the successful production of a hybridoma-secreting ovalbumin (OA)-specific murine IgE antibody. In this work, spleen and mesenteric lymph node cells from mice immunized 3 to 4 times with OA adsorbed on aluminum hydroxide gel (alum) were fused to myeloma cells. More than 2000 hybrid cell lines were screened and only one was found positive as demonstrated by the passive cutaneous anaphylaxis (PCA) test on rats. This indicates the low frequency of IgE-producing cells in immune mice. Subsequently, Bottcher et al.,[12] Eshhar et al.,[13] and Liu et al.[14] reported hybridomas secreting anti-2, 4-dinitrophenyl (DNP) murine IgE, and thus obtained sources for generating large amounts of homogeneous IgE antibody specific for a defined determinant. In the latter two studies, donor cells for fusion were obtained from an adoptive transfer protocol in which spleen cells from mice hyperimmunized with DNP-carrier protein conjugates were injected in sublethally irradiated mice that were then boosted with the antigen. This protocol is particularly advantageous in generating spleen cell populations with an exceptionally high frequency of DNP-specific IgE-secreting precursors (as well as cells of other Ig isotypes with anti-DNP specificity). This, in turn, resulted in a much higher frequency of IgE-secreting hybridomas than other protocols might have provided. For example, Liu et al. reported 2 out of the 58 hybrid

3

Table 1
MONOCLONAL ANTIBODIES AS USEFUL RESEARCH AND DIAGNOSTIC PROBES

Antigen	Application of mAb	Ref.
Intracellular and secretory peptides and proteins (hormones, enzymes, structural proteins, etc.)	Isolation of antigens Detection of antigens (research and clinic) Study of structure-function relationship	See sect. III
Cell surface antigens Receptors (e.g., Ig receptors, hormone receptors, etc.)	(Same as above) Study of expression and modulation of the receptor Characterization of disease states	See sect. III
Histocompatibility antigens	Isolation of the protein Establish the structure of the protein Tissue typing	2, 3
Tumor antigens	Isolation of proteins for structural studies Diagnosis Therapy	4
Differentiation antigens (on lymphocytes, monocytes, neurons, embryos, etc.)	Identification of unique antigens Study of the distribution of cell types Study of the development of cell types in developing tissues Isolation of various cell types Study of the function of various cell types Isolation of differentiation antigens and study of their functions	5, 6

Microorganisms (viruses, bacteria, and parasites)	Identification of surface antigens
	Isolation of antigens
	  For clinical use
	  For structural studies
	Diagnosis
	Therapy
		7–10

lines screened were secreting IgE and one of them became a permanent IgE-secreting cell line.[14]

The isolated IgE protein has been used to analyze the physicochemical characteristics of murine IgE.[14] It has a molecular weight of approximately 180,000 and a carbohydrate content of 13%, similar to those of human and rat IgE. The heavy chain has a mobility on SDS-PAGE similar to human and rat IgE heavy chain and, therefore, may also contain four constant region domains. The proteins have a high affinity for DNP. Association constants of $6.5 \times 10^7 \, M^{-1}$ and $1.4 \times 10^8 \, M^{-1}$ at 25°C were established for two separate antibodies, respectively.[13,14] More information about the structure and structure-function relationship of murine IgE should be generated in the future since a large amount of the protein can now be obtained from the hybridoma cell lines.

The hybridoma IgE has already been found useful to probe Fc receptors (FcR) of IgE (FcRε) on various cell types. Since IgE with anti-DNP specificity is available, indicator cells for a rosette-forming cell assay for detecting FcRε-bearing (FcRε+) cells can be readily prepared by derivatizing sheep red blood cells (SRBC) with trinitrophenyl (TNP) and then coating such cells with anti-DNP IgE. A very low number of FcRε+ lymphocyte was detectable in spleen, mesenteric lymph node, and thymus of normal mice. The number of FcRε+ lymphocyte was found to increase in mice infected with nematode, *Nippostrongylus Brasiliensis*,[15] or in mice carrying progressively growing IgE-secreting hybridoma cells.[93] Increased frequencies of FcRε+ lymphocytes were found in cultured lymphocytes that were either exposed to the monoclonal IgE or stimulated in two way mixed lymphocyte reaction.[15] FcRε+ lymphocytes were found in both B and T cell populations. These findings thus support observations made in the human and in the rat systems. Moreover, it was found that the induction of FcRε+ in lymphocytes can be suppressed by a material, suppressive factor of allergy (SFA)[15] that has previously been demonstrated to suppress IgE synthesis in vivo. Thus, the availability of murine monoclonal IgE has contributed to increasing our understanding of the murine IgE system and will obviously contribute even more to the understanding of regulation of IgE synthesis in the future.

The monoclonal IgE antibodies were demonstrated to mediate antigen-induced triggering of degranulation of mast cells and basophils in vivo and in vitro.[14] More recently a monoclonal IgE was used to demonstrate the presence of FcRε on a pure population of mouse mast cells grown out of bone marrow cells in vitro and the release of histamine when these cells were sensitized with IgE and triggered with anti-IgE.[16] Since monoclonal anti-DNP IgE has relatively high-binding affinity, it is now feasible to study the molecular mechanism of mast cell triggering when surface-bound IgE antibody molecules react with their specific ligand. Such studies should complement the previous studies performed in many laboratories using myeloma IgE-anti-IgE or polyclonal serum IgE-antigen systems.

Before monoclonal IgE became available, IgE-specific antibody reagents had been very difficult to obtain. Therefore, quantitation of antigen-specific IgE has relied largely on an in vivo bioassay, PCA. Both rabbit and goat anti-mouse IgE antibodies are now available and are specific for IgE after adsorption with normal mouse serum. With the use of anti-IgE reagents and monoclonal IgE, sensitive radioimmunoassays (RIA) both for total IgE and antigen-specific IgE have been developed.[14] Both assays employ flexible polyvinyl 96-well microtiter plates that are coated with either antigen or the IgG fraction from goat anti-mouse IgE serum for RIA for antigen-specific IgE and total IgE, respectively. After incubation with the test sample, adsorbed IgE proteins were detected with rabbit anti-mouse IgE antibodies followed by radiolabeled goat anti-rabbit IgG (GARG). Sensitivities of 10 to 100 pg/ml were obtained for both RIAs. An enzyme-linked immunosorbent assay (ELISA) for murine IgE has also been recently reported.[17]

In this assay, GARG conjugated with β-galactosidase was used instead of radiolabeled antibodies and the assay was developed with the substrate of the enzyme, o-nitrophenylgalactopyranoside. Sensitivity to detect 200 pg/ml of DNP-specific IgE has been obtained in this ELISA assay. Both RIA and ELISA have been found applicable for quantitating murine IgE in serum and can be expected to completely replace the PCA technique in the future.

A similar solid-phase RIA using ^{125}I-labeled goat anti-mouse IgE (GAME) antibodies with detection sensitivity of 0.5 ng/ml was reported by Kelly et al.[18] The GAME used was also obtained through immunization with purified hybridoma IgE.

B. Other Ig Classes

There is still considerable controversy on the existence of Fc receptor (FcR) for various Ig classes and subclasses on various cell types and their functions. FcR for almost all the classes and subclasses have been identified on lymphocytes, monocytes, and macrophages. These receptors are associated with at least four different functions: regulation of antibody synthesis by FcR-bearing lymphocyte, degranulation of mast cells and basophils, phagocytosis by macrophages, and antibody-dependent cytolysis of target cells. Questions of whether FcR for each class or subclass is a distinct entity, and which class or subclass of antibody mediates certain functions, have always existed. In the past, solutions to these questions have been approached by using either Ig purified from serum or myeloma proteins of known classes. The hybridoma technique has now provided homogeneous antibodies of defined specificity and Ig class and should facilitate these studies.

Diamond et al.[19] used anti-SRBC IgG_{2a} and IgG_{2b} monoclonal antibodies to examine FcR on macrophage-like cell lines and peritoneal macrophages. Since the antibodies used have known antigen-specificity, naturally occurring antigen-antibody complexes can be used and thus the ambiguities that arise when artificially aggregated Ig or heterogeneous antibodies are used can be avoided. It was concluded from these studies that IgG_{2a} and IgG_{2b} antigen-antibody complexes are bound to mouse macrophages and phagocytosed through functionally distinct FcR, thus confirming conclusions from previous studies using myeloma proteins.

Greenberg and Lydyard[20] used murine monoclonal IgG_1 and IgM anti-DNP antibodies to examine their ability to mediate cytolysis by effector cells. They found that BALB/c mouse spleen cells were able to kill trinitrophenyl (TNP)-coated SRBC via IgG_1 anti-DNP antibody. The cytotoxicity was inhibited by IgG, but not by IgM or IgA myeloma proteins, and IgG_{2a} was found to be more effective than IgG_1. On the other hand, three different IgM anti-DNP antibodies were found unable to mediate cytolysis of target cells by mouse effector cells. Similarly, Ralph et al.[21] used hybridoma antibodies of IgG_1, IgG_{2a}, IgG_{2b}, and IgG_3 subclasses of specificity to SRBC to study macrophage phagocytosis and lysis of erythrocytes. It was concluded that all classes of murine IgG antibody mediate these functions.

Studies of various FcR can also be benefited by hybridoma mAbs specific for the receptor proteins. Such studies are discussed in Section III.

III. mAbs SPECIFIC FOR RECEPTORS AND SOLUBLE PROTEINS

Hybridoma technology has brought a new dimension to biochemical research. mAb to many proteins have been reported. These mAbs provide tools for purification of proteins, probing the structure of proteins, studying structure-function relationships, detection of proteins in solutions by immunoassays, and detection of proteins in various tissues by immunocytochemistry.

There are many advantages of mAb over conventional polyclonal antibody such as:

1. Specificity. By virtue of cloning, each mAb is derived from a single clone of B cells and should have specificity for one determinant, or chemical structure, and other closely related structures. Therefore, if a mAb binds two different proteins or subunits, the presence of identical or closely related structures can be concluded. In contrast, one always has to worry about contaminants in a conventional antiserum before making such a conclusion.

2. The most attractive feature of hybridoma technique for producing mAb for use in biochemistry, or any area for that matter, is that one can start with crude or partially purified antigens for immunization. The antibody responses will be multispecific. However, the cloning and selection procedures replace the job necessary for purification of antigens that may be very difficult and sometimes even impossible. Furthermore, once a specific mAb is obtained, it can then be used for affinity purification of the specific protein of interest.

3. Once a stable clone-secreting desired mAb is obtained, it can be propagated in culture or passaged in appropriate animals to obtain a large quantity of ascites fluids. Antibodies can be easily purified and obtained in large quantitites. Batch variations that are often encountered with conventional antisera can be avoided.

In the following section, the authors would like to use a few examples to illustrate the above-mentioned points.

A. mAbs as Useful Reagents for Purification of Proteins

Before the usefulness of mAb in probing structure and function of proteins is discussed, it is appropriate to first illustrate point 2 mentioned above. The theoretical advantage of the hybridoma technology that allows the production of specific antibodies starting with crude antigens is best exemplified with mAb to human leukocyte interferon (IF) reported by Secher and Burke.[22] These investigators used as immunogen a preparation containing IF at a concentration of 0.1 to 1% of total proteins. Hybridoma cultures were screened for neutralization of the inhibitory activity of IF on viral RNA synthesis. Positive cultures were subcloned. Cultures were tested for the presence of secreted mouse Ig using a reverse plaque assay in addition to anti-IF activity. One clone was finally identified and isolated.

This report also serves as a good example that antibodies obtained starting with an impure antigen preparation can then be used to purify the antigen of interest. Furthermore, using the mAb and the purified antigen, an immunoassay can be developed for detection of the antigen. Using an immunoadsorbent composed of mAb to IF and a solid support, Secher and Burke[22] found that IF could be purified up to 5000-fold in a single step. mAb can, therefore, be used for large-scale purification of human leukocyte IF for clinical and research use.

An RIA for human IF was developed by Secher[23] using mAb. Polyclonal sheep anti-IF antibody was attached to polystyrene solid phase that was then incubated with an IF-containing sample. The adsorbed IF was then detected with ^{125}I-labeled mAb. The assay could be used to measure IF in human serum and IF concentrations of ≥ 50 U/ml^{-1} were readily measured. This type of assay should be able to replace the complex biological assays that are laborious and subject to inherent variability.

More recently, Staehelin et al.[24] also reported production of 13 hybridoma lines secreting mAb to the human leukocyte IFs. They found the mAbs exhibited different binding to purified IF species which is consistent with the structural multiplicity of the human leukocyte IFs. These mAbs will be useful as probes into structure of the proteins and for their purification and detection.

The success of obtaining mAb to IF and applying it to the isolation and detection of the protein should be a great encouragement to researchers concerned with lymphokines and monokines. Numerous lymphokine and monokine activities have been reported in the literature. The different names given to these activities are based on biological assay systems. It would not be surprising to find that many of these activities are exerted by the same or highly related molecule. Since the proteins are all present in very low concentrations in culture, purification of them has been very difficult. Therefore, establishment of chemical relatedness among different activities has been lacking. The availability of mAb will definitely facilitate the purification of various lymphokines and monokines and establish the chemical identity of each activity. Eventually, these mAbs should be useful for the study of the function of these biological factors. Furthermore, sensitive immunoassays can be developed for these proteins using mAbs similar to that developed for IF. These assays will be very useful in establishing the existence and the levels of these activities in physiological conditions. mAbs to several lymphokines including osteoclast-activating factor,[25,26] T cell replacing factor,[27] lymphocyte activiting factor (LAF or IL-1; Interleukin 1[28]) and T cell growth factor (TCGF or IL-2; Interleukin 2)[29] have already been prepared.

It is to be noted that various hybridomas secreting different lymphokines and monokines have been obtained (reviewed in Chapter 7). This should facilitate the partial purification of the relevant proteins to be used to produce mAb.

B. mAbs as Probes to Study Structure-Function Relationship of Soluble Proteins

A characteristic of mAb to proteins (or any complex antigen) that is hardly matched by polyclonal antibodies and that made it highly useful in investigations described in the next two subsections, is its monospecificity. A mAb, once the monoclonality is proved, reacts only with one kind of antigenic determinant. This is in contrast to conventional antisera that are polyspecific since they are composed of numerous antibodies each recognizing different determinants.

1. β-Galactosidase

An interesting example of use of mAb for probing structure and function of an enzyme concerns the case of β-galactosidase. Frackelton and Rotman[30] analyzed more than 300 cultures of hybridomas producing murine antibodies against β-D-galactosidase. Four types of functionally different mAbs were produced:

1. Activating. The mAb increases the enzymatic activity of a genetically defective β-D-galactosidase.
2. Inactivating. The mAb decreases the activity of the normal enzyme.
3. Protecting. The mAb prevents heat denaturation of normal enzyme.
4. Null. The mAb binds to the enzyme but does not exhibit any of the above three functions.

Analysis of the mAbs established that each of the four functions are attributable to distinct antibodies.

The inactivating mAbs are useful probes for the function of the enzyme. The possibility that one of the inactivating mAb inactivates by blocking the catalytic site was ruled out since the antibody did not affect the Km of the enzyme. Furthermore, binding of the substrate or a substrate analog did not affect binding of this mAb to the enzyme. The binding site of this type of mAb and its effect on the conformational structure of the enzyme is worth investigating.

Accolla et al.[31] also reported mAbs that mediate activation of genetically defective β-galactosidase. Three out of six mAbs established were found to activate defective enzymes produced by strains of *Escherichia coli* carrying Z-gene point mutations. Analysis of these mAbs provided direct evidence that the enzyme-activation reaction is a single-hit event in which one antibody site favors the correct conformation of one active center of the enzyme. Because each activating mAb is able to activate several, but not all point mutants tested, it was concluded that the correction of the genetic defect is produced by binding key sites of the protein three-dimensional structure rather than the sites affected by the mutation. mAbs to many other enzymes have been reported. Studies with these antibodies should provide interesting insights into the structure-function relationships of these enzymes in the near future.

2. Complement Components

mAbs made to a complement component, C3, turned out to be very useful for the study of the structure and function of this important protein, C3 is the central component of the complement system. It participates in the classical and the alternative pathways and has multiple biological activities. Tamerius et al.[32] have generated over 100 clones of hybridomas secreting mAbs to human C3b, a large fragment of C3. Twenty-four of the mAbs were analyzed for their activity for inhibiting the biological activities of C3b. It is known that C3b has sites for combination with Factor B to form the precursor of the alternative pathway C3 convertase and with Factor H (or β1H globulin) that leads to cleavage of C3b by the C3b inactivator. C3b also has a site for binding of properdin. By a radioassay, it was found that some mAbs inhibited binding of either one of Factor H or properdin to C3b, some inhibited both and some failed to inhibit at all. None of the mAbs inhibited binding of Factor B to C3b, although polyclonal anti-C3b did. With peptide mapping techniques, as described below for acetylcholine receptors (AChR), one should be able to relate structure and functions to a high definition. This is a good example of how mAb can provide a tool for researchers to localize regions responsible for certain functions. mAbs to human C3 have also been reported by Lachmann et al.[33] and Whitehead et al.[34]

C. mAbs as Probes to Study the Structure-Function Relationship of Biological Receptors

The monospecificity feature of mAb has also made it ideal to study biological receptors. Some examples are listed below.

1. Acetylcholine Receptor

mAb has been used extensively in the study of AChR. Five research groups have reported mAbs to AChR.[35-39] Gomez et al.[35] have obtained 11 mAbs to AChR of *Torpedo californica*. They can be grouped into four general categories of binding specificities: blockade only by α-bungarotoxin, partial blockade by various cholinergic ligands, increased titer in the presence of α-bungarotoxin and benzoquinonium chloride, and absence of effect by any ligand. James et al.[38] also reported mAbs directed against the neurotransmitter binding site of AChR that inhibits the binding of α-bungarotoxin. They have also obtained a mAb the binding of which is partially affected by the presence of the nicotinic agonist, carbamylcholine but not toxin. One possible explanation is that the antibody binds to a determinant affected by conformational changes induced in AChR by binding of the agonist. Lennon et al.[37] reported the use of mAbs to AChR for isolation of the receptor.

Tzartos and Lindstrom and co-workers[39–41] have generated a library of more than 70 clones secreting mAb to *Torpedo* AChR and have used these antibodies to characterize the structure of the receptor extensively. AChR consists of four glycoprotein subunits in the ratio of $\alpha_2\beta\gamma\delta$. By using these antibodies as probes it was concluded that a similar antigenic determinant is present on the α and β subunits and another similar determinant is present on both γ and δ subunits. This suggests the possibility of an evolutionary relationship between α and β subunits as well as between γ and δ. Many of the mAbs have been characterized by binding to proteolytically generated fragments of the α subunit by immunoprecipitation followed by gel electrophoresis.[40] These studies have provided resolution of structural features with a higher definition than has been available previously. Further studies with these mAbs and mAbs generated in other groups described above will undoubtedly provide detailed insights of the structure-function relationship of the receptor.

mAbs to α subunits can be one of two types. Depending on the distance of the determinant recognized by a mAb in two α subunits of the AChR monomer, the mAb can either bind two α subunits in the same molecule simultaneously or only cross-link two α subunits of different molecules. These two types of mAbs can be distinguished chemically. These studies provide information not only on the location of certain determinants but also on the antigenic modulation of receptors. A mAb of the second type was found to cross-react with receptors from fetal calf muscle and able to induce antigenic modulation of receptors in muscle cells in culture.[41] This suggests that muscle receptors also have two α subunits and that the antibody can cross-link the receptor in the plane of the membrane, thereby forming complexes that enhance endocytosis and increase the rate of receptor destruction. Unfortunately, mAbs of the first type are species-specific and therefore cannot be tested in the same system, although it would be expected that mAb that cross-link α subunits within a receptor cannot induce antigenic modulation.

mAb to AChR also provided some insight into the pathology of the autoimmune disease, myasthenia gravis. Myasthenia gravis is a disease that occurs as a consequence of an autoimmune response directed against the nicotinic AChR of the myoneural junction. The pathogenicity of anti-AChR antibodies has been documented by induction of the disease by passive transfer of sera from human to mouse and from rat to rat. Observations made by Lennon and Lambert,[42] Tzartos and Lindstrom,[39] and Richman et al.[43] demonstrated that the disease can be induced in experimental animals by anti-AChR mAbs that cause a defect of neurotransmission in these animals. These findings concluded that binding of a single molecular species of antibody reactive with a single antigenic determinant can result in all of the manifestation of an autoimmune disease. Furthermore, they established that neuromuscular transmission can be impaired by monospecific antibodies that do not inhibit the binding of neurotransmitter to its receptor site.

2. Ig FcR

In the previous example, donor mice were immunized with purified AChR or its subunits since chemistry of the purification had already been worked out. With the hybridoma technique one can use whole cells to immunize an animal and mAb obtained can be monospecific. This obviates the extensive adsorption necessary for conventional antibodies. Furthermore, new proteins on the cell surface can be discovered using this approach. (See Section IV for further discussion.)

Unkeless[44] reported a mAb to FcR on macrophages. Donor rats were primed with viable cells of the macrophage cell line J774 and boosted with a mixture of J774 and P388 D$_1$ (also a macrophage line) cells. The immunized rat spleen cells were then fused with mouse myelomas. Anti-FcR antibody-producing hybridomas were screened by inhibition of binding of IgG$_{2b}$-coated erythrocyte to J774 cells. The mAb inhibits the trypsin-resistant FcR (FcRII) that is specific for immune complexes of mouse IgG$_1$ and IgG$_{2b}$, but had no inhibitory effect on the trypsin-sensitive FcRI that binds monomeric IgG$_{2a}$. This is in agreement with the previous finding that IgG$_{2a}$ binds a receptor distinct from that binding aggregated IgG$_1$ and IgG$_{2b}$. When more mAbs are generated, each recognizing different determinants, it will be interesting to see whether some will inhibit both FcRI and FcRII whereas others will be specific for one receptor.

The mAb was found to bind to several lymphomas indicating the antigenic relatedness of FcR on lymphocytes and macrophages. In recent years FcR on lymphocytes has gained increasing attention. FcR to many Ig classes and subclasses have been identified on lymphocytes and studies have indicated that they may play important regulator roles in immune responses. Unkeless' report is the first to indicate the structural similarity of FcR on two different cell types. If one can generate a library of mAbs to these receptors, it will add enormously to understanding the structural relationship of these receptors to one another.

The mAb to FcRII was found useful for the purification of the receptor.[45] Two general types of polypeptides with electrophoretic mobilities of $\approx$60,000 and 47,000 mol wt were isolated from J774 cells. Similar broad bands ranging from 47,000 to 70,000 mol wt were isolated from various FcR-bearing cells of B, T, and null lymphocytes as well as macrophage origin. The isolated FcR exist as large aggregates that were shown to retain the binding activity. Interestingly, the isolated FcR bind not only IgG$_1$ and IgG$_{2b}$, but also IgG$_{2a}$. The authors suggested as possible explanations that the IgG$_{2a}$ FcR site is formed by aggregation of FcR, or formed by association of FcR with other membrane protein(s) present in smaller amounts and that these associations are abolished when the cells are treated with trypsin.

mAbs to FcR for IgE (FcRϵ) on rat basophilic leukemia (RBL) cells have also been reported.[46] These mAbs inhibit the binding of rat IgE to RBL cells and inhibit the IgE-mediated histamine release. Interestingly, the antibody does not cause release of histamine from RBL cells when added either alone or followed by rabbit anti-mouse Ig. It has been reported that polyclonal anti-FcRϵ could cause triggering of histamine release from normal mast cells or RBL by cross-linking of FcRϵ on the cell surface. Therefore, it would be very important to establish whether the failure of triggering by the mAb is due to no effective cross-linking of FcRϵ as a result of either low affinity of the antibody to the receptor or geometrical reasons, or that triggering induced by certain anti-FcRϵ antibodies is site-specific. It would be useful to obtain a number of mAbs with and without triggering capacity.

3. Other Systems

An interesting application of the mAb to study cellular activation has been reported by Beachy and Czech.[47] They have produced mAbs against rat adipocyte plasma membranes. About 30% of mAbs that bind plasma membranes can mimic insulin action to stimulate the oxidation of glucose to CO_2. It is known that patients suffering from certain insulin-resistant diabetes have autoantibodies to insulin receptors that block insulin binding and mimic the action of insulin on stimulation of glucose transport. This activity requires the bivalency of the Ig molecules and may involve cross-linking of insulin receptors. Therefore, it will be of interest to know the mechanism of the activation caused by the insulinomimetic mAbs. Establishment of antigenic molecules recognized by the insulinomimetic and nonfunctional mAbs, the reason for the lack of activity of the latter group of mAbs, and the modulation of membrane molecules during activation caused by the mAbs will add significantly to the understanding of cellular activation.

Most of the hormone and neurotransmitter receptors are present at low concentrations in tissues. This has hindered the purification and molecular characterization of these receptors. With the development of the hybridoma technique, it becomes relatively easy to obtain specific mAbs to various receptors. These mAbs can be used for purification and characterization of the receptors. Therefore, fast progress in research studies on receptors can be expected. mABs to β-adrenergic receptors[48] and estrogen receptors[49] have already been reported.

D. mAbs as Probes to Study Multiprotein Complexes

In the last three sections mAbs each made to one protein of interest was discussed. When a group of related proteins is of interest, the hybridoma technique may have the unique potential of providing mAbs to each of the components in a single experiment. The feasibility of obtaining mAbs to each component of a multiprotein complex using the complex as the immunizing agent has been tested with *Escherichia coli* 50S ribosome.[50] Total 50S ribosomal proteins were used to immunize donor mice. Four clones were analyzed, two having specificity for L5 and the other two directed against L20. Since all ribosomal proteins are highly immunogenic when tested separately, it is yet to be seen whether one can obtain mAbs to other subunits. Nevertheless, hybridoma technology certainly has a potential for generating mAbs against a group of antigens in a single experiment. The mAbs should be useful for detection and identification of individual ribosomal proteins without the problem of possible contamination by nonspecific Ab. The most promising use of these mAbs is in the extension of the analysis of ribosome structure by immunoelectron microscopy.

In another example,[51] total nuclear protein from the embryonic *Drosophila melanogaster* cell line and crude hydroxyapatite fractions were used for immunization of mice. By immunofluorescence, 58 cultures of 311 showed a highly selective staining pattern on polytene chromosomes from the salivary glands of *D. melanogaster* third instar larvae. Eight of these cultures were cloned and further characterized. They can be distinguished as staining of active regions, staining of phase dark bands, or staining of mast interbands. Antigens that these mAbs are directed against have been identified by electrophoresis.

IV. IDENTIFICATION OF CELL SURFACE MARKERS BY mAbs

A general review of mAbs would not be complete without at least a brief discussion of application of mAbs to the fascinating area of research on cell differentiation. Because of the many features of mAbs discussed above, the hybridoma technique is ideal in searching for unique cell surface antigens representing a cell population at a distinct stage of differentiation. To approach this goal, one uses a population of cells or tissues to immunize appropriate animals. After the preparation of hybridomas, those secreting antibodies to the cells of interest are then selected and a library of mAbs can be established. These mAbs can then be tested for their specificities to various cell populations by an immunofluorescence technique or immunoassay. If a mAb is specific to certain cells, it can be extremely useful as discussed below. The use of mAbs in the study of developing cell surfaces has been elegantly reviewed by Milstein and Lennox.[52]

In immunology, this approach has turned out to be remarkably productive in the study of human T lymphocytes. A number of mAbs have been generated, each recognizing distinct subsets of human T cells. These mAbs have been very useful in studies on the regulatory network of the human immune system, as reviewed in Chapter 4 of this volume. Studies of differentiation antigens on murine- and rat-lymphocytes have also been reviewed.[5,6]

The potential usefulness of hybridoma technology in the study of complex neurobiology has also been appreciated. Barnstable[53] reported the production of mAbs against a membrane preparation from adult rat retina. Seven mAbs were obtained. These mAbs were found to react with rat photoreceptor cell surface, glial cells, or other types of neuronal cells. Zipser and McKay[54] reported a library of mAbs reacting with nerve cords in the leech. Twenty mAbs reacting with specific neurons were studies in great detail. They include antibodies against sensory neurons, motor neurons, as well as numerous undifferentiated cells. mAbs against chicken embryo retina cells[55] and against astrocyte subclasses in mouse cerebellum[56] have also been discussed. These antibodies will be extremely useful for study of the distribution of particular cell types in the intact organism, study of the development of particular cell types in the intact organism, study of the development of particular cell types in the developing tissues, separation of various cell types and study of the function of separated cells, and isolation of identified cell antigens that may be intimately related to particular cellular functions or cell–cell recognition.

In the field of developmental biology, mAbs have been applied to study spermatogenesis,[57,58] the development of the embryo,[59,60] and the development of myoblasts.[61] These studies will clearly lead to exciting findings in the future.

Finally, it is appropriate to recognize the potential tie of the hybridoma technology with the recombinant DNA technology. mAbs to a unique antigen, as described above, can be used to identify in vitro translation products from messenger RNA (mRNA) isolated from a cell population. The corresponding mRNA can then be cloned. Specific antibodies will be very useful in the selection of specific cDNA clones. The isolated cDNA can then be used to study the expression and the regulation of the expression of the relevant gene. Furthermore, the amino acid sequence of the protein can be derived from the nucleotide sequence of the cDNA.

V. mAbs AS DIAGNOSTIC PROBES

Hybridoma technique has a great promise for production of mAbs useful for clinical diagnostic tests. Compared to conventional antibodies, mAbs have at least the following advantages for use in diagnosis:

High specificity. Contamination of a reagent by antibodies against impurities in the immunizing antigens, frequently a problem with conventional antisera, is ruled out.
Ease of purification. In the hybridoma technique, cloning itself can be considered a purification process. Once a hybridoma cell line is cloned and proven to be monoclonal, the mAb product must be specific for a single determinant. Whether this mAb is useful or not depends on whether it is specific for the antigen of interest and not other antigens that may have a similar determinant. Extensive adsorption often necessary for conventional Abs is not necessary. Hybridoma cells can be propagated in pristane-primed animals, and the ascites fluid so obtained contains a large quantity of desired mAb. An antibody preparation of reasonable purity can be easily obtained by ammonium sulfate precipitation and, if necessary, DEAE ion-exchange chromatography. Of course, if the antigen is readily available, an affinity purification will provide even purer reagents.

Unlimited supply of standardized reagents. Once a stable hybridoma cell line is established, almost unlimited quantities of mAb can be prepared. Therefore, a long-term supply of reagents of consistent properties (homogeneity, specificity, and affinity) can be assured. This will therefore guarantee reproducible results within a single laboratory and comparable results from different laboratories.

mAbs that are useful diagnostically and are commercially available are still limited in number. However, many mAbs reported in the literature have potential usefulness. Selected examples are discussed in the following sections.

A. Detection of Human Peptides and Proteins

Determination of α-fetoprotein (AFP) in maternal serum and in amniotic fluid during pregnancy has proved to be an important tool in prenatal diagnosis of spina bifida and congenital nephrosis. Production of AFP by germ cell tumors and primary liver cancer is utilized to monitor cancer patients. Uotila et al.[62] and Tsung et al.[63,64] reported anti-AFP-mAbs. The former group[65] recently reported a two-site sandwich enzyme immunoassay for human AFP. In this method, one mAb is immobilized on a microtiter plate test sample and another mAb labeled with horseradish peroxidase are added simultaneously to the wells. After incubation and washing, the plate is developed with the substrate of the enzyme, o-phenylenediamine. A sensitivity to detect 1 ng of AFP has been obtained. Since two mAbs bind to different site of AFP, they do not compete for binding. Use of the mAb on both sites of the ''sandwich'' also makes this assay highly specific. This rapid, simple, specific, and sensitive assay should be useful in diagnosis and follow-up of liver cancer and teratocarcinoma as well as in prenatal diagnosis of a number of fetal malformations.

RIA for human growth hormone (hGH) using mAb has been reported.[66] The concentrations of hGH in human serum samples were determined with mAb and the values showed a high degree of correlation with those obtained by polyvalent antibodies. Finally, monoclonal anti-human IgE is available commercially and should become useful in immunoassay of human IgE in the diagnosis of allergy.

B. Detection of Membrane Proteins

Many disease states are related to changes in the membrane proteins on various cell types. Antibodies to these proteins should be very useful for diagnosis and understanding the nature of the diseases. The use of mAbs in this respect is nicely demonstrated in the studies of thrombasthenia. Thrombasthenia is a congenital platelet disorder characterized by a normal platelet count, prolonged bleeding time, abnormal clot retraction, and absent platelet aggregation in response to ADP, thrombin, and epinephrine. It has been found by two-dimensional gel electrophoresis that two glycoproteins (IIb and IIIa) are present in reduced amounts in the patient. Because several proteins migrate similarly to these proteins in electrophoresis, quantitation of their amounts has been difficult. Furthermore, these glycoproteins have not been isolated. McEver et al.[67] obtained several hybridomas from spleen cells of mice immunized with human platelets. One of the cell lines was found to secrete an antibody that binds to a protein on normal but not thrombasthenic platelets. This protein was isolated from a solubilized membrane using an immunoadsorbent made of the mAb and found to be a complex of glycoproteins IIb and IIIa. Studies with this mAb have enabled quantitation of the number of glycoprotein IIb—IIIa complexes on normal platelet membranes, demonstrated that thrombasthenic homozygotes lack and heterozygotes have a partial deficiency of this complex, and made possible isolation of this membrane protein that may be required for normal platelet aggregation and clot retraction.

C. Immunodiagnosis of Tumors

Hybridoma antibodies have been used extensively in detection of surface antigens on tumor cells including melanoma, neuroblastoma, colon carcinoma, and carcinoembryonic antigens, among others.[4] These mAbs, due to their specificities, have served as excellent reagents for isolation of relevant antigens and will be useful for the structural studies of these tumor antigens. These mAbs should also have potential for use in diagnosis, prognosis, and therapy of tumors (see Chapter 4).

An interesting approach for producing useful mAbs against tumor antigens has been reported by Schlom et al.[68] Lymphocytes from lymph nodes obtained at mastectomy in breast cancer patients were fused with murine nonproducer myeloma cells to obtain human-mouse hybridoma cultures that synthesize human mAbs. Hybridoma cultures (52) synthesizing either human IgG or human IgM have been obtained from lymph nodes of 13 patients. Several of the human mAbs demonstrate preferential binding to human mammary tumor cells. As these authors pointed out, it will be of interest to determine if staining with mAb can be used as an adjunct to the detection of small populations of metastatic mammary carcinoma cells in lymph node removed at mastectomy, and if the level of expression of the antigen on primary or metastatic mammary tumor cells can be used as a useful prognostic indicator. Since human-mouse interspecies hybrids have a high frequency of human chromosomal loss, if this approach proves to be clinically useful, there will no doubt be application of human-human hybridomas in this direction.

mAbs to human estrogen receptor (ER) have been reported.[49] It has been known for some time that about 20 to 30% of patients with metastatic breast cancer obtain remission after hormone treatment. Recently, it has been found that the metastatic breast cancer tissue containing ER is of predictive value in identifying patients most likely to respond to treatment with hormones. Therefore, an important potential application of mAbs to ER is for the simple immunoradiometric determination of ER in human breast cancers as a guide to therapy.

In the future, increasing application of mAb in nuclear medicine will be seen, especially in the patient-imaging technique in the establishment of the presence or absence of malignant diseases and tumor localization. In the past, images of both primary tumor and metastases in man have been successful by using ^{125}I- (or ^{131}I-) labeled Ig from adsorbed specific goat antisera. These results strongly support the possibility of using radiolabeled antibodies for the detection of tumors and metastases, even those located deep within the body. Progress in this area has been hampered by the unavailability of suitable antibodies to give sufficient target-to-nontarget contrast for imaging, and the difficulty of reproducible preparation and purification of antitumor antibodies. With the successful development of mAb to many tumor antigens, this technique should be significantly improved. In mice, it has already been demonstrated that ^{125}I-labeled mAb to teratocarcinoma can be used to localize the tumor by external X-ray scintigraphy.[69,70]

D. Immunodiagnosis of Viral, Bacterial, and Parasitic Infections

mAbs have proven extremely useful in studies of microorganisms. Numerous mAbs to viral, bacterial, and parasitic antigens have been reported. Those for viral and bacterial antigens have been reviewed.[7-10] These mAbs are useful for the detection, isolation, and characterization of surface antigens and are expected to be useful toward the production of vaccines. Examples of efforts toward development of diagnostic methods for infections using mAbs are discussed below.

1. Immunodiagnosis of Hepatitis B (HBs)

A sensitive RIA using a high-affinity IgM anti-HBs mAb has been reported.[71] Solid beads are coated with a mAb. ^{125}I-labeled IgM-anti-HBs mAb and test sample are added to the coated beads at the same time and the mixture is incubated for 2 hr at 45°C. The beads are washed and the radioactivity measured. The lower limit of this assay is reported to be ≈100 ± 30 pg. It is interesting that IgM used in both sites of the "sandwich" is the same mAb indicating that the mAb must be directed against a highly represented epitope on HBs Ag. Compared to available commercial radioassays, preliminary studies have shown the IgM-IgM assay to have increased sensitivity that improved the determination of a HBs Ag-associated determinant in acute hepatitis and post-transfusion hepatitis.

2. Immunoassay for Streptococcal Antigen

Nahm et al.[72] reported evaluation of mouse mAb to streptococcal group A carbohydrate in a diagnostic laboratory. A total of 262 isolates of β-hemolytic streptococci were classified with commercial and the mAb to group A carbohydrate by using immunofluorescence and Lancefield precipitin tests. Both monoclonal and commercial antibodies gave the same reactivity in the precipitin test. However, in the fluorescence assay, commercial antibodies gave both false-positive and false-negative results, in contrast to the mAb that gave the same reactivity as seen in the precipitin test. These results suggest that monoclonal reagents may be superior to conventional antisera.

Enzyme-linked monoclonal antibody inhibition assay (ELMIA) for detection of group B streptococcal (GBS) antigen has been reported.[73] Bacteria are fixed on a microtiter plate and sample and serial dilutions of hybridoma supernatant containing anti-type III GBS are added to the wells. After incubation and washing, peroxidase-labeled anti-mouse IgG is added. The assay is finally developed with the substrate of the enzyme as usual. The concentration of the antigen in test samples is reversely proportional to the anti-mouse IgG bound. The ELMIA-detected streptococcal antigen at a concentration of 10 ng/ml and was found to be more sensitive and specific than currently used immunodiagnostic tests. Using this assay, type III GBS antigen was detected in cerebrospinal fluid specimens from 11 culture-proven cases of GBS meningitis and in the knee aspirate from an infant with GBS septic arthritis. Five spinal fluid specimens from meningitis due to other bacterial pathogens and 10 other control samples were negative.

3. Immunodiagnosis of Parasitic Infections

Understanding of metazoan and protozoan parasitic diseases and development of preventive and therapeutic methods for these diseases are definitely a great challenge to modern biomedical research. Immunological approaches have played important roles in the studies of these diseases. Such studies have the goals of:

1. Identification and Characterization of Parasite Surface Antigens: These antigens are expected to be useful for development of vaccines to parasitic infections.
2. Development of Specific Antibodies to Parasites: These antibody reagents are useful for detection, characterization, and isolation of surface antigens and for development of immunodiagnostic tests for parasitic infections.

These studies have progressed slowly in the past. Purification of antigens had been very difficult due to the lack of specific probes and specific antibodies had been very difficult to obtain. The immunodiagnostic tests had, therefore, suffered from the problems of low sensitivity and inadequate specificity.

The hybridoma technology has brought a new dimension to the study of parasites. Now, one can hope to obtain a large quantity of a mAb of desired specificity that can then be used to purify the specific antigen. A detailed general procedure for obtaining hybridomas specific for a parasite has been outlined.[74] mAbs to gamete,[75] sporozoite,[76,77] and merozoite[78–80] stages of malaria parasites have already been reported. They have proven useful for characterization of surface antigens and inhibition of parasite growth in vitro and in vivo. mAbs to other parasites such as *trypanosome,*[81,82] *toxoplasma,*[83–85] *Schistosome,*[86] and *Theileria*[87] parasites have also been reported and have been used in the immunochemical characterization of surface antigens.

Reports on immunodiagnostic tests utilizing mAbs are still limited in the literature. Following are a few examples illustrating efforts in this direction.

Mitchell et al.[88] developed a prototype immunodiagnostic assay using chronic infection with the larval cestode, *Mesocestoides corti,* in mice as a model system. Spleens and lymph nodes of mice infected for four months with *M. corti* were fused with a myeloma line to obtain hybridomas. A group of mAbs, most likely from the same clone, was obtained. The mAb was used to develop a solid-phase competitive RIA for detection of antiparasite antibodies in mouse sera. In this assay, the test serum is analyzed for its capacity to inhibit the binding of ^{125}I-labeled mAb to *M. corti* antigen extract coated on microtiter plates. The assay is reported to be highly sensitive and specific for *M. corti* infection. In large-scale experiments, no false-positive results were detected.

Craig et al.[89] have obtained a mAb specific for *Taenia hydatigena* larval antigens. A similar RIA as described above was devised as an immunodiagnostic test for experimental *T. hydatigena* infection in sheep.

Araujo et al.[90] reported the preparation of mAbs to *Toxoplasma gondii* and the use of mAb in an ELISA to detect the parasite antigens in peritoneal fluid of mice and in sera from humans acutely infected with *T. gondii.* In this assay, samples are incubated in microtiter plates containing mAb coated to the plastic surface and the bound antigens detected with enzyme-labeled IgG from rabbit antitoxoplasma serum. Four of the six mAbs were able to detect antigens of toxoplasma serum. Although the assay is highly specific, it was found that conventional polyclonal antibody reagents gave more satisfactory results.

It seems, therefore, that much effort will be required for development of highly sensitive and specific immunoassays for diagnosis of various parasitic infections in the future. We have no doubt that such a goal is being actively pursued in many laboratories in the world. For the detection of antiparasite antibodies, it seems that an assay similar to radioallergosorbent test (RAST), or related enzyme assays, for detection of antiallergen IgE in human serum would be useful. In this approach, antigens should be purified for use in the solid-phase. Various mAbs that are now available or forthcoming should facilitate the isolation of antigens. For detection of antigens, approaches using two-site sandwich RIAs or enzyme immunoassays as described above for α-fetoprotein and hepatitis B would be most promising.

Finally, it is worth mentioning that human–human hybridomas producing mAbs of defined antigenic specificity have been reported.[91,92] These hybridomas can be obtained by fusion of human peripheral blood lymphocytes and appropriate human myeloma cells. Therefore, a variety of mAbs to many pathogens can potentially be obtained by using lymphocytes from patients. Besides the obvious therapeutic potential, these mAbs will be useful in diagnosis. For example, many parasites are species-specific and mouse antibodies produced against a certain parasite may not recognize the same antigen recognized by human. For this reason, preparation of human–human hybridomas secreting human mAbs using peripheral blood lymphocyte derived from infected patients would be a useful direction.

VI. CONCLUSION

From the examples discussed above it is clear that hybridoma technology is a very powerful one to provide useful mAb reagents for research and clinical diagnosis. Indeed, this technology is revolutionizing immunology as well as biological and medical sciences, as evidenced by over 600 publications related to hybridoma-derived mAbs first introduced only six years ago. It should also be clear from discussions in this chapter and other chapters of this book that a great deal of effort should be invested in producing, screening, and characterizing mAbs before they become useful reagents. However, once a stable hybridoma cell line is established, the supply of the mAb can almost be unlimited. This is in contrast to the conventional polyclonal antibodies which are limited much of the time to use in the laboratory that produces the reagent due to the limitation of the antisera and the antigens used for immunization. It is for this reason that one would expect to see many of the useful mAb reagents become available to researchers working in various scientific disciplines tackling problems that may not even be the original purposes for preparing the hybridomas. Therefore, we can expect to see more and more fruitful and exciting research applying mAbs in the future.

ACKNOWLEDGMENTS

The authors are grateful for the expert assistance of Beverly Burgess, Rebecca Mead, and Lucy Gunnill in the preparation of this manuscript. This is publication no. 2496 from the Immunology Departments, Research Institute of Scripps Clinic, La Jolla, Calif. The authors' work cited herein was supported by NIH grant AI-13874.

REFERENCES

1. **Köhler, G. and Milstein, C.,** Continuous cultures of fused cells secreting antibody of predefined specificity, *Nature (London)*, 256, 495, 1975.
2. **Möller, G., Ed.,** *Immunological Reviews, Hybrid Myeloma Monoclonal Antibodies Against MHC Products,* Vol. 47, Munksgaard, Copenhagen, 1979.
3. **McKearn, T. J., Smilek, D. E., and Fitch, F. W.,** Rat-mouse hybridomas and their application to studies of the major histocompatibility complex, in *Monoclonal Antibodies-Hybridomas: A New Dimension in Biological Analysis,* Kennett, R. H., McKearn, T. J., and Bechtol, K. B., Eds., Plenum Press, New York, 1980, 219.
4. **Kennett, R. H., Jonak, Z. L., and Bechtol, K. B.,** Monoclonal antibodies against human tumor-associated antigens, in *Monoclonal Antibodies-Hybridomas: A New Dimension in Biological Analysis,* Kennett, R. H., McKearn, T. J., and Bechtol, K. B., Eds., Plenum Press, New York, 1980, 155.
5. **Ledbetter, J. A., Goding, J. W., Tokuhisa, T., and Herzenberg, L. A.,** Murine T-cell differentiation antigens detected by monoclonal antibodies, in *Monoclonal Antibodies–Hybridomas: A New Dimension in Biological Analysis,* Kennett, R. H., McKearn, T. J., and Bechtol, K. B., Eds., Plenum Press, New York, 1980, 235.
6. **Mason, D. W., Brideau, R. J., McMaster, W. R., Webb, M., White, R. A. H., and Williams, A. F., Monoclonal antibodies that define T–lymphocyte subsets in the rat,** in *Monoclonal Antibodies–Hybridomas: A New Dimension in Biological Analysis,* Kennett, R. H., McKearn, T. J., and Bechtol, K. B., Eds., Plenum Press, New York, 1980, 251.
7. **Nowinski, R. C., Stone, M. R., Tam, M. R., Lostrom, M. E., Burnette, W. N., and O'Donnell, P. V.,** Mapping of viral proteins with monoclonal antibodies. Analysis of the envelope proteins of murine leukemia viruses, in *Monoclonal Antibodies–Hybridomas: A New Dimension in Biological Analysis,* Kennett, R. H., McKearn, T. J., and Bechtol, K. B., Eds., Plenum Press, New York, 1980, 295.
8. **Gerhard, W., Yewdell, J., Frankel, M. E., Lopes, A. D., and Staudt, L.,** Monoclonal antibodies against influenza virus, in *Monoclonal Antibodies–Hybridomas: A New Dimension in Biological Analysis,* Kennett, R. H., McKearn, T. J., and Bechtol, K. B., Eds., Plenum Press, New York, 1980, 317.
9. **Koprowski, H. and Wiktor, T.,** Monoclonal antibodies against rabies virus, in *Monoclonal Antibodies–Hybridomas: A New Dimension in Biological Analysis,* Kennett, R. H., McKearn, T. J., and Bechtol, K. B., Eds., Plenum Press, New York, 1980, 335.
10. **Polin, R. A.,** Monoclonal antibodies against streptococcal antigens, in *Monoclonal Antibodies–Hybridomas: A New Dimension in Biological Analysis,* Kennett, R. H., McKearn, T. J., and Bechtol, K. B., Eds., Plenum Press, New York, 1980, 353.

11. **Böttcher, I., Hammerling, G., and Kapp, J. F.,** continuous production of monoclonal mouse IgE antibodies with known allergenic specificity by a hybrid cell line, *Nature (London),* 275, 761, 1978.

12. **Böttcher, I., Ulrich, M., Hirayama, N., and Ovary, Z.,** Production of monoclonal mouse IgE antibodies with DNP specificity by hybrid cell lines, *Int. Arch. Allergy Immunol.,* 61, 248, 1980.

13. **Eshhar, Z., Ofarim, M., and Waks, T.,** Generation of hybridomas secreting murine reaginic antibodies of anti-DNP specificity, *J. Immunol.,* 124, 775, 1980.

14. **Liu, F.-T., Bohn, J. W., Ferry, E. L., Yamamoto, H., Molinaro, C. A., Sherman, L., Klinman, N. R., and Katz, D. H.,** Monoclonal dinitrophenyl-specific murine IgE antibody: preparation, isolation and characterization, *J. Immunol.,* 124, 2728, 1980.

15. **Chen, S.-S., Bohn, J. W., Liu, F.-T., and Katz, D. H.,** Murine lymphocytes expressing receptors for IgE (FcRε). I. Conditions for inducing FcRε⁺ lymphocytes and inhibition of the inductive events by suppressive factor of allergy (SFA), *J. Immunol.,* 127, 166, 1981.

16. **Razin, E., Cordon-Cardo, C., and Good, R. A.,** Growth of a pure population of mouse mast cells *in vitro* with conditioned medium derived from concanavalin A-stimulated splenocytes, *Proc. Natl. Acad. Sci. U.S.A.,* 78, 2559, 1981.

17. **Hill, P. and Liu, F.-T.,** A sensitive enzyme-linked immunosorbent assay for the quantitation of antigen-specific murine immunoglobulin E, *J. Immunol. Methods,* 45, 51, 1981.

18. **Kelly, K. A., Lang, G. M., Bundesen, P. G., Holford-Strevens, B., Bottcher, I., and Schon, A. H.,** The development of a radioallergosorbent test (RAST) for murine IgE antibodies, *J. Immunol. Methods,* 39, 317, 1980.

19. **Diamond, B., Bloom, B. R., and Scharff, M. D.,** The Fc receptors of primary and cultured phagocytic cells studied with homogeneous antibodies, *J. Immunol.,* 121, 1329, 1978.

20. **Greenberg, A. H. and Lydyard, P. M.,** Observations of IgG1 anti-DNP hybridoma-mediated ADCC and the failure of three IgM anti-DNP hybridomas to mediate ADCC, *J. Immunol.,* 123, 861, 1979.

21. **Ralph, P., Nakoinz, I., Diamond, B., and Yelton, D.,** All classes of murine IgG antibody mediate macrophage phagocytosis and lysis of erythrocytes, *J. Immunol.,* 125, 1885, 1980.

22. **Secher, D. S. and Burke, D. C.,** A monoclonal antibody for large scale purification of human leukocyte interferon, *Nature (London),* 285, 446, 1980.

23. **Secher, D. S.,** Immunoradiometric assay of human leukocyte interferon using monoclonal antibody, *Nature (London),* 290, 501, 1981.

24. **Staehelin, T., Durrer, B., Schmidt, J., Takacs, B., Stocker, J., Misgiano, V., Stahli, C., Rubinstein, M., Levy, W. P., Hershberg, R., and Pestka, S.,** Production of hybridomas secreting monoclonal antibodies to the human leukocyte interferons, *Proc. Natl. Acad. Sci. U.S.A.,* 78, 1848, 1981.

25. **Luben, R., Mohler, M., and Nedwin, G.,** Production of hybridomas secreting monoclonal antibodies against the lymphokine osteoclast activating factor, *J. Clin. Invest.,* 64, 337, 1979.

26. **Luben, R. A. and Mohler, M. A.,** *In vitro* immunization as an adjunct to the production of hybridomas producing antibodies against the lymphokine osteoclast activating factor, *Mol. Immunol.,* 17, 635, 1980.

27. **Hübner, L., Schimpl, A., and Wecker, E.,** Partial characterization and purification of murine T helper cell replacing factor (TRF)--III, *Mol. Immunol.,* 17, 591, 1980.

28. **Bühler, H. P. and Blaser, K.,** Production of hybridoma secreting monoclonal antibodies against lymphocyte activating factor (interleukin 1), *Behring Inst. Mitt.,* 67, 226, 1980.

29. **Gillis, S. and Henney, C. S.,** The biochemical and biological characterization of lymphocyte regulatory molecules. VI. Generation of a B cell hybridoma whose antibody product inhibits interleukin 2 activity, *J. Immunol.,* 126, 1978, 1981.

30. **Frackelton, A. R., and Rotman, B.,** Functional diversity of antibodies elicited by bacterial β-D-galactosidase-monoclonal activating, inactivating, protecting and null antibodies to normal enzyme, *J. Biol. Chem.,* 255, 5286, 1980.

31. **Accolla, R. S., Cina, R., Montesoro, E., and Celada, F.,** Antibody-mediated activation of genetically defective *E. coli* β-galactosidases by monoclonal antibodies produced by somatic cell hybrids, *Proc. Natl. Acad. Sci. U.S.A.,* 78, 2478, 1981.

32. **Tamerius, J. D., Pangburn, M. K., and Müller-Eberhard, H. J.,** Selective inhibition of functional sites of cell-bound C3b by hybridoma-derived antibodies, *J. Immunol.,* 128, 512, 1982.

33. **Lachmann, P. J., Oldroyd, R. G., Milstein, C., and Wright, B. W.,** Three rat monoclonal antibodies to human C3, *Immunology,* 41, 503, 1980.

34. **Whitehead, A. S., Sim, R. B., and Dodmer, W. F.,** A monoclonal antibody against human complement component C3: the production of C3 by human cells *in vitro, Eur. J. Immunol.,* 11, 140, 1981.

35. **Gomez, C. M., Richman, D. P., Berman, P. W., Burres, S. A., Arnason, B. G. W., and Fitch, F. W.,** Monoclonal antibodies against purified nicotinic acetylcholine receptor, *Biochem. Biophys. Res. Commun.,* 88, 575, 1979.

36. **Moshlyro, D., Fuchs, S., and Eshhar, Z.,** Monoclonal antibodies against defined determinants of acetylcholine receptor, *FEBS Lett.,* 106, 389, 1979.

37. **Lennon, V. A., Thompson, M., and Chen, J.,** Properties of nicotinic acetylcholine receptors isolated by affinity chromatography on monoclonal antibodies, *J. Biol. Chem.,* 255, 4395, 1980.

38. **James, R. W., Kato, A. C., Rey, M. J., and Fulpures, B. W.,** Monoclonal antibodies directed against the neurotransmitter binding site if nicotinic acetylcholine receptor, *FEBS Lett.,* 120, 145, 1980.

39. **Tzartos, S. J. and Lindstrom, J. M.,** Monoclonal antibodies used to probe acetylcholine receptor structure: localization of the main immunogenic region and detection of similarity between subunits, *Proc. Natl. Acad. Sci. U.S.A.,* 77, 755, 1980.

40. **Gullick, W. J., Tzartos, S., and Lindstrom, J.,** Monoclonal antibodies as probes of acetylcholine receptor structure. I. Peptide mapping, *Biochemistry,* 20, 2173, 1981.

41. **Conti-Tronconi, B., Tzartos, S., and Lindstrom, J.,** Monoclonal antibodies as probes of acetylcholine receptor structure. II. Binding to native receptor, *Biochemistry,* 20, 2181, 1981.

42. **Lennon, V. A. and Lambert, F. H.,** Myasthenia gravis induced by monoclonal antibodies to acetylcholine receptors, *Nature (London),* 285, 238, 1980.

43. **Richman, D. P., Gomez, C. M., Berman, P. W., Burres, S. A., Fitch, F. W., and Arnason, B. G. W.,** Monoclonal anti-acetylcholine receptor antibodies can cause experimental myasthenia, *Nature (London),* 286, 738, 1980.

44. **Unkeless, J. C.,** Characterization of a monoclonal antibody directed against mouse macrophage and lymphocyte Fc receptor, *J. Exp. Med.,* 150, 580, 1979.

45. **Mellman, I. S., and Unkeless, J. C.,** Purification of a functional-mouse Fc receptor through the use of a monoclonal antibody, *J. Exp. Med.,* 152, 1048, 1980.

46. **Basciano, L. K., Berenstein, E. H., Fox, P. C., and Siraganian, R. P.,** A monoclonal antibody to the IgE receptor on rat basophilic leukemia cells, *Fed. Proc. Fed. Am. Soc. Exp. Biol.,* 40, 968, 1981.

47. **Beachy, J. C. and Czech, M. P.,** Production of insulinomimetic antibodies against rat adipocyte membrane by hybridoma cells, *J. Supra mol. Struct.,* 13, 447, 1980.

48. **Fraser, C. M. and Venter, J. C.,** Monoclonal antibodies to β-adrenergic receptors: use in purification and molecular characterization of β-receptors, *Proc. Natl. Acad. Sci. U.S.A.,* 77, 7034, 1980.

49. **Greene, G. L., Nolan, C., Engler, J. P., and Jensen, E. V.,** Monoclonal antibodies to human estrogen receptor, *Proc. Natl. Acad. Sci. U.S.A.,* 77, 5115, 1980.

50. **Shen, V., King, T. C., Kumar, V., and Daughterty, B.,** Monoclonal antibodies to *E. coli* 50 S ribosomes, *Nucl. Acid Res.,* 8, 4639, 1980.

51. **Saumweber, H., Symmons, P., Kabisch, R., Will, H., and Bonhoeffer, F.,** Monoclonal antibodies against chromsomal proteins of *Drosophila melanogaster:* establishment of antibody producing cell lines and partial characterization of corresponding antigens, *Chromosoma,* 80, 253, 1980.

52. **Milsten, C. and Lennox, E.,** The use of monoclonal antibody techniques in the study of developing cell surface, *Curr. Topics Develop. Biol.,* 14(II), 1, 1980.

53. **Barnstable, C. J.,** Monoclonal antibodies which recognize different cell types in the rat retina, *Nature (London),* 286, 231, 1980.

54. **Zipser, B. and McKay, R.,** Monoclonal antibodies distinguish identifiable neurons in the leech, *Nature (London),* 289, 549, 1981.

55. **Eisenbarth, G. S., Walsh, F. S., and Nirenberg, M.,** Monoclonal antibody to a plasma-membrane antigen of neurons, *Proc. Natl. Acad. Sci. U.S.A.,* 76, 4913, 1979.

56. **Lagenaur, C., Sommer, I., and Schachner, M.,** Subclass of astroglia in mouse cerebellum recognized by monoclonal antibody, *Develop. Biol.,* 79, 367, 1980.

57. **Bechtol, K. B., Brown, S. C., and Kennett, R. H.,** Recognition of differentiation antigens of spermatogenesis in the mouse by using antibodies from spleen cell myeloma hybrids after syngeneic immunization, *Proc. Natl. Acad. Sci. U.S.A.,* 76, 363, 1979.

58. **Myles, D. G., Primokoff, P., and Belleve, A. R.,** Surface domains of the guinea pig sperm defined with monoclonal antibodies, *Cell,* 23, 433, 1981.

59. **Solter, D. and Knowles, B. B.,** Monoclonal antibody defining a stage-specific mouse embryonic antigen (SSEA-1), *Proc. Natl. Acad. Sci. U.S.A.,* 75, 5565, 1978.

60. **Bruler, P., Rabinet, C., Kemler, R., and Jacob, F.,** Monoclonal antibodies against trophectoderm-specific markers during mouse blastocyte formation, *Proc. Natl. Acad. Sci. U.S.A.,* 77, 4113, 1980.

61. **Lee, H. U. and Kaufmann, S. J.,** Use of monoclonal antibodies in the analysis of myoblast development, *Develop. Biol.,* 81, 81, 1981.

62. **Uotila, M., Engvall, E., and Ruoslahti, E.,** Monoclonal antibodies to human alpha fetoprotein, *Mol. Immunol.,* 17, 791, 1980.

63. **Tsung, Y. K., Milunsky, A., and Alpert, E.,** Secretion by a hybridoma of antibodies against human alpha fetoprotein, *N. Engl. J. Med.,* 302, 180, 1980.

64. **Tsung, Y. K., Milunsky, A., and Alpert, E.,** Derivation and characterization of a monoclonal hybridoma antibody specific for human alpha fetoprotein, *J. Immunol. Methods,* 39, 363, 1981.

65. **Uotila, M., Ruoslahti, E. and Engvall, E.,** Two-site sandwich enzyme immunoassay with monoclonal antibodies to human alpha fetoprotein, *J. Immunol. Methods,* 42, 11, 1981.

66. **Bundesen, P. G., Drake, R. G., Kelley, K., Worsley, Z. G., Friesen, H. G., and Sehon, A. H.,** Radioimmunoassay for human growth hormone using monoclonal antibodies, *J. Clin. Endocrinol.,* 51, 1472, 1980.

67. **McEver, R. P., Baenziger, N. L., and Najerus, P. W.,** Isolation and quantitation of the platelet membrane glycoprotein deficient in thrombasthenia using a monoclonal hybridoma antibody, *J. Clin. Invest.,* 66, 1311, 1980.

68. **Scholm, J. Wunderlich, D., and Teramoto, Y. A.,** Generation of human monoclonal antibodies reactive with human mammary carcinoma cells, *Proc. Natl. Acad. Sci. U.S.A.,* 77, 6841, 1980.

69. **Ballou, B., Levine, G., Hakala, T. R., and Solter, D.,** Tumor location detected with radioactively labeled monoclonal antibody and external scintigraphy, *Science,* 206, 844, 1979.

70. **Levine, G., Ballou, B., Reiland, J., Solter, D., Gumerman, L., and Hakala, T.,** Localization of I-131-labeled tumor-specific monoclonal antibody in the tumor-bearing BALB/c mouse, *J. Nucl. Med.,* 21, 570, 1980.

71. **Wands, J. R., Carlson, R. J., Schoemaker, H., Isselbacher, K. J., and Zurawski, V. R., Jr.,** Immunodiagnosis of hepatitis-B with high-affinity IgM monoclonal antibodies, *Proc. Natl. Acad. Sci. U.S.A.,* 78, 1214, 1981.

72. **Nahm, M. H., Murray, P. R., Clevinger, B. L., and Davie, J. M.,** Improved diagnostic accuracy using monoclonal antibody to group A streptococcal carbohydrate, *J. Clin. Microbiol.,* 12, 506, 1980.

73. **Polin, R. A. and Kennett, R.,** Use of monoclonal antibodies in an enzyme-linked inhibition assay for rapid detection of streptococcal antigen, *J. Pediatr.,* 97, 540, 1980.

74. **Pearson, T. W., Pinder, M., Roelants, G. E., Santosh, K. K., Lundin, L. B., Mayor-Withey, K. S., and Hewett, R. S.,** Methods for derivation and detection of anti-parasite monoclonal antibodies, *J. Immunol. Methods,* 34, 141, 1980.

75. **Rener, J., Carter, R., Rosenberg, Y., and Miller, L. H.,** Anti-gamete monoclonal antibodies synergistically block transmission of malaria by preventing fertilization in the mosquito, *Proc. Natl. Acad. Sci. U.S.A.,* 77, 6797, 1980.

76. **Potocnjak, P., Yoshida, N., Nussenzweig, R. S., and Nussenzweig, V.,** Monovalent fragment (Fab) of monoclonal antibodies to a sporozoite surface antigen (Pb 44) protect mice against malarial infection, *J. Exp. Med.,* 151, 1504, 1980.

77. **Yoshida, N., Nussenzweig, R. S., Potocnjak, P., Nussenzweig, V., and Aikawa, M.,** Hybridoma produces protective antibodies directed against the sporozoite stage of malaria parasite, *Science,* 207, 71, 1980.

78. **Freeman, R. R., Trejdosiewicz, A. J., and Cross, G. A. M.,** Protective monoclonal antibodies recognising stage-specific merozoite antigens of a rodent malaria parasite, *Nature (London),* 284, 366, 1980.

79. **Perrin, L. H., Ramirez, E., Erhsiang, L., and Lambert, P. H.,** Plasmodium-falciparum characterization of defined antigens by monoclonal antibodies, *Clin. Exp. Immunol.,* 41, 91, 1980.

80. **Perrin, L. H., Ramirez, E., Lambert, P. H., and Miescher, P. A.,** Inhibition of *P. falciparum* growth in human erythrocytes by monoclonal antibodies, *Nature (London),* 289, 301, 1981.

81. **Pearson, T. W., Kar, S. K., McGuire, T. C., and Lundin, L. B.,** Trypanosome variable surface antigens: studies using two-dimensional gel electrophoresis and monoclonal antibodies, *J. Immunol.,* 126, 823, 1981.

82. **Lyon, J. A., Pratt, J. M., Travis, R. W., Doctor, B. P., and Olenick, J. G.,** Use of monoclonal antibody to immunochemically characterize variant-specific surface coat glycoprotein from *Trypanosoma rhodesiense, J. Immunol.,* 126, 134, 1981.

83. **Handman, E., Goding, J. W., and Remington, J. S.,** Detection and characterization of membrane antigens of *Toxoplasma gondii, J. Immunol.,* 124, 2578, 1980.

84. **Sethi, K. K., Endo, T., and Brandis, H.,** Hybridomas secreting monoclonal antibody with specificity for *Toxoplasma gondii, J. Parasitol.,* 66, 192, 1980.

85. **Handman, E. and Remington, J. S.,** Serological and immunochemical characterization of monoclonal antibodies to *Toxoplasma gondii, Immunology,* 40, 579, 1980.

86. **Verwarede, C., Grzych, J. M., Bazin, H. Capron, M., and Capron, A.,** Production of anti-*Schistosoma mansoni* monoclonal antibodies. Preliminary study of their biological activities, *C. R. Acad. Sci. Ser. D.,* 289, 725, 1979.

87. **Pinder, M. and Hewett, R. S.,** Monoclonal antibodies detect antigenic diversity in *Theileria parva* parasites, *J. Immunol.,* 124, 1000, 1980.

88. **Mitchell, G. F., Cruise, K. M., Chapman, C. B., Anders, R. F., and Howard, M. C.,** Hybridoma antibody immunoassays for the detection of parasitic infection. Development of a model system using a larval cestode infection in mice, *Aust. J. Exp. Biol. Med. Sci.,* 57, 287, 1979.
89. **Craig, P. S., Mitchell, G. F., Cruise, K. M., and Rickard, M. D.,** Hybridoma antibody immunoassays for the detection of parasitic infection—attempts to produce an immunodiagnostic reagent for a larval taenid cestode infection, *Aust. J. Exp. Biol. Med. Sci.,* 58, 339, 1980.
90. **Araujo, F. G., Handman, E., and Remington, J. S.,** Use of monoclonal antibodies to detect antigens of *Toxoplasma gondii* in serum and other body fluids, *Infect. Immun.,* 30, 12, 1980.
91. **Olsson, L. and Kaplan, H. S.,** Human–human hybridomas producing monoclonal antibodies of pre-defined antigenic specificity, *Proc. Natl. Acad. Sci. U.S.A.,* 77, 5429, 1980.
92. **Croce, C. M., Linnenbach, A., Hall, W., Steplewski, Z., and Koprowski, H.,** Production of human hybridoma secreting antibodies to measles virus, *Nature (London),* 288, 488, 1980.
93. **Chen, S.-S. et al.,** Unpublished results.

Chapter 2

mAbs AS PROBES OF PROTEIN STRUCTURE: MOLECULAR DIVERSITY AMONG THE ENVELOPE GLYCOPROTEINS (gp70s) OF THE MURINE RETROVIRUSES

Henry L. Niman and John H. Elder

TABLE OF CONTENTS

I.   Introduction 24
      A.   Background 24
      B.   gp70s Comprise a Multigene Family of Proteins with
            Recognitive Functions 24
      C.   Technical Considerations Regarding mAbs 24

II.   Procedures for Immunizations and Subsequent Fusions 25
      A.   Choice of Immunogen 25
      B.   Immunization and Fusion 25
      C.   Conditions and Procedures for Assay of Hybridomas 26

III.   Initial Characterization of Hybridomas 27
      A.   Binding Assays with Rauscher Virus 27
      B.   Binding Assays with Other Murine Retroviruses 28
      C.   Surface Fluorescence 28
      D.   Immune Precipitation and Glycosylation 28
      E.   Immune Precipitation of gp70 Breakdown Products 29

IV.   Generation of a Linear Map of Hybridoma Binding Sites 29
      A.   Immune Precipitation Patterns of ''Natural
            Breakdown'' Fragments 29
      B.   Peptide–Mapping the Fragments 29
      C.   Orienting the Hybridoma Reactivities 30
      D.   The Generation of PEC–MAP 32
      E.   Defining the 19 Domains 38
      F.   Localization of the 19 Domains 38

V.   Constraints on the Tertiary Structure of gp70 41
      A.   Distribution of Antibody–Binding and Enzyme–
            Cleavage Sites 41
      B.   Localization of the Regions Affected by Glycosylation 42
      C.   Location of P15e Binding Sites 44
      D.   Localization of Surface Immunofluorescence 46
      E.   Reactivity Against Other Related Retroviruses 46

VI.   Concluding Remarks 49

Acknowledgments 49

References 50

I. INTRODUCTION

A. Background

Protein chemists, immunologists, and other followers of evolutionary divergence have traditionally used antisera as a tool to measure the relative relationships of various protein species. Typically, antisera raised against one member of a family of proteins would be used in a competitive assay to determine not only a quantitation, but also relatedness to other members of that particular family. Although useful, the approach had certain limitations, primarily dictated by the heterologous antisera used in the assay. Since an immunological response could be considered a competition reaction, such antisera could be biased as to antigenic sites recognized and could vary greatly from one antiserum to another. In effect, the heterosera was assumed to recognize antigenic sites in a uniform manner along the molecule and thus give an accurate reflection of protein relatedness. Clearly, this simplistic approach was born of necessity rather than experimental proof and determination of antigenic bias was difficult. With advent of the mAb technology, however, the cells producing the family of antibodies raised against a particular antigen could be separated.[23] This breakthrough has allowed for more detailed experiments regarding the molecular diversity of a multigene family of proteins as well as probing the structure of the protein itself. The following is a summation of the authors' analyses of the molecular structure of the retroviral glycoprotein gp70 using mAbs. Reported here are the procedures that have worked well in the authors' system and should apply equally well to the study of other proteins.

B. gp70s Comprise a Multigene Family of Proteins with Recognitive Functions

Retroviral gp70 is an interesting molecule for a variety of reasons. The molecule dictates the host range, interference, and neutralization properties of the virus that indicates gp70 possesses recognition functions. As might be expected from such a molecule, gp70 exhibits extensive polymorphism[21,8] rivaling that of the Ig family and is the primary vehicle by which these viruses diverge. gp70 is interesting from a developmental standpoint because it is encoded by genes endogenous to the mouse and is expressed during development at various sites of differentiation in the absence of other viral constituents.[37,40,5,24] Furthermore, structurally distinct gp70s are expressed at different sites[10] and it has been suggested that gp70 be classified as a differentiation antigen.[36] Finally, alteration in gp70 via recombination[7,38,32,15,2,33,9,4,26,18] may play a role in generating highly leukemogenic retroviruses[19,16,43,18,42] from innocuous parental viruses endogenous to the mouse. The recombined gp70s have also been found in the tumor tissues of the mice.[31,41] Thus, gp70 is an ideal molecule for structural analysis with mAbs. These reagents offer precise tools for dissecting gp70 at the submolecular level. Furthermore, they offer a means to study the relationship of discrete regions of the molecule relative to each member of the multigene family.

C. Technical Considerations Regarding mAbs

mAbs, by their specificity for a single antigenic site, can be used to probe protein structure in ways not readily accomplished by conventional antisera. Furthermore, the homogeneity of these antibodies provides very discrete physiochemical properties that aid in their purification as well as in release of antigen when used as immunoadsorbents. However, negative results must be viewed with caution because each mAb recognizes a single antigenic determinant and the activity can be affected by minor changes in conformation, glycosylation, or assay conditions. Thus, because of their monoclonality, and furthermore, because each preparation is of a single isotype, hybridomas warrant

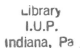

several technical considerations usually ignored in uses of heterologous antisera. These considerations include the following:

1. How specific is the antibody binding?
   - Is the assay sufficiently discriminatory?
   - Is the assay biased?
2. What is the avidity of the antibody?
   - Can the resultant antigen–antibody reaction be dissociated by high salt treatments generally considered as washing steps in heterosera–directed precipitations?
   - Does the antigen–antibody complex demand more stringent conditions than usually employed for heterosera?
3. What is the isotype of the antibody?
   - Will it bind to the current vehicle used in immune precipitations: Staph. Protein A?
   - Is there selective pressure against certain isotypes in the assay system?
4. How available is the antigenic site recognized by each mAb?
   - Again, is selection imposed on a family of antibodies by the assay methods?
   - How may these properties be used to advantage?
5. How many monoclonals were produced against the antigen in question?
   - Is the number biased by technical considerations or by the relative antigenicity of the given protein?
   - Do the antibodies reflect an accurate sample of the immune response?
   - Does the response vary as to method used in antigen presentation?

In the following section, the authors will outline procedures that were successful in their studies and answer the questions posed above as they apply to their experience.

II. PROCEDURES FOR IMMUNIZATIONS AND SUBSEQUENT FUSIONS

A. Choice of Immunogen

In preliminary studies, the authors attempted to elicit immune responses against gp70 using purified virus, virus–infected cells, and purified gp70. Not unexpectedly, the best results were obtained using the purified molecule. The latter immunogen also allowed accurate determination of the amount of material injected and thus did not suffer from the variability in specific antigen concentrations encountered with virus or virus–infected cells. The host response to virus or tumor invasion (i.e., regressor antibodies) could not be directly analyzed by the panel of antibodies raised against the purified molecule. However, it was found that the immune response to various regions of gp70 was enhanced and thus a large panel of structural probes was produced for uses described below.

B. Immunization and Fusion

The authors chose to immunize the 129 mouse because this strain of mouse is not viremic (although gp70 is expressed, as below) and congenic mice for G_{IX} determinants found on some gp70s, were available. Both G_{IX+} and G_{IX-} mice were immunized. Since G_{IX+} mice are high in endogenous gp70 expression and G_{IX-} are low, it was reasoned that the immune response might be greater in the latter due to possible tolerance in the former. However, the immunization protocol produced readily detectable antibodies to gp70 within three weeks in both G_{IX^+} and G_{IX^-} mice. The mice were immunized with 50 μg of gp70 in a 1:1 mixture of PBS and complete Freund's adjuvant given s.c. or i.p. Two weeks later an additional 50 μg in 5 mg/ml alum was given i.p. One week later the mice were bled and assayed for anti–gp70 activity. Although the original procedures did not call for antibody assay, the authors found that many laborious and expensive failures in their early experiences were simply due to insufficient immunization. The serum is routinely assayed prior to fusion. The authors waited one to two months for the activity to decrease and then immunized with 50 μg gp70 given i.v. Five days later, the spleens were removed for subsequent fusion.

The SP-20 hypoxanthine–aminopterin–thymidine (HAT)–sensitive myeloma cell line was used for fusion.[35] This line had two main advantages for the authors' study in that it does not secrete its own Ig, thus facilitating isotype analysis and subsequent purification and it does not produce retroviruses, found to be the case with both the P–3 and 45.6 cell lines. Spleen cells were prepared by pushing the spleen through a stainless steel screen. After the large clumps had settled out of the mixture, the cells were removed and pelleted, followed by resuspension in ammonium chloride (0.1 M, 0.01 M Tris pH 7.2) to lyse the red blood cells. The spleen cells from one mouse were mixed with 2×10^7 SP-20 cells grown in the presence of 10^{-4} M 8-azaguanine. The SP-20 cells were washed with minimum essential media (MEM) supplemented with 10% fetal calf serum (FCS) followed by a wash with MEM. The myeloma/spleen cell mixture was pelleted, spread in a conical centrifuge tube, and resuspended in 200 μl of 30% polyethylene glycol (PEG) to facilitate fusion. For unclear reasons, the efficiency of fusion was increased when the PEG solution was made up at least 1 month prior to use. The exposure to PEG was 8 min including centrifugation for 4 min beginning 2 min after PEG addition. The PEG was aspirated and the cell pellet was transferred to a T–25 tissue culture flask in MEM supplemented with 10% FCS. After overnight incubation (37°C, 10% CO_2), the cells were pelleted and resuspended in 200 ml HMT (MEM supplemented with 10% FCS, 10^{-4} M hypoxanthine, 10^{-6} M methotrexate, and 1.6×10^{-5} M thymidine). The suspension was dispensed into 16 microtiter plates (96–well). Plates were fed with one drop of HT (HMT without methotrexate) at weekly intervals. Macroscopic colonies (first evident around 12 to 14 days) were transferred to 24–well plates to equalize cell densities for subsequent assay.

C. Conditions and Procedures for Assay of Hybridomas

For purposes of minimizing the cost, labor, and time required as well as maximizing the success of a fusion, an accurate and discriminatory assay system must be employed. These procedures must be thoroughly worked out prior to the start of a fusion, since a successful fusion will produce thousands of clones and only 1 to 15% of these clones will produce the desired antibody. The assay system should include the closest possible negative control. For this assay, the gp70 of purified Rauscher virus was presented by methanol–fixation of dried virus in 96–well microtiter plates. Subsequent testing of positive supernatants revealed a dependency upon the method of antigen presentation if the antigen or antibody was at limiting concentrations. When the antigen concentration was low or the antisera was titrated, many hybridomas would show a marked preference for either plates presenting methanol–fixed virus that presumably exposes hydrophobic determinants or plates presenting virus-bound by raising the pH to 9.5 in aqueous buffer that presents the molecule in a more native state. The authors were able to detect hybridomas that displayed a wide spectrum of binding activities because high concentrations of gp70 in a virus–binding assay system were used. Others have employed immunofluorescence and immune precipitation to assay for the presence of antibodies. However, as will be shown below, the latter two procedures are informational but provide a biased view of the antibody population.

Supernatants were assayed in a binding assay that employed a radioactive signal. Rauscher virus was diluted with PBS to a concentration of 0.1 mg/ml. 25 μl were added per well. The solution was dried onto the bottom of the 96-well plate by incubation overnight at 37°C. 50 μl of methanol was added for 5 min at 25°C. Nonspecific binding sites were blocked with 1% bovine serum albumin (BSA) in PBS by incubating for 4 hr at 37°C. 25 μl of tissue culture supernatant was added to each well for 16 hr at 25°C. The plates were washed 10 times with PBS. A rabbit anti–mouse Ig sera was then added for 4 hr at 37°C. After washing with PBS, 25 μl of ^{125}I–affinity purified GARG was added. After incubation for 16 hr at 25°C the plates were aspirated and dried prior to cutting and counting in a gamma counter. Each of the positive clones was tested for its isotype. The supernatants were assayed as described above except an antisera specific for only one class of heavy chain was used in place of the rabbit anti-Ig sera. Over 100 of the non–IgM supernatants were stable and positive for the virus–coated plate. These supernatants were also tested against a virus that was bound to the microtiter plates by raising the pH to 9.5 and incubating for 16 hr at 25°C in a moist chamber. The buffer was removed and the plates were blocked for nonspecific binding as described above. Positive cell lines were cloned by endpoint dilution and cells were seeded into 96–well plates with a 1:1 mixture of HT and media conditioned by the hybridoma. Macroscopic colonies were transferred to 24–well plates and assayed with a binding assay. The assay employing a radioactive signal was replaced with an ELISA assay. In this assay the rabbit anti-mouse Ig sera was replaced with rabbit anti–mouse λ and κ sera. The immunoaffinity goat anti–rabbit sera was conjugated to glucose oxidase. The presence of glucose oxidase was detected by adding 50 μl 0.1 M phosphate pH 6.0, 1.2% glucose (mutorotated) 10 μg/ml horseradish peroxidase and 100 μg/ml ABTS dye. The optical density at 414 nm was read using a microscanner.

III. INITIAL CHARACTERIZATION OF HYBRIDOMAS

The authors' primary concern was to partition the hybridomas obtained by as many criteria as possible. By doing so, monoclonal reactivity reacted against unique determinants as well as functional criteria for further experimentation could be established. The approach was to assay the monoclonals under a variety of conditions including differential binding to virus treated with methanol or high pH, reacting with viruses other than Rauscher virus, immune precipitating native and deglycosylated gp70, as well as surface immunofluorescing virus-infected cells.

A. Binding Assays with Rauscher Virus

The initial screening of the tissue culture supernatants used R–MuLV methanol fixed to 96–well microtiter plates. Because fairly high concentrations of virus were used, the authors were able to detect a very heterogeneous population of mAbs. About 15% of the 2000 wells had binding activity that was 3 to 30 times that of either a negative control plate (BSA or pelleted FCS instead of virus) or virus–coated wells containing nonbinding antibody. In addition to these 300 positive wells, about 10% of the clones had high binding to the negative control plate. These hybridomas generally secreted IgM antibodies.

The 300 positive clones were also tested for the isotype of the secreted Ig. This analysis indicated that approximately 50% of the clones secreted IgM antibodies. These clones were frozen and not tested further. Of the remaining 150 clones, approximately 100 were stable and specific for Rauscher gp70. The heavy chain frequencies of these clones were 64%γ_1, 26%γ_{2a}, 3%γ_{2b}, 3%γ_3, 2%α, 2%ε while the light chain frequencies were 95% κ and 5% λ. This analysis suggested that the panel of hybridomas was fairly heterogeneous but did not discriminate between many different hybridomas binding either discrete or nondiscrete numbers of determinants.

To further characterize the antibodies, the antigen was presented two different ways on the 96–well plates. Virus was either dried onto the plate and fixed with methanol or adsorbed to the plate by raising the pH to 9.5. The binding activity was titered using serial two–fold dilutions and the binding was detected with the ELISA assay described above. The titers of the supernatant ranged from undetectable binding to titers >2040. Hybridomas demonstrating a differential titer of >4 were scored as showing a preference for antigen presentation. This titer difference could be >256. 44% of the hybridomas showed preference for methanol–fixed virus, 19% preferred pH 9.5 pretreated virus and 38% had differential titers of ≤4. This analysis further confirmed the heterogeneity of the hybridoma clones and pointed out the necessity of a broadly reactive screening assay.

B. Binding Assays with Other Murine Retroviruses

To further differentiate the binding sites of these antibodies, they were reacted with some common laboratory strains of murine leukemia virus. The binding activity of the mAb was determined by reacting the tissue culture supernatant with virus presented on methanol–fixed and pH 9.5 plates. The highest degree of relatedness (91%) was found with Friend virus (F–MuLV). A Rauscher–derived recombinant (R-MCF) that had mink cell focus–inducing properties was found to react with 42% of the mAbs. Moloney virus (M–MuLV) reacted with 27% of the antibodies while the endogenous ecotropic virus of AKR mice (AKv2) reacted with only 8% of the mAbs. Once again the differential reactivity patterns suggested the mAb panel was very heterogeneous.

C. Surface Fluorescence

To further characterize the binding sites of the mAbs, the tissue culture supernatant was used in an indirect surface fluorescence assay. Rauscher–infected cells were incubated with hybridoma tissue culture supernatants. Antibody–binding was labeled with a fluoresceinated rabbit anti–mouse IgG probe and visualized with a fluorescein–activated cell sorter. This analysis indicated that about 50% of the mAbs would surface fluoresce virus–infected cells while 50% would not. There was a significant but not universal correlation between a positive signal on a pH 9.5 plate and surface fluorescence that was expected since the pH 9.5 plate presents more hydrophilic residues.

D. Immune Precipitation and Glycosylation

The authors reacted the tissue culture supernatant of the various cell lines with ^{125}I–labeled, NP40–disrupted Rauscher virus to determine what proportion of the anti–gp70 hybridomas would facilitate immune precipitation. All of the mAbs that gave a precipitation pattern higher than background levels reacted with gp70. There was a great deal of heterogeneity in the amount of gp70 precipitated and several mAbs appeared very weak or unreactive in the immunoprecipitation assay although they reacted well with virus presented in the microtiter plates.

To determine if this poor reactivity was due to glycosylation, the supernatants were reacted with ^{125}I–labeled Rauscher virus that had been treated with a deglycosidase that had been isolated in this laboratory.[12] This reagent reduces the apparent molecular weight of the gp70 molecule to 55,000 daltons although the entire protein backbone appears to be intact as judged by peptide mapping and reactivity with the mAbs (see below). A comparison of the efficiency of precipitation of native or deglycosylated gp70 indicated most of the mAbs exhibited a preference. 15% of the mAbs precipitated the native molecule more efficiently than deglycosylated gp70. 50% of the hybridomas reacted better with the deglycosylated molecule while 35% reacted equally well with either presentation. Thus, although many of the antibodies reacted poorly with the native gp70 molecule, the deglycosylated gp70 was readily precipitated. This assay further pointed out the heterogeneity of the antibodies in the authors' panel.

E. Immune Precipitation of gp70 Breakdown Products

When preparing ^{125}I–labeled Rauscher virus it was noted that gp70 would ''naturally'' begin to degrade after incubation for 16 hr at room temperature. When the mAbs were reacted with this partially degraded material, different mAbs would precipitate different fragments. In addition, several of the mAbs that produced weak immune precipitation of the native molecule would readily precipitate a gp70 fragment indicating the binding was sterically hindered by the tertiary structure of the native gp70 molecule. These data again pointed out the heterogeneity of the monoclonal panel. In addition it pointed out the need for a broadly reactive screening procedure that would not select against various determinants because of the method of antigen presentation.

The above assays indicated that most, if not all, of the hybridoma cell lines recognized different determinants. The numbers, however, did not tell much about the molecular nature of gp70, since it was not known where on the molecule the monoclonals reacted. For example, the authors knew that 50% facilitated immunofluorescence, but the real issue was where these exposed regions were on the gp70 molecule. A linear map of gp70 binding sites was generated, as described below.

IV. GENERATION OF A LINEAR MAP OF HYBRIDOMA BINDING SITES

A. Immune Precipitation Patterns of "Natural Breakdown" Fragments

Since it was noted that gp70 would naturally begin to degrade after incubation for 16 hr at room temperature and mAbs are directed against a single antigenic determinant, it seemed reasonable that if a mAb were reacted against this mixture, the gp70 fragment that contained the hybridoma–binding site, as well as the native molecule, would be precipitated. Figure 1 demonstrates the precipitation patterns obtained with these antibodies. A goat anti–gp70 sera produced a complex pattern (lane A) when reacted with virus preparation that had gp70 breakdown products. The pattern was much simpler when mAbs were used. Lane B is the pattern of a hybridoma that was called a P–45/34 reactor[26] because in addition to gp70, fragments of Mr 45,000 (P–45) and 34,000 (P–34) daltons were precipitated. Lane C is the precipitation pattern of a P–45–only reactor that contains the P–45 fragment in addition to gp70. The third pattern produced by the mAb panel is represented in lane D. In addition to gp70, a minor fragment of Mr 42,000 (P–42) and a major fragment of Mr 32,000 (P32) was precipitated. Hybridomas that produced this pattern were called P–32 reactors. Thus the panel of hybridomas produced three readily distinguishable patterns when reacted with gp70 breakdown products.

B. Peptide–Mapping the Fragments

To investigate the relationship of the gp70 fragments to each other and the parental gp70 molecule, the precipitated material was subjected to two–dimensional peptide fingerprinting as shown in Figure 2. The peptides of P–45 (Figure 2B) are a subset of gp70 (Figure 2A) and the peptides of P–34 (Figure 2C) are a subset of P–45. The two peptides of P–45 marked with arrows (Figure 2B) are missing or greatly reduced in

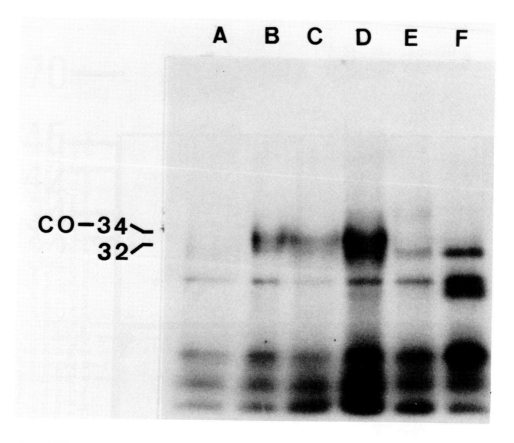

FIGURE 3. Immunoprecipitation of collagenase–generated R–MuLV gp70 fragments. R–MuLV was digested with collagenase at a concentration which was 10–fold higher than described.[28] The antibody sources were preimmune rabbit (4621) sera (lane A), sera of the rabbit (4621) immunized with synthetic pentadecapeptide Tyr–Gln–Ala–Leu–Asn–Leu–Thr–Ser–Pro–Asp–Lys–Thr–Gln–Glu–Cys (lane B), cell lines R_105E06 (lane C), R_116C12 (lane D), R_206B08 (lane E), and R_109E11 (lane F). The primary gp70 fragments were 34,000 daltons (C0–34) seen in lanes B,C,D, and 32,000 daltons (C0–32) seen in lane F. The 29,000 dalton fragment in lane F was not characterized.

(lane F).[26] Thus the "natural" breakdown P–32 fragment represents the N–terminal portion of gp70 (not P–45 and P–34 as originally described),[26] while P–34 represents the C–terminal portion of gp70 (not P–32 as originally described).[26] The peptide mapping and antisynthetic peptide precipitation data explain the "natural" breakdown fragment precipitation patterns of the three groups of hybridomas. Since P–34 represents the carboxyl portion of P–45, the mAbs that bind to this region of gp70 precipitate both P–34 and P–45. Those hybridomas that react with the central portion of gp70 (between P–34 and P–32) precipitate only the P–45 fragment. The monoclonals that bind to the amino portion of gp70 precipitate P–32 and the minor band of P–42. As will be shown below, the 45–only hybridomas also, in fact, bind P–42 but because it is present in much lower amounts than P–45, its presence was not readily detected in the "natural" breakdown digest.

D. The Generation of PEC–MAP

The panel of mAbs could now be classified into three reactivity patterns based upon immune precipitation of gp70 "natural breakdown" products but the authors did not

31

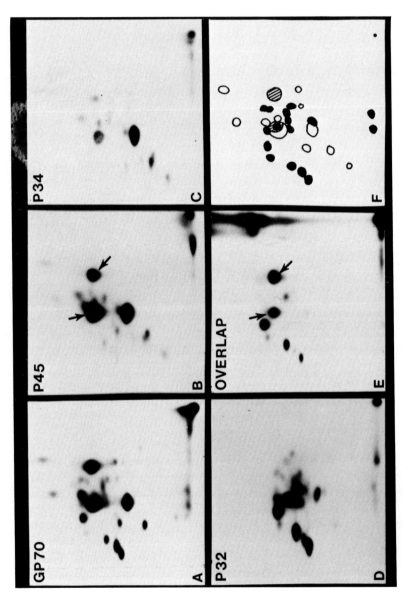

FIGURE 2. Two–dimensional separation of chymotryptic peptides of R–MuLV gp70 and natural breakdown products. Gp70 and breakdown fragments were treated as described.[26] (A) Total R–MuLV gp70, (B) P–45 immunoprecipitated by R_206B08, (C) P–34 immunoprecipitated by R_101D09, (D) P–32 immunoprecipitated by R_209C11, (E) Mr 55,000 fragment generated by V8 protease, and (F) composite drawing of gp70 peptides indicating relative contribution of the various fragments. Closed circles, derived from P–32; open circles, shared by P–45 and P–34; crosshatched circles, lost from P–45 (arrows in B), in transition to P–34 (C), and present in the V8 overlap fragments (arrows in E).

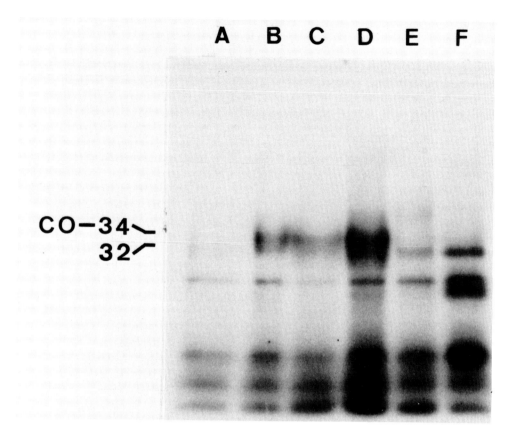

FIGURE 3. Immunoprecipitation of collagenase–generated R–MuLV gp70 fragments. R–MuLV was digested with collagenase at a concentration which was 10–fold higher than described.[28] The antibody sources were preimmune rabbit (4621) sera (lane A), sera of the rabbit (4621) immunized with synthetic pentadecapeptide Tyr–Gln–Ala–Leu–Asn–Leu–Thr–Ser–Pro–Asp–Lys–Thr–Gln–Glu–Cys (lane B), cell lines $R_1$05E06 (lane C), $R_1$16C12 (lane D), $R_2$06B08 (lane E), and $R_1$09E11 (lane F). The primary gp70 fragments were 34,000 daltons (C0–34) seen in lanes B,C,D, and 32,000 daltons (C0–32) seen in lane F. The 29,000 dalton fragment in lane F was not characterized.

(lane F).[26] Thus the "natural" breakdown P–32 fragment represents the N–terminal portion of gp70 (not P–45 and P–34 as originally described),[26] while P–34 represents the C–terminal portion of gp70 (not P–32 as originally described).[26] The peptide mapping and antisynthetic peptide precipitation data explain the "natural" breakdown fragment precipitation patterns of the three groups of hybridomas. Since P–34 represents the carboxyl portion of P–45, the mAbs that bind to this region of gp70 precipitate both P–34 and P–45. Those hybridomas that react with the central portion of gp70 (between P–34 and P–32) precipitate only the P–45 fragment. The monoclonals that bind to the amino portion of gp70 precipitate P–32 and the minor band of P–42. As will be shown below, the 45–only hybridomas also, in fact, bind P–42 but because it is present in much lower amounts than P–45, its presence was not readily detected in the "natural" breakdown digest.

D. The Generation of PEC–MAP

The panel of mAbs could now be classified into three reactivity patterns based upon immune precipitation of gp70 "natural breakdown" products but the authors did not

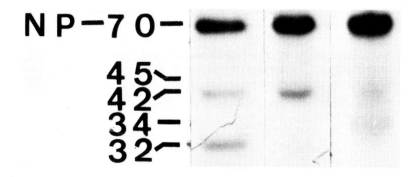

FIGURE 4. Contaminating protease PEC–MAP of R–MuLV gp70. R–MuLV was digested by protease present in dilute NP–40 preparations as described.[28] The cell lines secreting the mAbs were $R_2$06E04 (lane A), $R_1$05A06 (lane B), and $R_1$10H06 (lane C). NP–32 were present only in lane A. NP–42 was precipitated in lanes A and B while NP–45 was rather diffuse and present in lane B and C. NP–34 was also light and diffuse and present only in lane C.

know if the hybridomas recognized several determinants in each region, or if several hybridomas recognized a single determinant. The approach taken to begin to answer this question was to cleave the gp70 with a variety of proteases that cleaved at specific residues. This information would clarify the distribution of the determinants and would also put certain restrictions on the tertiary structure on the gp70 molecule because the authors chose to subject the molecule to limited proteolysis. This technique was called PEC–MAP. This stands for Partial Enzymatic Cleavage–Monoclonal Antibody Precipitation.

To try to reproduce the "natural" degradation originally observed, the ^{125}I–labeled was incubated with the 0.5% NP–40 solution used to disrupt the virus. Immune precipitation of this preparation resulted in three major precipitation patterns shown in Figure 4. The hybridomas that had been mapped towards the carboxyl end of the molecule (P–45/34 reactors) produced a pattern similar to natural breakdown (lane C). They precipitated molecules of approximately 45,000 daltons (NP–45) and 34,000 daltons (NP–34). Both of these fragments were rather diffuse on the gel. The hybridomas that mapped in the center (lane B) of gp70 (P45–only reactors) precipitated the diffuse NP–45 as well as a sharp band migrating slightly faster (NP–42). In lane A the amino–binding antibodies (P–32 reactors) precipitated NP–42 and a 32,000 dalton fragment (NP–32). Thus, a 20 min incubation with the dilute NP–40 mixture produced fragments that were similar to those of natural breakdown. The difference between this preparation and natural breakdown was the relative amount of the 42,000 dalton fragment. In the "natural breakdown" preparation P–42 had been further degraded to P–32, resulting in only a very minor amount of P–42 being present in the precipitations. In the NP–40 preparation, approximately equal amounts of NP–42 and NP–32 were present. Thus, although the precipitation patterns were somewhat different, the number of domains was still only three.

The immune precipitation patterns obtained with a virus preparation cleaved with α–chymotrypsin (chymotrypsin PEC–MAP) is shown in Figure 5. This time there were four major precipitation patterns. The amino reactors again precipitated 42,000 (CT–42) and 32,000 (CT–32) dalton fragments (Figures 4A and B) but a subset of these hybridomas also precipitated a 12,000 dalton fragment (CT–12, Figure 4B). The hybridomas that bound to the center of gp70 again precipitated a 42,000 dalton fragment (CT–42). In addition a minor fragment of approximately 20,000 daltons (CT–20) was precipitated

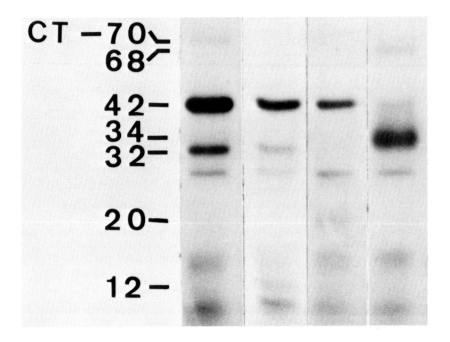

FIGURE 5. α–chymotrypsin PEC–MAP of R–MuLV gp70. R–MuLV was digested by α-chymotrypsin as described.[28] The cell lines secreting the mAbs were R$_2$06E04 (lane A), R$_2$09C11 (lane B), R$_1$05A06 (lane C), and R$_1$01D09 (lane D). The band, (CT–68) migrating slightly faster than CT–70, was seen only with carboxyl–binding hybridomas precipitating α-chymotrypsin generated fragments and probably represents dimers of CT–34 (lane D). CT–42 was present in lanes A to C, CT–32 was precipitated in lanes A and B, while only lane B had CT–12 and only lane D had CT–20.

by these hybridomas (Figure 4C). The carboxyl reactors again precipitated a 34,000 dalton fragment (CT–34) but the 45,000 dalton fragment was not present (Figure 4D).

The penicillinase PEC–MAP was similar to that of chymotrypsin except the amino reactors could not be divided. The amino reactors (Figure 6, lane A) precipitated a fragment of 42,000 daltons (PE–42) and a 32,000 dalton fragment (PE–32). The hybridomas that bound to the center of gp70 precipitated PE–42 (lane B). The carboxyl reactors (lane C) only precipitated a fragment of approximately 34,000 daltons (PE–34). This fragment was light and diffuse. Although these patterns were similar to the chymotrypsin PEC–MAP, the sites of cleavage were slightly different as will be described below.

The elastase PEC–MAP (Figure 7) demonstrated two cleavage sites around the junction of P–45 and P–32. In addition, a hybridoma that appears to be dependent somewhat upon the configuration of the fragments gave a unique precipitation pattern. Again the amino reactors precipitate a 32,000 (EL–32) dalton fragment (lane A). A small region of gp70 appears to be removed because a number of the P–32– and P–45–only reactors do not recognize any of the elastase–generated gp70 fragments (lane B) although fragments of 32,000 (lane A) and 45,000 daltons (lanes C to E) are present. The carboxyl reactors and most of the hybridomas that bound to the center of gp70 (lanes C to E) precipitated a fragment of approximately 45,000 daltons. The carboxyl reactors generally precipitated fragments of 36,000 (EL–36) and 34,000 (EL–34) daltons (lane E). The hybridoma that appears to be affected by the configuration of the fragments produced a pattern (lane D) that involved only EL–45 and EL–36. This pattern cannot be

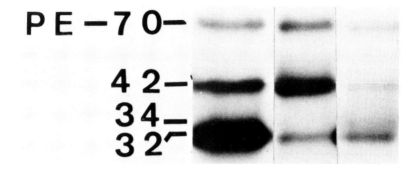

FIGURE 6. Penicillinase PEC–MAP of R–MuLV gp70. R–MuLV was digested by penicillinase as described.[28] The cell lines secreting the mAbs were R₂06E04 (lane A), R₂06B08 (lane B), and R₂03F09 (lane C). PE–42 was precipitated in lanes A and B while PE–32 was seen only in lane A. PE–34 was diffuse, light, and seen only in lane C.

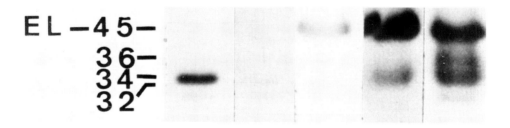

FIGURE 7. Elastase PEC–MAP of R–MuLV gp70. R–MuLV was digested by elastase as described.[28] The cell lines secreting the mAbs were R₂13A10 (lane A), R₁11GO2 (lane B), R₂16A09 (lane C), R₂02G12 (lane D), and R₁09C11 (lane E). EL–45 and EL–34 were readily precipitated in lanes D and E while EL–36 was seen only in lane E. Lane C contained only EL–45. Lane B did not reveal any gp70 fragment while lane A contained only EL–32.

explained without involving a conformational argument. The hybridoma cannot map at the far carboxyl end of gp70 because of its V8 PEC–MAP (see below). It also cannot map just past the amino end of EL–36 because R₁10DO5 precipitated EL–36 and mapped to the amino side of R₂02G12. Thus, conformation constraints are the most likely explanation for the lack of reactivity with EL–36. The explanation is supported by the lack of reactivity of this mAb with deglycosylated gp70.

The clostripain PEC–MAP (Figure 8) contains a 55,000 dalton fragment (CL–55) in addition to fragments that are similar to those described above. CL–55 (lanes B to E) is recognized by all hybridomas except a subset of amino reactors (lane A). The remaining fragments are similar to those described in NP40 PEC–MAP and elastase PEC–MAP. The carboxyl reactors (lane E) generally recognize a 45,000 dalton (CL–45), 38,000 dalton (CL–38), and 34,000 dalton (CL–34) fragment. The exception again is R₂02G12 (lane D) that precipitates CL–45 and CL–34, but not CL–38. The hybridomas that bind in the center precipitate CL–45 and CL–42 (lane C) while the amino reactors precipitate CL–42 and CL–32 (lanes A and B).

The trypsin PEC–MAP (Figure 9) is similar to that of clostripain with certain exceptions. Again, the 42,000 dalton fragment is precipitated by hybridomas that bind to the amino and central portions of gp70 (lanes A to D). Again, a 53,000 dalton fragment (TR–53) is precipitated by all hybridomas (lanes C to F), except a subset of

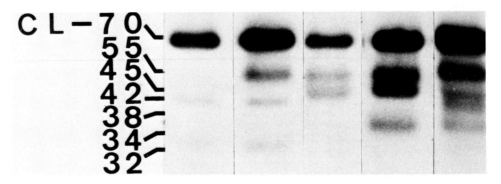

FIGURE 8. Clostripain PEC–MAP of R–MuLV gp70. R–MuLV was digested by clostripain as described.[28] The cell lines secreting the mAbs were $R_2$06E04 (lane A), $R_1$09E11 (lane B), $R_1$11G02 (lane C), $R_2$02G12 (lane D), and $R_1$12F10 (lane E). CL–55 was seen in lanes B to E. CL–42 was present in lanes A to C while CL–32 was present only in lanes A and B. CL–45 began in lane C and continued through lanes D and E. CL–34 was present in lanes D and E while CL–38 was present only in lane E.

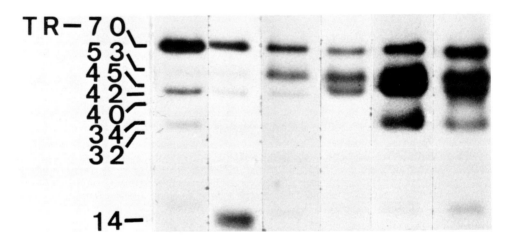

FIGURE 9. Trypsin PEC–MAP of R–MuLV gp70. R–MuLV was digested by trypsin as described.[28] The cell lines secreting the mAbs were $R_2$06E04 (lane A), $R_1$10B06 (lane B), $R_1$09E11 (lane C), $R_1$11G02 (lane D), $R_2$02G12 (lane E), and $R_1$10H06 (lane F). TR–53 was present in lanes C to F. TR–45 was present in lanes D to F, while TR–42 was in lanes A to D. TR–40 was present only in lane A while TR–34 was in lanes E and F.

amino reactors (lanes A and B). The 45,000 dalton fragment is precipitated by hybridomas that bind on the carboxyl and central portions of gp70 (lanes D to F). A 40,000 dalton fragment (TR–40) is precipitated by all carboxyl reactors (lane F) except R_2O2G12 (lane E). The 34,000 dalton fragment is precipitated by the carboxyl reactors (lanes E and F) while the 32,000 dalton fragment is precipitated by the amino reactors (lanes A to C). A unique fragment is evident with hybridoma $R_1$10B06 that precipitates a fragment (lane B) of approximately 14,000 daltons (TR14).

The collagenase PEC–MAP (Figure 10) is similar to the trypsin map with respect to the fragments recognized by large groups of the hybridoma panel. The 53,000 dalton fragment (CO–53) is precipitated by all hybridomas (lanes B to D) except a subset of amino reactors (lane A). The 45,000 dalton fragment (CO–45) is precipitated by the central– and carboxyl–binding hybridomas (lanes C and D). The 42,000 dalton fragment begins in the amino end of gp70 and extends to the center (lanes B to D). The

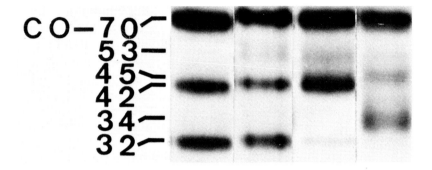

FIGURE 10. Collagenase PEC–MAP of R–MuLV gp70. R–MuLV was digested by collagenase as described.[28] The cell lines secreting the mAbs were R$_2$06E04 (lane A), R$_1$09E11 (lane B), R$_1$05A06 (lane C), and R$_1$10H06 (lane D). CO–53 was present in lanes B to D. CO–45 was precipitated in lanes C and D while CO–42 was present in lanes A to C. CO–34 was present only in lane D while CO–32 was present in lanes A and B.

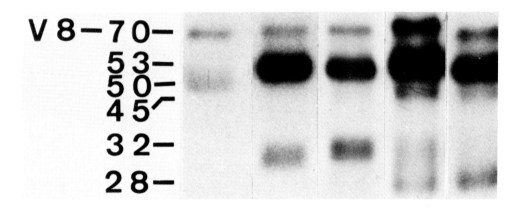

FIGURE 11. V8–protease PEC–MAP or R–MuLV gp70. R–MuLV was digested by V8 protease as described.[28] The cell lines secreting the mAbs were R$_2$06E04 (lane A), R$_1$05A06 (lane B), R$_1$01B01 (lane C), R$_1$10H06 (lane D), and R$_1$12F10 (lane E). V8–53 was precipitated in lanes B to E. V8–45 is a minor component seen in lanes C to E. V8–32 was precipitated in lanes B to D while V8–28 was present in lanes D and E. V8–50 was seen only in lane A indicting either an unusual configuration that prevents many of the monoclonals from binding, heavy glycosylation resulting in aberrant migration, or another molecule that contains the carboxyl portion gp70 but binds to the mAbs only after V8 cleavage.

34,000 dalton fragment is precipitated by carboxyl reactors (lane D) while the 32,000 dalton fragment is precipitated by the amino reactors (lanes A and B).

The V8 protease PEC–MAP (Figure 11) is unique. The 53,000 dalton fragment V8–53 again begins in the amino third of the molecule and extends through a subset of carboxyl reactors (lanes B to E). However, the amino reactors that do not recognize V8–53 do bind a fragment (lane A) of approximately 50,000 daltons (V8–50). Since this molecule is only recognized by a subset of amino reactors it either has an unusual configuration that precludes binding by the other amino reactors as well as the central reactors, or is heavily glycosylated and consequently has a slower migration rate, and only cleavage by V8 protease allows recognition by this panel of mAbs. Immune precipitation of deglycosylated fragments and peptide mapping should resolve these possibilities. The V8 cleavage also produces a minor peptide of approximately 45,000 daltons recognized by central and carboxyl–binding hybridomas (lanes C to F). The 32,000 dalton fragment (lanes B to D) represents the center of gp70 and spans the cleavage sites that generate the 34,000 and 32,000 dalton fragments seen in the other digests. A subset of the amino reactors (lane B) and carboxyl reactors (lane D) as well as central binders, (land C) precipitate V8–32. Another subset of the carboxyl reactors binds the 28,000 dalton fragment (lanes D and E).

E. Defining the 19 Domains

A compilation of the PEC–MAP of the 51 mAbs are listed in Table 1. The precipitation pattern produced by each hybridoma is listed. On the basis of these patterns it is possible to define 19 domains on the gp70 molecule. The domains differed either because the fragments precipitated were different or a similar fragment was precipitated in one digest and not another. The hybridomas in domain I precipitated V8–50 as well as the various 42,000 and 32,000 dalton fragments produced by all of the digests except V8. They did not precipitate TR–14 or CT–12 as was found with the domain II hybridoma. Domain III hybridomas failed to precipitate TR–14 although they still bound CT–12. The domain IV hybridoma was the same as domain III except it also precipitated CL–55. The domain V hybridoma had the same fragment reactivities as IV except it also precipitated TR–53. The domain VI hybridoma did not bind V8–50 or CT–12 although it did bind V8–32 and CO–53. The domain VII hybridoma precipitated CL–45 at the expense of EL–32 and CL–32. The domain VIII hybridoma bound TR–45 but did not bind TR–32. The domain IX hybridoma bound NP–45 at the expense of NP–32. Similarly, the domain X hybridoma bound CO–45 but did not bind CO–32. Domain XI hybridomas no longer bound CT–32 or PE–32 but did bind CT–20. Domain XII hybridomas are the same as those in domain XI except V8–45 was precipitated. The domain XIII hybridomas precipitate EL–45 in addition to those fragments precipitated by the domain XII hybridomas. The domain XIV hybridoma precipitated CT–34 and CO–34 at the expense of CT–42 and CT–20. The Domain XV hybridoma precipitated NP–34, PE–34, EL–36, EL–34, CL–38, CL–34, and TR–40 at the expense of CO–42, TR–42, CL–42, PE–42, and NP–42. The domain XVI hybridoma no longer precipitated EL–36, CL–38, and TR–40, but TR–34 was precipitated. The domain XVII hybridomas were the same as the domain XV hybridoma except TR–34 was precipitated. The domain XVIII hybridomas were the same as the domain XVII hybridomas except V8–28 precipitated. The domain XIX hybridomas were the same as XVIII except V8–32 was no longer precipitated.

F. Localization of the 19 Domains

The localization of the 19 domains is somewhat hampered by the altered mobility of glycosylated fragments as well as conformational constraints which the fragments may have. To help visualize the location of the domains, the 39 gp70 fragments are listed in Table 2. The fragments are denoted by the respective enzyme abbreviations and by a number representing the apparent molecular weight ($\times 10^{-3}$) on SDS–PAGE (left hand column). These molecular weights are inaccurate in most instances due to glycosylation and the length of the line defining each fragment dictated by the number of hybridoma domains that they encompass. To partially correct for the effects of glycosylation gp70 was cleaved and the mixture deglycosylated after inhibiting the proteolytic activity with EDTA, PMSF, and heat. The mixture was subjected to SDS–PAGE, electrophoresed onto nitrocellulose paper, and incubated with hybridoma supernatants. The results of this analysis indicated the mobility of the fragments originating from the amino end of gp70 were slightly affected by the sugars removed by the deglycosidase. The fragments that mapped in the center of gp70 were not altered

Table 1
PRECIPITATION PATTERNS OF ANTI R–MULV gp70 HYBRIDOMAS

Name[a]	Domain	V8[b]	TR	EL	CL	NP	PE	CT	CO
R₂11D10	I	A[c]	A	A	A	A	A	A	A
R₂01F01		A	A	A	A	A	A	A	A
R₁05B05		A	A	A	A	A	A	A	A
R₂04F07		A	A	A	A	A	A	A	A
R₂03G01		A	A	A	A	A	A	A	A
R₂06E04		A	A	A	A	A	A	A	A
R₁13H03		A	A	A	A	A	A	A	A
R₁04C07		A	A	A	A	A	A	A	A
R₁10B06	II	A	B	A	A	A	A	B	A
R₂03D11	III	A	A	A	A	A	A	B	A
R₂09C11		A	A	A	A	A	A	B	A
R₁04D05		A	A	A	A	A	A	B	A
R₁13A10	IV	A	A	A	B	A	A	B	A
R₂03E11	V	A	C	A	B	A	A	B	A
R₁09E11	VI	B	C	A	B	A	A	A	B
R₂05F06	VII	B	C	B	C	A	A	A	B
R₁04E05	VIII	B	D	B	C	A	A	A	B
R₂02A09	IX	B	D	B	C	B	A	A	B
R₁08B03	X	B	D	B	C	B	A	A	C
R₁01H11	XI	B	D	B	C	B	B	C	C
R₁12G02		B	D	B	C	B	B	C	C
R₁11G02		B	D	B	C	B	B	C	C
R₁05A06		B	D	B	C	B	B	C	C
R₁12CO2		B	D	B	C	B	B	C	C
R₁11C12		B	D	B	C	B	B	C	C
R₁15H06	XII	C	D	B	C	B	B	C	C
R₁01G11		C	D	B	C	B	B	C	C
R₂06B08	XIII	C	D	C	C	B	B	C	C
R₂16A09		C	D	C	C	B	B	C	C
R₁04D01		C	D	C	C	B	B	C	C
R₁01B01		C	D	C	C	B	B	C	C
R₁15G12	XIV	C	D	C	C	B	B	D	D
R₁10D05	XV	C	D	E	E	C	C	D	D
R₂02G12	XVI	C	E	D	D	C	C	D	D
R₁16C12	XVII	C	F	E	E	C	C	D	D
R₂03F09		C	F	E	E	C	C	D	D
R₁10E12		C	F	E	E	C	C	D	D
R₂02G09		C	F	E	E	C	C	D	D
R₂13G07		C	F	E	E	C	C	D	D
R₂11A03	XVIII	D	F	E	E	C	C	D	D
R₁10G05		D	F	E	E	C	C	D	D
R₁06F09		D	F	E	E	C	C	D	D
R₁04C10		D	F	E	E	C	C	D	D
R₁15G05		D	F	E	E	C	C	D	D
R₁10H06		D	F	E	E	C	C	D	D
R₁01D09	XIX	E	F	E	E	C	C	D	D
R₁09C11		E	F	E	E	C	C	D	D

Table 1 (continued)
PRECIPITATION PATTERNS OF ANTI R–MULV gp70 HYBRIDOMAS

Name[a]	Domain	V8[b]	TR	EL	CL	NP	PE	CT	CO
$R_1$12F10		E	F	E	E	C	C	D	D
$R_1$05E06		E	F	E	E	C	C	D	D
$R_1$06B03		E	F	E	E	C	C	D	D
$R_1$11B04		E	F	E	E	C	C	D	D

[a]Nomenclature of hybridomas has been described.

[b]Enzyme abbreviations are as follows: V8 (*S. aureus* V8 protease), TR (TPCK trypsin), EL (elastase), CL (clostripain), NP (contaminating protease in NP–40 solution), PE (penicillinase), CT (α–chymotrypsin), CO (collagenase).

[c]Letter refers to precipitation pattern shown from respective enzymes in Figures 4 to 11.

Table 2

LOCALIZATION OF GP70 FRAGMENTS

DOMAIN[b]

FRAGMENT[a]: I II III IV V VI VII VIII IX X XI XII XIII XIV XV XVI XVII XVIII XIX

Fragments listed:
V8-50, CL-32, EL-32, TR-32, NP-32, CO-32, CT-32, PE-32, CT-42, CO-42, TR-42, CL-42, PE-42, NP-42, CT-12, TR-14, CT-20, V8-32, CL-55, TR-53, CO-53, V8-53, CL-45, TR-45, NP-45, CO-45, V8-45, EL-45, CO-34, CT-34, NP-34, PE-34, EL-36, EL-34, CL-38, CL-34, TR-40, TR-34, V8-28

[a]First two characters refer to enzyme used to generate fragments (abbreviations defined in legend to Table 1). Number after dash refers to apparent molecular weight (fragments shown in Figures 4 to 11).

[b]Domain defined by precipitation patterns listed in Table 1.

in mobility while those fragments originating from the carboxyl end of gp70 were most affected in mobility. For example, the amino fragments CT–32, TR–32, and TR–14 had Mr 25,000, 27,000, and 12,000 daltons, respectively. In contrast, the fragment representing the center of gp70, CT20, was not electrophoretically altered by treatment with deglycosidase. Those fragments containing the central and amino portions of gp70 (CT–42, TR–42, V8-32) had Mr 40,000, 40,000, and 25,000 daltons, respectively, while those fragments representing the carboxyl portion of gp70 (V8–55, TR–45,

TR–34, CT–34, and V8–28) had Mr 38,000, 27,000, 15,000, 14,000, and 12,000 daltons, respectively. These molecular weights are probably still slightly altered. When the fragments are added up, they result in a total of 55 to 60,000 daltons. Since nucleotide sequence analysis[34] indicates the true molecular weight of gp70 to be closer to 47,000 daltons, the authors have localized the cleavage site using a 55,000 dalton molecule and reduced all fragments by 15% to approximate the 47,000 dalton deglycosylated gp70 molecule.

Domain I maps approximately within the first 2000 daltons of the deglycosylated gp70 molecule because of the lack of reactivity with both CT–12 and TR–14, representing a large portion of amino end of the molecule not present in the various 55,000 to 53,000 dalton fragments. Domain II is represented by the TR–14 fragment and should map between 6 to 12,000 daltons from the amino end of the molecule. Domain III is represented by precipitation of CT–12, but not TR–14, and thus maps at the carboxyl end of CT–12 (approximately 12,000 to 14,000 daltons from the amino end of gp70). Domains IV and V map at the amino end of the various 55,000 to 53,000 dalton fragments or approximately 14,000 daltons from the amino end of gp70. Domain VI maps between the amino end of these 55,000 to 53,000 dalton fragments and the carboxyl end of the various 32,000 dalton fragments or between 14,000 to 18,000 daltons from the amino end of gp70. Domains VII to XII are defined by the various 32,000 dalton fragments originating from the amino end of gp70, representing 18,000 to 20,000 daltons of protein. Domain XIII is represented by CT–20, representing about 17,000 daltons of protein, placing domain XIII between 20,000 to 34,000 daltons from the amino end of gp70. Domain XIV and XV map at the end of the various 34,000 dalton fragments or approximately 34,000 daltons from the amino end. Domain XVI and XVII map between the amino end of the 34,000 dalton fragments and the amino end of V8–28 or between 34,000 and 38,000 daltons from the amino end of gp70. Domain XVIII should map near the amino end of V8–28 because only one fragment of the approximately 28,000 daltons is precipitated. Domain XIX is defined by V8–28, mapping in the final 9000 daltons.

V. CONSTRAINTS ON THE TERTIARY STRUCTURE OF gp70

Once the linear array of antigenic sites was determined, the data regarding reactivity characteristics described above could be evaluated in a more concise manner. The following is a summary of what can now be said about discrete regions of the gp70 molecule.

A. Distribution of Antibody–Binding and Enzyme–Cleavage Sites

A linear map of the enzyme-cleavage sites (symbols) as well as the antibody–binding site domains is presented in Figure 12. The enzyme–cleavage sites are clustered in three areas. Five cleavages are seen at three distinguishable sites approximately 14,000 daltons from the amino end. Cleavages (9) are made at 7 distinguishable sites approximately 17,000 daltons from the amino end and 7 of the 8 enzyme preparations cleave at 3 distinguishable sites approximately 34,000 daltons from the amino end. Thus, as one would expect, certain regions of gp70 are more susceptible to partial proteolytic attack than others. Since the domains are predominantly defined by the enzyme–cleavage sites, the authors were able to subdivide certain regions more than others. For example, domain XIII comprises approximately 15,000 daltons in the center of gp70 whereas domains VII to XII are all clustered in a relatively small region around 17,000 daltons from the N–terminus. These domains could be defined because several antigenic sites in this region were recognized by these hybridomas. Thus, the data indicate a corre-

PROTEASE CLEAVAGE SITES

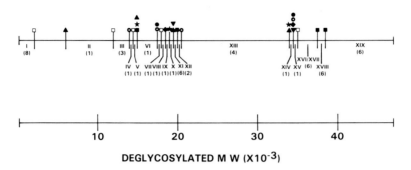

FIGURE 12. Linear map of 19 mAb–binding domains and protease cleavage sites of Rauscher virus gp70. The molecular weight of deglycosylated gp70 was estimated by sequence analysis to be Mr 47,000.[34] Map location of antibody–binding domains (Roman numerals with number of hybridomas that bind in those domains within parentheses) and enzyme cleavage sites (symbols) were determined by the size of the various deglycosylated fragments. The enzyme symbols are, *S. aureus* V8 protease (■), TCPK trypsin (□), elastase (●), clostripain (O), contaminating protease in NP–40 solution (◆), penicillinase (▼), α-chymotrypsin (▲), collagenase (★).

lation exists between highly antigenic sites and availability to partial proteolysis. In addition to the highly antigenic site at approximately 17,000 daltons from the amino end of gp70, sites of high antigenicity are found within the first 2000 daltons from the amino end of gp70 as well as approximately 37,000 daltons from the amino end of the molecule.

B. Localization of the Regions Affected by Glycosylation

To further the structural analysis of gp70 the mAbs were mapped with respect to glycosylation effects that were described above. The partially deglycosylated molecule will react differentially with the panel of mAbs. Figure 13 displays five different immune precipitation patterns produced by the mAbs. Certain mAbs do not immune precipitate either native or deglycosylated gp70 (lane A). Some hybridomas precipitate the native gp70 more efficiently than deglycosylated gp70 (lane C). Other hybridomas precipitate gp70 only after deglycosylation (lane B) or to a greater extent after carbohydrate is removed (lanes D and E). Finally, other mAbs precipitate native and deglycosylated gp70 equally well (lane F).

The hybridomas that mapped (Figure 14) in the amino portion (domain I to XII) of the molecule were strongly affected by the presence or absence of the glycosidic residues. 74% of these hybridomas precipitated the deglycosylated molecule more or less efficiently than the native molecule. Two of the four hybridomas that mapped in the center of gp70 (domain XIII) precipitated the deglycosylated gp70 more efficiently than the native molecule. In contrast, of the hybridomas that mapped in the carboxyl portion of the molecule (domains XIV to XIX), only 35% were affected by deglycosylation. This distribution of epitopes affected by the glycosidic residues contrasts with the altered mobility of the deglycosylated fragments. The fragments that are altered most by removal of glycosidic residues map in the carboxyl portion of the molecule. In addition, most of the possible glycosylation sites are found in this carboxyl region.[34]

The glycosidic residues that map in the carboxyl region may affect epitopes in the amino region because of the tertiary structure of the gp70. Since the gp70 molecule has a hydrophobic leader sequence as well as a hydrophobic region in p15e that is initially

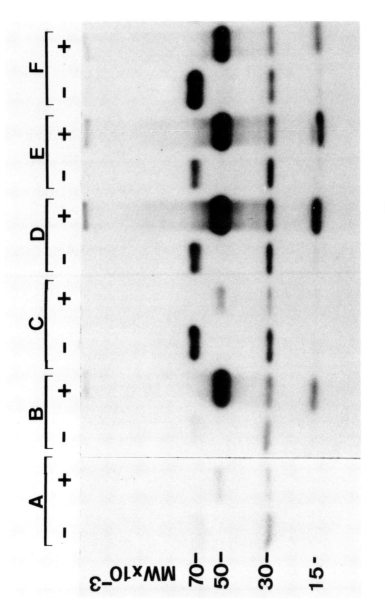

FIGURE 13. Differential immunoprecipitates of native and deglycosylated gp70. ^{125}I–gp70 was deglycosylated (from total virus) by an endoglycosidase isolated in this lab.[12] The deglycosylated gp70 has an apparent molecular weight of 49,000 daltons and is devoid of carbohydrate by periodic acid–Schiffs staining and by loss of all [^{3}H] mannose and [^{3}H]–glucosamine label. (−) native gp70 and (+) deglycosylated gp70. The cell lines secreting the mAbs were, None (lane A), R$_1$01H11 (lane B), R$_2$02D06 (lane C), R$_2$03F09 (lane D), R$_1$01D09 (lane E), and R$_2$06E04 (lane F).

EFFECT OF DEGLYCOSYLATION ON MONOCLONAL ANTIBODY ACTIVITY

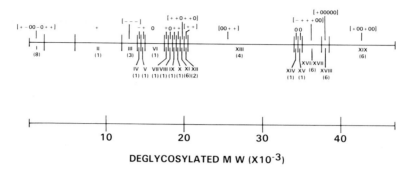

DEGLYCOSYLATED M W (X10⁻³)

FIGURE 14. Linear map of 19 mAb–binding domains and sites affected by deglycosylation. Map derivation is explained in legend to Figure 12. (−) Immune precipitation of native gp70 was more efficient than deglycosylated gp70. (+) Immune precipitation of native gp70 was less efficient than deglycosylated gp70. (O) Immune precipitation of deglycosylated gp70 was similar to that of native gp70.

linked to the carboxyl end of gp70,[34] the molecule may form a looped structure similar to that of HA$_1$ and HA$_2$ of influenza.[44] This structure may be stabilized by the association of the carboxyl glycosidic residues with the amino end of gp70. This possibility is strengthened by the binding activities of the hybridomas that are affected by the glycosidic residues. The affected hybridomas that map in domains I to VII have higher binding titers on antigen presented in a more native state (pH 9.5 plates vs. methanol–fixed plates). Of the 12 hybridomas that map in this region, 8 bind the native gp70 more efficiently than denatured gp70 while only 1 binds denatured gp70 more efficiently. In contrast, 4 of the 9 hybridomas that map in domains IX to XIII prefer denatured gp70 while none bind native gp70 more efficiently. The preference for denatured gp70 is even more striking in domains XIV to XIX where 5 of the 6 hybridomas bind denatured gp70 more efficiently and none prefer native gp70. These results suggest the hybridomas affected by glycosidic residues in the carboxyl portion of the molecule map near the sterically hindering glycosidic residues while those hybridomas that map in the amino portion of the molecule are affected by the tertiary structure of the molecule that may be stabilized by those glycosidic residues that are covalently linked to the carboxyl end of the molecule.

C. Location of p15e–Binding Sites

The other protein encoded by the envelope gene of the retroviruses is p15e which is produced C–terminal to gp70 in the envelope precursor and is disulfide–bonded to gp70 in the intact virion.[30] Due to disulfide linkage, antibodies to p15e will typically also precipitate gp70 and vice versa. To determine the region of gp70 that was associated with p15e, partial enzymatic cleavages were performed as described above and fragments were precipitated with αp15e hybridomas.[29] Thus, after reduction, the fragment pattern should be indistinguishable from hybridomas precipitated by mAbs to gp70 that react in the same region of the molecule. Figure 15 shows two representative precipitations. Lane A is the immune precipitation pattern of a carboxyl–binding anti–gp70 hybridoma reacted with Rauscher virus digested with trypsin. Lane B is the pattern produced by an anti–p15e hybridoma reacted against the same digest. The patterns are identical with the exception of an enhancement of a band migrating slightly slower than p15 that may represent p15e. Since hybridomas that map in domains XVII to XIX all

45

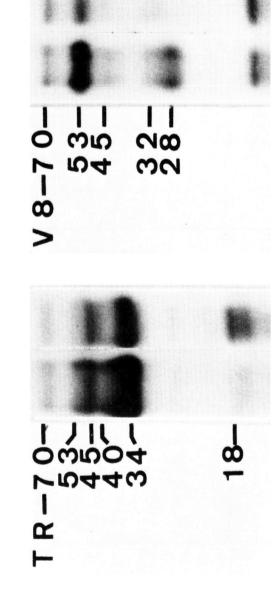

FIGURE 15. Trypsin and V8 protease PEC–MAP of gp70 defining p15e–binding site. R–MuLV was digested with trypsin (lane A and B) or V8 protease (lane C and D) as described.[28] The cell lines secreting the mAbs were R₂11A03 (lane A), 19V111E8 (lane B), R₁04C10 (lane C), and 19–F8 (lane D). Lanes B and D display the precipitation patterns of 2 of the 3 αp15(e) hybridomas. The third αp15(e) (9E8) produced identical patterns. The sera were ascites fluid that had been diluted with MEM supplemented with 10% FCS to a ratio of 1/1000 for 9E8 and 19–VIII–E8 or 1/100 for 19-F8. Lanes A and B contain all TR fragments listed with lane B showing an enhancement of TR–18. Lanes C and D contain V8–53, V8–45, and V8–32. The latter two bands were light in lane D but overexposure of the gel readily showed these two bands. V8–28 was present only in lane C.

produce this pattern on trypsin digests, a gp70 hybridoma that maps in domain XVIII is compared to a p15e hybridoma on a V8 digest (lanes C and D). The anti–gp70 pattern (lane C) contains V8–28. This is readily precipitated by hybridomas that map in domains XVIII and XIX (see Figure 11). This fragment is clearly absent in the p15e pattern (lane D) indicating p15e is disulfide linked to gp70 within domain XVII.

The location of the p15e binding site suggests a mechanism for the incomplete processing of the gp70 precursor in mink cell foci (MCF) recombinants that are generated by recombination within gp70.[19,7,32,26] The amino portion of the molecule is denoted by a xenotropic virus (grows preferentially in cells of heterologous species) while the carboxyl portion is contributed by an ecotropic (grows preferentially in murine cells of a heterologous species) gp70.[27] MCFs originating from quite distinctive ecotropic viruses have very similar yet distinguishable xenotropic sequences[11] that originate in an open reading frame on the 5′ of gp70 coding sequences and end in the carboxyl third of the gp70 molecule. MCF recombinants found in the AKR strain of mice process the gp70–p15e polyprotein at a slower rate than either ecotropic or xenotropic viruses isolated from this same strain.[13] This poorly processed precursor protein is also found on the preleukemic thymocytes of these mice.[14] The recombination site for the Rauscher MCFs is located between domains XVIII and XIV.[26,27] Since the p15e binding site (domain XVII) and polyprotein processing site (the end of domain XIX) are ecotropic in nature, the poor cleavage of the gp70–p15e) polyprotein may be due to a processing enzyme that has a xenotropic specificity. This activity can be coded by the sequences located in the open reading frame on the 5′ side of sequences coding for gp70.[34] Examination of various Moloney and AKR tumors has revealed new restriction sites in this region.[41,31]

D. Localization of Surface Immunofluorescence

The construction of the linear map now allowed the localization of the hybridomas that did and did not produce surface fluorescence. The molecule generally displayed clusters of fluorescence. Half of the hybridomas in domain I had strong surface fluorescence while half had weak or no fluorescence. The remainder of the amino end (domain II to III) had weak or no surface fluorescence. Since most of these activities were affected by glycosylation, it is probable that the glycosidic residues either sterically or allosterically block the antibody molecule from binding. The small region (about 20,000 daltons from the amino end of the molecule) that contained the highest concentration of protease sites as well as hybridoma–binding sites (domain VII to XII) had the most (10 of the 12 hybridomas) surface fluorescence. Low or no fluorescence was also clustered around domain XVII. This diminished fluorescence activity was probably due to the glycosidic residues that map in this region as well as p15e. The final carboxyl domain also contained some highly accesible antibody–binding sites.

E. Reactivity Against Other Related Retroviruses

Friend, Moloney, Rauscher, AKv2, and Rauscher MCF represent the common laboratory strains of retroviruses that produce different diseases in mice. Friend, Moloney, and Rauscher form the FMR group because of similar mouse cells tropism. All three can grow in either NIH–Swiss or BALB/c–derived cells. The three viruses are generally not considered to be endogenous to the mouse. AKv virus is endogenous to AKR mice and is also an ecotropic virus. Friend, Moloney, Rauscher, and AKv can all recombine with a xenotropic gp70 to give rise to a virus with an expanded host range that can produce mink cell foci (MCF). Friend and Rauscher MCFs have been isolated from crythroleukemias[39,42] while AKR and Moloney MCFs have been isolated from T cell lymphomas.[19,43]

The relatedness between the Rauscher gp70 and that of the above four viruses was

Table 3
VIRUS REACTIVITIES OF ANTI–R–MuLV gp70 HYBRIDOMAS

Gp70 map distance	domain	name	R–MCF	F–MuLV	M–MuLV	AKv2
0—2	I	$R_2$11D10($\kappa\gamma_1$)	−	+	−	−
		$R_2$01F01($\kappa\gamma_{2a}$)	−	+	−	−
		$R_1$05B05($\kappa\gamma_1$)	−	−	+	−
		$R_2$04F07($\kappa\gamma_1$)	−	+	−	−
		$R_2$03G01($\kappa\gamma_3$)	−	−	−	−
		$R_2$06E04($\kappa\gamma_1$)	−	−	−	−
		$R_1$13H03($\kappa\gamma_1$)	−	+	−	−
		$R_1$04C07($\kappa\gamma_{2b}$)	−	+	−	−
6—12	II	$R_1$10B06($\kappa\gamma_1$)	−	+	−	−
12—14	III	$R_2$03D11($\kappa\gamma_1$)	−	−	+	−
		$R_2$09C11($\kappa\gamma_{2b}$)	−	−	+	−
		$R_1$04D05($\kappa\gamma_1$)	−	+	+	−
14—18	IV	$R_2$13A10($\kappa\gamma_1$)	−	+	+	−
18	V	$R_1$03E11($\kappa\gamma_1$)	−	+	+	−
18	VI	$R_1$09E11($\kappa\gamma_1$)	−	+	+	+
18	VII	$R_2$05F06($\kappa\gamma_{2b}$)	−	+	+	−
18	VIII	$R_1$04E05($\kappa\varepsilon$)	−	+	−	−
18	IX	$R_2$02A09($\kappa\gamma_1$)	−	+	−	−
18	X	$R_1$08B03($\kappa\gamma_1$)	−	+	−	−
18	XI	$R_1$01H11($\kappa\gamma_1$)	−	+	−	−
		$R_1$12G02($\kappa\gamma_1$)	−	+	−	−
		$R_1$11G02($\kappa\gamma_1$)	−	+	−	−
		$R_1$05A06($\kappa\gamma_{2a}$)	−	+	−	−
		$R_1$12C02($\kappa\gamma_1$)	−	+	−	−
		$R_1$11C12($\kappa\gamma_1$)	−	+	−	−
18	XII	$R_1$15H06($\kappa\gamma_1$)	−	+	−	−
		$R_1$01G11($\kappa\gamma_1$)	+	+	−	−
18—34	XIII	$R_2$06B08($\kappa\gamma_{2a}$)	−	+	+	−
		$R_2$16A09($\kappa\gamma_1$)	−	+	−	−
		$R_1$04D01($\kappa\gamma_1$)	−	+	−	−
		$R_1$01B01($\kappa\gamma_1$)	−	+	−	−
34	XIV	$R_1$15G12($\kappa\gamma_1$)	+	+	−	−
34	XV	$R_1$10D05($\kappa\alpha$)	+	+	+	+
34—38	XVI	$R_2$02G12($\kappa\gamma_{2a}$)	−	+	−	−
34—38	XVII	$R_1$16C12($\kappa\gamma_3$)	+	+	−	−
		$R_2$03F09($\kappa\gamma_{2b}$)	+	+	−	+
		$R_1$10E12($\kappa\gamma_1$)	+	+	−	−
		$R_2$02G09($\kappa\gamma_{2a}$)	+	+	−	−
		$R_2$13G07($\kappa\gamma_1$)	+	+	−	−
38	XVIII	$R_2$11A03($\kappa\gamma_1$)	+	+	−	−
		$R_1$10G05($\kappa\gamma_1$)	+	+	−	−
		$R_1$06F09($\kappa\gamma_1$)	+	+	+	−
		$R_1$04C10($\kappa\gamma_1$)	+	+	−	−
		$R_1$15G05($\kappa\gamma_{2a}$)	+	+	−	−
		$R_1$10H06($\kappa\gamma_{2a}$)	+	+	−	−
38—47	XIX	$R_1$01D09($\kappa\gamma_1$)	+	+	−	−
		$R_1$09C11($\kappa\gamma_{2a}$)	+	+	−	−
		$R_1$12F10($\kappa\gamma_{2a}$)	+	+	−	−
		$R_1$05E06($\kappa\gamma_1$)	+	+	−	−
		$R_1$06B03($\kappa\gamma_{2a}$)	+	+	−	−
		$R_1$11B04($\kappa\gamma_{2a}$)	+	+	+	−

[a]Map distance was determined by the size of the various precipitation fragments and was based upon deglycosylated gp70 being Mr 47,000.
[b]Domains are defined in Table 1.
[c]Nomenclature has been described.[26]
[d]Origin of viruses has been described.[27]

Table 4
PERCENT HOMOLOGY WITH RAUSCHER gp70 HYBRIDOMAS

Domain	No.	R–MCF	F–MuLV	M–MuLV	AKV2
I–VII	(22)	5	73	64	5
VIII–XIII	(16)	6	100	6	0
XIV–XIX	(28)	96	100	11	14

Note: Fifteen additional hybridomas have been tested for binding activity. Although these hybridomas could not be precisely located due to glycosylation or conformational constraints, the binding site could be restricted to one of the three regions grouped above. The additional hybridomas which map between domains I to VII are $R_1$09C12 ($\lambda\gamma_{2a}$), $R_1$16D12 (Kϵ), $R_1$13A11 (Kγ_1), $R_1$15F07 (Kγ_1), $R_2$14D01 (Kγ_1), $R_1$16G07 (Kγ_{2a}). The hybridoma in domains VIII to XIII is $R_2$05E06 (Kγ_1). XIV to XIX contain $R_2$04G08 (Kγ_1), $R_1$10G02 (Kγ_{2a}), $R_1$12C07 (Kγ_1), $R_2$02E07 (Kγ_1), $R_2$04F07 (Kγ_1), $R_2$04G05 (Kγ_1), $R_1$08C08 (Kγ_{2a}), $R_1$12H06 ($\lambda\gamma_1$).

assayed in a virus–binding assay utilizing methanol–fixed and pH 9.5 plates.[28] The Rauscher gp70 molecule displayed three different reactivity patterns (Table 3) based upon mAb reactivity. The N–terminal portion of Rauscher gp70 (domain I to VII), has a high degree of homology with F–MuLV and M–MuLV. In contrast, the C–terminal portion (domain XIV to XIX) has homology with F–MuLV and R–MCF, but has virtually no relationship to M–MuLV. Moreover, the center of the gp70 molecule (domains VII to XII) generally has homology only with F–MuLV. This reactivity almost certainly represents the nonframework determinants of gp70 because of the limited reactivity of the mAbs. The mAb reactivities indicate AKv2 gp70 is quite divergent from R–MuLV: only 8% of the hybridomas reacted (Table 4). In contrast, F–MuLV gp70 contained a high degree of homology (91%) throughout the molecule. However, M–MuLV gp70 displayed a different pattern of reactivity. Only 27% of the monoclonals recognized M–MuLV gp70 determinants and most were clustered toward the N–terminus of the molecule representing 67% of the antigenic sites recognized in domains I to VII. The R–MCF recombinant, on the other hand, showed homology (96%) with the C–terminal portion of gp70 (domains XIV to XIX). The localization of homology suggests recombinations have occurred but does not prove any specific mechanism. The differential activities of the three section gp70 suggests the molecule may be generated by multiple recombinational events similar to those involved in the formation of Ig heavy chains.[3,22,25] Such a mechanism would explain the extreme heterogeneity found in the gp70 family. This type of recombination would also explain the homologies seen in various gp70. The gp70s in the FMR group all have a similar amino end as shown by peptide mapping and mAb reactivity. This modular assortment of gp70 fragments is also evident when various MCF viruses are compared.[11] The chymotryptic peptide maps of Rauscher (R319), AKR (247), and Moloney (MP 2) demonstrate that although each MCF has homology with the carboxyl end of its distinctive ecotropic parent, the amino 32,000 dalton fragments are remarkably similar. Similar substitutions were observed with other recombinants including AKR–13, AKV–1–36, AKV–2–34, Graffi (wild mouse ecoderived recombinant) as well as gp70s of HRS strain recombinants. Restriction analysis of tumors originating in strains of mice expressing AKR[31] and Moloney[41] ecotropic virus further substantiates this substitution in the amino portion of gp70. This restriction mapping as well as heteroduplex mapping[2,6,1] and mAb reactivities[26,27] indicate the amino 60 to 75% of gp70 has been substituted with xenotropic information. Based upon the reactivity with the Rauscher hybridomas the Rauscher,

Friend, Moloney, and AKR MCFs fall into two categories. Rauscher and Friend are indistinguishable in the ecotropic region (domains XIV to XIX) of MCFs while both are quite distinct from Moloney and AKR. Rauscher and Friend MCFs have both been isolated from erythroleukemias while Moloney and AKR MCFs have been isolated from T cell lymphomas. These correlations further implicate the viral gp70 in the targeting the cell type at risk for transformation.

VI. CONCLUDING REMARKS

The authors have described the isolation and characterization of a panel of mAbs directed against the major envelope glycoprotein of Rauscher murine leukemia virus. This analysis has revealed a heterogeneous group of determinants recognized by these hybridomas. Differential activities were demonstrated against the antigen presented in a variety of ways that points out the necessity of a large panel of monoclonals to make generalizations about the biochemistry or biology of determinants recognized by mAbs. The most useful method for discriminating the different specificities of the panel was obtained by generating a linear map of the binding sites through a technique that employs immune precipitation of gp70 fragments generated by partial proteolysis. This technique verified the heterogeneity seen in various assays and was useful in placing restraints on the tertiary configuration of the molecule.

The linear map also provided a framework for investigating the expression of this molecule on normal and abnormal differentiating tissues. Since this molecule is expressed on normal tissues in the absence of virus production, one mechanism for generating proliferative disease would involve inappropriate expression of the gp70 molecule. To further understand the mechanisms involved in these disease processes, normal tissues will be examined for the expression of various segments of gp70. The tissue distribution of this expression as well as the inhibition of tumor growth by mAbs will help understand the mechanisms involved in the generation of the viruses oncopotential.

Although the above study was directed at questions of interest to the murine retrovirus field, the approaches outlined here are equally applicable to other studies of protein structure and divergence. It is hoped that these studies may contribute to a generalized approach to the subdivision of mAb reactivities.

ACKNOWLEDGMENTS

We gratefully acknowledge helpful discussions with and use of laboratory facilities provided by Dr. Richard Lerner. We also thank Drs. Thomas Shinnick and J. Gregor Sutcliffe for providing results prior to publication. We appreciate the p15e mAbs provided by the laboratory of Dr. Robert Nowinski and the antisynthetic peptide provided by the laboratory of Dr. J. Gregor Sutcliffe. We thank Diane Schloeder, Douglas Bingham and Paula Eisenhart for excellent technical assitance.

The research was supported in part by NIH Grants CA 25803–02 and CA 25533–02, American Cancer Society Grant BC–267, a National Institutes of Health Training Grant T32 GM 07437 (HLN), and a Cancer Research Institute Fellowship (JHE). This is publication no. 2522 from the Research Institute of Scripps Clinic.

REFERENCES

1. **Bosselman, R. A., Van Guensven, L. J. L. D., Vogt, M., and Verma, I. M.** Genome organization of retroviruses. VI. Heteroduplex analysis of ecotropic and xenotropic sequences of Moloney mink cell focus–reducing viral RNA obtained by either a cloned isolate or a thymome cell line, *J. Virol.*, 32, 968, 1979.

2. **Chien, Y., Verma, I. M., Shih, T. Y., Scolnick, E. M., and Davidson, N.,** Heteroduplex analysis of the sequence relations between the RNAs of "mink cell focus–inducing" (MCF) and murine leukemia viruses, *J. Virol.*, 28, 352, 1978.

3. **Davis, M. M., Calame, K., Early, D. W., Levait, D. L., Joho, R., Weissman, I. L., and Hood, L.,** An immunoglobulin–heavy chain gene is formed by at least two recombinational events, *Nature (London)*, 283, 733, 1980.

4. **Devare, S. G., Rapp, U. R., Todaro, G. J., and Stephenson, J. R.,** Acquisition of oncogenicity by endogenous mouse type C viruses; effects of variations in *env* and *gag* genes. *J. Virol.*, 28, 457, 1978.

5. **Del Villano, B. C., Nave, B., Croker, B. P., Lerner, R. A., and Dixon, F. J.,** The oncornavirus glycoprotein gp69/71: a constituent of the surface of normal and malignant thymocytes, *J. Exp. Med.*, 141, 172, 1975.

6. **Donoghue, D. J., Rothenberg, E., Hopkins, N., Baltimore, D., and Sharp, P. A.,** Heteroduplex analysis of the nonhomology region between Moloney MuLV and the dual host range derivative HIX virus, *Cell*, 14, 959, 1978.

7. **Elder, J. H., Gautsch, J. W., Jensen, F. C., Lerner, R. A., Hartley, J. W., and Rowe, W. P.,** Biochemical evidence that MCF murine leukemia viruses are envelope (env) gene recombinants, *Proc. Natl. Acad. Sci. U.S.A.*, 74, 4676, 1977a.

8. **Elder, J. H., Jensen, F. C., Bryant, M. L., and Lerner, R. A.,** Polymorphism of the major envelope glycoprotein (gp70) of murine C–type viruses: virion associated and differentiation antigens encoded by a multi–gene family, *Nature (London)*, 267, 23, 1977b.

9. **Elder, J. H., Jensen, F. C., Gautsch, J. W., Lerner, R. A., and Vogt, M.,** Structural analysis of the surface glycoproteins (gp70s) of recombinant murine C–type viruses: evidence for envelope gene recombination, in *Advances in Comparative Leukemia Research*, Bentvelzen, P., et al., Eds., Elsevier/North Holland, Amsterdam, 1978, 156.

10. **Elder, J. H., Gautsch, J. W., Jensen, F. C., Lerner, R. A., Chused, T. M., Morse, H. C., Hartley, J. W., and Rowe, W. P.,** Differential expression of two distinct xenotropic viruses in NZB mice, *Clin. Immunol. Immunopathol.*, 15, 493, 1980.

11. **Elder, J. H. and Niman, H. L.,** Structural homologies in the substituted portions of envelope gene recombinant retroviruses, submitted.

12. **Elder, J. H.,** unpublished observations.

13. **Famulari, N. G. and Jelalian, K.,** Cell surface expression of *env* gene polyprotein in dual tropic mink cell focus-forming murine leukemia virus, *J. Virol.*, 30, 720, 1979.

14. **Famulari, N. G., Tung, J.-S., O'Donnell, P. V., and Fleissner, E.,** Murine leukemia virus *env*-gene expression in preleukemic thymocytes and leukemia cells of AKR strain mice, *Cold Spring Harbor Symp. Quant. Biol.*, 44, 1281, 1979.

15. **Fischinger, P. J., Frankel, A. E., Elder, J. H., Lerner, R. A., Ihle, J. N., and Bolognesi, D. P.,** Biological, immunological, and biochemical evidence that HIX virus is a recombinant between Moloney leukemia virus and murine xenotropic C type virus, *Virology*, 90, 241, 1978.

16. **Fischinger, P. J., Ihle, J. N., deNoronha, F., and Bolognesi, D. P.,** Oncogenic and immunogenic potential of cloned HIX viruses in mice and cats, *Med. Microbiol. Immunol.*, 164, 119, 1977.

17. **Fischinger, P. J., Ihle, J. N., Levy, J.-P., Bolognesi, D. P., Elder, J. H., and Schafer, W.,** Recombinant murine leukemia viruses and protective factors in leukemogenesis, *Cold Spring Conf. Cell Proliferation*, Cold Spring Harbor Laboratory, 70, 989, 1980.

18. **Green, N., Hiai, H., Elder, J. H., Schwartz, R. S., Khiroya, R. H., Thomas, C. Y., Tsichlis, P. N., and Coffin, J. M.,** Expression of leukemogenic recombinant viruses associated with a recessive gene in HRS/J mice, *J. Exp. Med.*, 152, 249, 1980.

19. **Hartley, J. W., Wolford, N. K., Old, L. J., and Rowe, W. P.,** A new class of murine leukemia virus associated with development of spontaneous lymphomas, *Proc. Natl. Acad. Sci. U.S.A.*, 74, 789, 1977.

20. **Henderson, L. E., Copeland, T. D., Smythers, G. W., Marquardt, H., and Oroszlan, S.,** Amino–terminal amino acid sequence and carboxyl–terminal analysis of Rauscher murine leukemia virus glycoproteins, *Virology*, 85, 319, 1978.

21. **Hino, S., Stephenson, J. R., and Aaronson, S. A.,** Radioimmunoassays for the 70,000–molecular–weight glycoproteins of endogenous mouse type C viruses: viral antigen expression in normal mouse tissues and sera, *J. Virol.*, 18, 933, 1976.

22. **Kataska, T., Kawakami, T., Takahashi, N., and Honjo, T.,** Rearrangement of immunoglobulin γ–chain gene and mechanism for heavy–chain class switch, *Proc. Natl. Acad. Sci. U.S.A.,* 77, 919, 1980.

23. **Kohler, G. and Milstein, C.,** Continuous cultures of fused cells secreting antibody of predefined specificity, *Nature (London),* 256, 495, 1975.

24. **Lerner, R. A., Wilson, C. P., Del Villano, B. C., McConahey, P. J., and Dixon, F. J.,** Endogenous oncornaviral gene expression in adult and fetal mice: quantitative, histological and physiologic studies of the major viral glycoprotein, gp70, *J. Exp. Med.,* 143, 151, 1976.

25. **Maki, R., Traunecher, A., Sakano, H., Roeder, W., and Tonegawa, S.,** Exon shuffling generates an immunoglobulin heavy chain gene, *Proc. Natl. Acad. Sci. U.S.A.,* 77, 2138, 1980.

26. **Niman, H. L. and Elder, J. H.,** Molecular dissection of Rauscher virus gp70 by using monoclonal antibodies: localization of acquired sequences of related envelope gene recombinants, *Proc. Natl. Acad. Sci. U.S.A.,* 77, 4524, 1980.

27. **Niman, H. L. and Elder, J. H.,** Independent assortment of murine retrovirus gp70 domains as demonstrated by monoclonal antibodies, submitted.

28. **Niman, H. L. and Elder, J. H.,** Structural analysis of Rauscher virus gp70 using monoclonal antibodies: sites of antigenicity and p15(E) linkage, submitted.

29. **Nowinski, R. C., Lostrom, M. E., Tam, M. R., Stone, M. R., and Burnetter, W. N.,** The isolation of hybrid cell lines producing monoclonal antibodies against the p15(E) protein of murine leukemia viruses, *Virology,* 93, 111, 1979.

30. **Pinter, A. and Fleissner, E.,** The presence of disulfide-linked gp70-p15(E) complexed in AKR murine leukemia virus, *Virology,* 83, 222, 1977.

31. **Quint, W., Quax, W., van der Putten, H., and Berns, A.,** Characterization of AKR murine leukemia virus sequences in AKR mouse substrains and structure of integrated recombinant genomes in tumor tissues, *J. Virol.,* 39, 1, 1981.

32. **Rommelaere, J., Faller, D. V., and Hopkins, N.,** Characterization and mapping or RNase T1–resistant oligonucleotides derived from the genomes of AKV and MCF murine leukemia viruses, *Proc. Natl. Acad. Sci. U.S.A.,* 75, 495, 1978.

33. **Shih, T. Y., Weeks, M. O., Troxler, D. H., Coffin, J. M., and Scolnick, E. M.,** Mapping host range–specific oligonucleotides within genomes of the ecotropic and mink cell focus–inducing strains of Moloney murine leukemia virus, *J. Virol.,* 26, 71, 1978.

34. **Shinnick, T. M., Lerner, R. A., and Sutcliffe, J. G.,** Nucleotide sequence of Moloney murine leukemia virus, *Nature (London),* 293, 543, 1981.

35. **Shulman, M., Wilde, C. D., and Kohler, G.,** A better cell line for making hybridomas secreting specific antibodies, *Nature (London),* 276, 269, 1978.

36. **Stockert, E., Old, L. J., and Boyse, E. A.,** The GIX system: a cell surface allo-antigen associated with murine leukemia virus; implications regarding chromosomal integration of the viral genome, *J. Exp. Med.,* 133, 1334, 1971.

37. **Strand, M., Lilly, F., and August, J.,** Host control of endogenous murine leukemia virus gene expression: concentration of viral proteins in high and low leukemia mouse strains, *Proc. Natl. Acad. Sci. U.S.A.,* 71, 3682, 1974.

38. **Troxler, D. H., Lowry, D., Hawk, R., Young, H., and Scolnick, E. M.,** Friend strain of spleen focus–forming virus is a recombinant between ecotropic murine type C virus and the env region of xenotropic type C virus, *Proc. Natl. Acad. Sci. U.S.A.,* 74, 4671, 1977.

39. **Troxler, D. H., Yuan, E., Linemeyer, D., Ruscetti, S., and Scolnick, E. M.,** Helper–independent mink cell focus–inducing strain of Friend murine type C virus: potential relationship to the origin of replication–defective spleen focus forming virus, *J. Exp. Med.,* 148, 639, 1978.

40. **Tung, J.-S., Vitetta, E. S., Fleissner, E., and Boyse, E. A.,** Biochemical evidence linking the GIX thymocyte surface antigen to the gp69/71 envelope glycoprotein of murine leukemia virus, *J. Exp. Med.,* 141, 198, 1975.

41. **van der Putten, H., Quint, W., van Raaij, J., Maanday, E. R., Verma, I. M., and Berns, A.,** M–MuLV induced leukemogenesis: interpretation and structure of recombinant proviruses in tumors, *Cell,* 24, 729, 1981.

42. **Van Guensven, L. J. L. D. and Vogt, M.,** Rauscher "mink cell focus–inducing" (MCF) virus causes erythroleukemia in mice: its isolation and properties, *Virology,* 101, 376, 1980.

43. **Vogt, M.,** Properties of a "mink cell focus-inducing" MCF virus from spontaneous lymphoma lines of BALB/c mice carrying Moloney leukemia virus as an endogenous virus, *Virology,* 93, 226, 1979.

44. **Wilson, J. A., Skekel, J. J., Wiley, D. C.,** Structure of the haemoglutinin membrane glycoprotein of influenza virus at 3Å resulution, *Nature (London),* 289, 366, 1981.

I. INTRODUCTION

The concept that regulation of immune responses (Ir) occurs through cellular interactions restricted by recognition of ''self''-determinants is an established tenet of immunology. Although initial theories maintained that recognition of ''self''-determinants
would stimulate an immune response and lead to a state of autoimmunity,[1,2] it is now
clear that recognition of certain ''self''-determinants is in fact necessary for the initiation, expression, and modulation of normal immune function. This requirement for
''self''-recognition in the expression of immunity was emphasized by the now classic
experiments of Zinkernagle and Doherty. These investigators demonstrated that effective T cell-mediated cytotoxicity of virally infected cells required not only recognition
of antigenic determinants expressed by the virus, but also membrane determinants displayed by the virally infected cell that are coded for by genes in the K and D region
of the murine major histocompatibility complex (MHC).[3-5] Although this phenomenon
was demonstrated for T cells capable of lysing virally infected cells, comparable recognition of ''self''-MHC determinants has been demonstrated using cytotoxic cells with
specificity for chemically modified target cells or target cells displaying minor transplantation antigens.[5-8]

''Self''-recognition is also necssary for the induction of reactivity among proliferating
and helper T cells. For example, activation of helper T cells requires that they not only
distinguish nominal determinants inherent in conventional antigen but also determinants
displayed by antigen-presenting cells. In contrast to the ''self''-gene products recognized by effector cytotoxic cells, helper and proliferating cells discern products of genes
in the immune response associated region of the MHC.[9-14]

Recently, it has become clear that recognition of another set of ''self''-determinants
is crucially required for interactions involved in the control of immune reactivity. The
network theory of Jerne postulates that the immune system communicates through a
network in which the language for communication requires recognition of idiotypes
(Id) inherent in secreted antibodies or cell surface antigen receptors.[15] This theory has
been supported by studies demonstrating that exogenous administration of anti-Id can
modulate delayed hypersensitivity reactions and antibody production in an antigen-specific fashion.[16-19] In addition, interactions between Id and anti-Id have been shown to
be involved in the control of normal immune reactivity to exogenous antigens.[20,21]

Thus, it is clear that recognition of certain ''self''-determinants by immunocompetent
cells is required for immunologic homeostasis, and that at least three distinct classes
of cell surface molecules are identified by interacting cells. This principle of ''self''-
recognition assures specificity in the induction and effector phases of the immune response and in modulation of the immune response by restricting cellular interactions
to those cells bearing the appropriate surface structures.

One in vitro correlate of the ''self''-recognition principle is the autologous mixed
lymphocyte reaction (AMLR). The AMLR is the proliferation of T cells when they are
appropriately cultured with autologous non-T cells in the absence of added antigen or
lectin.[22,23] Since the proliferation is induced by autologous cells, the AMLR appears
to be an in vitro manifestation of ''self''-recognition. However, the precise nature of
the stimulating cell, the function of the responsive T cells, the nature of the signal that
induces proliferation, and the relevance of this in vitro ''self''-recognition to cognitive
interactions occurring among immunocompetent cells in vivo are not clear. For example, B cells,[23-25] null cells,[26,27] dendritic cells,[28] and classical macrophages (Mφ)[25,26,29]
have each been claimed to be capable of serving as stimulators in the AMLR. While
some investigators indicate that suppressive influences are generated during the
AMLR,[26,30-33] others have reported that the responding T cells mediate help.[25,34] Blocking experiments utilizing antibodies,[29,35] including F(ab)$'_2$ fragments,[24] with specificity

I. INTRODUCTION

The concept that regulation of immune responses (Ir) occurs through cellular interactions restricted by recognition of "self"-determinants is an established tenet of immunology. Although initial theories maintained that recognition of "self"-determinants would stimulate an immune response and lead to a state of autoimmunity,[1,2] it is now clear that recognition of certain "self"-determinants is in fact necessary for the initiation, expression, and modulation of normal immune function. This requirement for "self"-recognition in the expression of immunity was emphasized by the now classic experiments of Zinkernagle and Doherty. These investigators demonstrated that effective T cell-mediated cytotoxicity of virally infected cells required not only recognition of antigenic determinants expressed by the virus, but also membrane determinants displayed by the virally infected cell that are coded for by genes in the K and D region of the murine major histocompatibility complex (MHC).[3-5] Although this phenomenon was demonstrated for T cells capable of lysing virally infected cells, comparable recognition of "self"-MHC determinants has been demonstrated using cytotoxic cells with specificity for chemically modified target cells or target cells displaying minor transplantation antigens.[5-8]

"Self"-recognition is also necssary for the induction of reactivity among proliferating and helper T cells. For example, activation of helper T cells requires that they not only distinguish nominal determinants inherent in conventional antigen but also determinants displayed by antigen-presenting cells. In contrast to the "self"-gene products recognized by effector cytotoxic cells, helper and proliferating cells discern products of genes in the immune response associated region of the MHC.[9-14]

Recently, it has become clear that recognition of another set of "self"-determinants is crucially required for interactions involved in the control of immune reactivity. The network theory of Jerne postulates that the immune system communicates through a network in which the language for communication requires recognition of idiotypes (Id) inherent in secreted antibodies or cell surface antigen receptors.[15] This theory has been supported by studies demonstrating that exogenous administration of anti-Id can modulate delayed hypersensitivity reactions and antibody production in an antigen-specific fashion.[16-19] In addition, interactions between Id and anti-Id have been shown to be involved in the control of normal immune reactivity to exogenous antigens.[20,21]

Thus, it is clear that recognition of certain "self"-determinants by immunocompetent cells is required for immunologic homeostasis, and that at least three distinct classes of cell surface molecules are identified by interacting cells. This principle of "self"-recognition assures specificity in the induction and effector phases of the immune response and in modulation of the immune response by restricting cellular interactions to those cells bearing the appropriate surface structures.

One in vitro correlate of the "self"-recognition principle is the autologous mixed lymphocyte reaction (AMLR). The AMLR is the proliferation of T cells when they are appropriately cultured with autologous non-T cells in the absence of added antigen or lectin.[22,23] Since the proliferation is induced by autologous cells, the AMLR appears to be an in vitro manifestation of "self"-recognition. However, the precise nature of the stimulating cell, the function of the responsive T cells, the nature of the signal that induces proliferation, and the relevance of this in vitro "self"-recognition to cognitive interactions occurring among immunocompetent cells in vivo are not clear. For example, B cells,[23-25] null cells,[26,27] dendritic cells,[28] and classical macrophages (Mφ)[25,26,29] have each been claimed to be capable of serving as stimulators in the AMLR. While some investigators indicate that suppressive influences are generated during the AMLR,[26,30-33] others have reported that the responding T cells mediate help.[25,34] Blocking experiments utilizing antibodies,[29,35] including F(ab)$'_2$ fragments,[24] with specificity

Chapter 3

USE OF mAbs TO PROBE THE FUNCTION AND SPECIFICITY OF CELLS PARTICIPATING IN THE AUTOLOGOUS MIXED LYMPHOCYTE REACTION (AMLR)*

Bruce Richardson, ** **Perrie Hausman, Howard Raff, and John Stobo** **

TABLE OF CONTENTS

I. Introduction 54

II. Materials and Methods 55

III. Results 55
    A. Heterogeneity Among Cells Capable of Stimulating
        in the AMLR 55
    B. Heterogeneity Among Responder Cells 58
    C. Function of Mac-120$^+$ Mϕ and T-29$^+$ T Cells 60

IV. Discussion 66

Acknowledgments 68

References 68

* Supported in part by U.S.P.H.S. Grant A.I. 14104. Part of this work was performed in fulfillment of a Ph.D. degree (Hausman).
**Dr. Richardson is a Research Associate and Dr. Stobo is an Investigator of the Howard Hughes Medical Institute.

22. **Kataska, T., Kawakami, T., Takahashi, N., and Honjo, T.,** Rearrangement of immunoglobulin γ–chain gene and mechanism for heavy–chain class switch, *Proc. Natl. Acad. Sci. U.S.A.,* 77, 919, 1980.

23. **Kohler, G. and Milstein, C.,** Continuous cultures of fused cells secreting antibody of predefined specificity, *Nature (London),* 256, 495, 1975.

24. **Lerner, R. A., Wilson, C. P., Del Villano, B. C., McConahey, P. J., and Dixon, F. J.,** Endogenous oncornaviral gene expression in adult and fetal mice: quantitative, histological and physiologic studies of the major viral glycoprotein, gp70, *J. Exp. Med.,* 143, 151, 1976.

25. **Maki, R., Traunecher, A., Sakano, H., Roeder, W., and Tonegawa, S.,** Exon shuffling generates an immunoglobulin heavy chain gene, *Proc. Natl. Acad. Sci. U.S.A.,* 77, 2138, 1980.

26. **Niman, H. L. and Elder, J. H.,** Molecular dissection of Rauscher virus gp70 by using monoclonal antibodies: localization of acquired sequences of related envelope gene recombinants, *Proc. Natl. Acad. Sci. U.S.A.,* 77, 4524, 1980.

27. **Niman, H. L. and Elder, J. H.,** Independent assortment of murine retrovirus gp70 domains as demonstrated by monoclonal antibodies, submitted.

28. **Niman, H. L. and Elder, J. H.,** Structural analysis of Rauscher virus gp70 using monoclonal antibodies: sites of antigenicity and p15(E) linkage, submitted.

29. **Nowinski, R. C., Lostrom, M. E., Tam, M. R., Stone, M. R., and Burnetter, W. N.,** The isolation of hybrid cell lines producing monoclonal antibodies against the p15(E) protein of murine leukemia viruses, *Virology,* 93, 111, 1979.

30. **Pinter, A. and Fleissner, E.,** The presence of disulfide-linked gp70-p15(E) complexed in AKR murine leukemia virus, *Virology,* 83, 222, 1977.

31. **Quint, W., Quax, W., van der Putten, H., and Berns, A.,** Characterization of AKR murine leukemia virus sequences in AKR mouse substrains and structure of integrated recombinant genomes in tumor tissues, *J. Virol.,* 39, 1, 1981.

32. **Rommelaere, J., Faller, D. V., and Hopkins, N.,** Characterization and mapping or RNase T1–resistant oligonucleotides derived from the genomes of AKV and MCF murine leukemia viruses, *Proc. Natl. Acad. Sci. U.S.A.,* 75, 495, 1978.

33. **Shih, T. Y., Weeks, M. O., Troxler, D. H., Coffin, J. M., and Scolnick, E. M.,** Mapping host range–specific oligonucleotides within genomes of the ecotropic and mink cell focus–inducing strains of Moloney murine leukemia virus, *J. Virol.,* 26, 71, 1978.

34. **Shinnick, T. M., Lerner, R. A., and Sutcliffe, J. G.,** Nucleotide sequence of Moloney murine leukemia virus, *Nature (London),* 293, 543, 1981.

35. **Shulman, M., Wilde, C. D., and Kohler, G.,** A better cell line for making hybridomas secreting specific antibodies, *Nature (London),* 276, 269, 1978.

36. **Stockert, E., Old, L. J., and Boyse, E. A.,** The GIX system: a cell surface allo-antigen associated with murine leukemia virus; implications regarding chromosomal integration of the viral genome, *J. Exp. Med.,* 133, 1334, 1971.

37. **Strand, M., Lilly, F., and August, J.,** Host control of endogenous murine leukemia virus gene expression: concentration of viral proteins in high and low leukemia mouse strains, *Proc. Natl. Acad. Sci. U.S.A.,* 71, 3682, 1974.

38. **Troxler, D. H., Lowry, D., Hawk, R., Young, H., and Scolnick, E. M.,** Friend strain of spleen focus–forming virus is a recombinant between ecotropic murine type C virus and the env region of xenotropic type C virus, *Proc. Natl. Acad. Sci. U.S.A.,* 74, 4671, 1977.

39. **Troxler, D. H., Yuan, E., Linemeyer, D., Ruscetti, S., and Scolnick, E. M.,** Helper–independent mink cell focus–inducing strain of Friend murine type C virus: potential relationship to the origin of replication–defective spleen focus forming virus, *J. Exp. Med.,* 148, 639, 1978.

40. **Tung, J.-S., Vitetta, E. S., Fleissner, E., and Boyse, E. A.,** Biochemical evidence linking the GIX thymocyte surface antigen to the gp69/71 envelope glycoprotein of murine leukemia virus, *J. Exp. Med.,* 141, 198, 1975.

41. **van der Putten, H., Quint, W., van Raaij, J., Maanday, E. R., Verma, I. M., and Berns, A.,** M–MuLV induced leukemogenesis: interpretation and structure of recombinant proviruses in tumors, *Cell,* 24, 729, 1981.

42. **Van Guensven, L. J. L. D. and Vogt, M.,** Rauscher "mink cell focus–inducing" (MCF) virus causes erythroleukemia in mice: its isolation and properties, *Virology,* 101, 376, 1980.

43. **Vogt, M.,** Properties of a "mink cell focus-inducing" MCF) virus from spontaneous lymphoma lines of BALB/c mice carrying Moloney leukemia virus as an endogenous virus, *Virology,* 93, 226, 1979.

44. **Wilson, J. A., Skekel, J. J., Wiley, D. C.,** Structure of the haemoglutinin membrane glycoprotein of influenza virus at 3Å resulution, *Nature (London),* 289, 366, 1981.

for Ia determinants suggest that recognition of these "self"-determinants is required to initiate T cell proliferation. However, one study demonstrates that the stimulating determinants may be different from classical Ia antigens.[36] Finally, no studies have yet demonstrated that the AMLR indeed occurs in vivo or that the T cell proliferation noted in vitro represents immunologic recognition involved in either the induction or controlled expression of in vivo immune reactivity. The latter point is crucial. If the AMLR represents only an in vitro curiosity, the phenomena is biologically trivial.

The authors approach to determining the immunologic relevance of the AMLR has been to dissect the reaction, examine the nature of the stimulating and responder cells, and ask if these cells that participate in the AMLR include cells that would be expected to interact in an immunologic reaction in vivo. To do this, somatic cell hybridization has been utilized to produce mAbs specific for cells reacting in the AMLR. Although several of the questions posed above remain unanswered, the studies reported here support the concept that at least a portion of the "self"-recognition manifested by the AMLR occurs among immunologically relevant T and non-T cells.

II. MATERIALS AND METHODS

The majority of the methods and reagents used have been described in previous publications.[37–41] The following is a brief description of the most important technical points of the studies presented here.

In general, responding cells consisted of E rosette-positive populations (90 ± 4% T, 4% - 2% esterase-positive cells) while stimulating populations consisted of E rosette-negative cells (10% T, 40 ± 5% Ig positive and 30 ± 8% esterase-positive cells). Stimulator cells were further fractionated into adherent cell-enriched populations (95% esterase-positive, 90% phagocytic) by 2, 1 hr adherences onto polystyrene petri dishes in the presence of 10% nonheat-inactivated autologous serum. Nonadherent cells were removed by vigorous pipetting while adherent cells were removed with xylocaine (12 mM). All cultures were performed in the presence of 5 to 10% heat-inactivated serum that was autologous to the responding cell, and each AMLR was tested at two ratios of responder to stimulator cells (1:1 and 2:1). Reactivity was measured by the incorporation of tritiated thymidine into DNA and was assayed at two times (day 6 and day 8) after the initiation of culture. Results are presented as maximal reactivities.

Two mAbs, produced by the fusion of immune spleen cells from BALB/c mice with the NS-1 myeloma line were used. Mac-120 is a monocyte specific κ, μ Ig. T-29 is a T cell-specific κ, γ$_{2b}$. The antibodies were purified by lentil-lectin affinity chromatography or selective elution from a Staph Protein A column, respectively. To cytolytically remove cells reactive with either reagent, a sandwich technique (i.e. mouse mAb followed by rabbit anti-mouse Ig) and rabbit complement was used.

Negative selection with BURD and light was performed by the addition of 3 μg/ml of BURD at two successive times of culture. 12 hr after the last addition of BURD, the cells were exposed to cool white light at room temperature for 2 hr.

In a panning technique to positively select cells reactive with the Mac-120 antibody, adherent cells were allowed to bind at 23°C for 1 hr to a bacteriologic petri dish that had been previously coated with purified antibody. The adherent cells were removed with xylocaine. (Mφ do not adhere to noncoated bacteriologic petri dishes when incubated at 23°C).[42]

III. RESULTS

A. Heterogeneity Among Cells Capable of Stimulating in the AMLR
As indicated in the introduction, B cells, Mφ, null cells, and dendritic cells each

Table 1
AMLR TO B AND Mφ POPULATIONS

| Responder T | Stimulator Populations | | | |
| | B | | Mφ | |
	CPM	SI	CPM	SI
Exp. 1	5,886	7.8	1,700	2.3
2	29,123	29.0	4,075	4.0
3	19,976	16.0	8,636	7.7
4	24,800	11.0	10,837	4.9
5	8,659	32.0	7,149	26.0
Mean SI ± SE	15.94 ± 4.2		4.7 ± 1.0	

Note: 100,000 T-enriched cells were cultured in 10% HAS with 100,000 and 50,000 autologous B cells or Mφ for 6 to 9 days. Reactivity was measured by the incorporation of ^{3}H-TdR into DNA during the last 18 hr of culture. Results are expressed as the maximal CPM of cultures containing responders and stimulators or as the maximal SI for 5 individual experiments.

have been claimed to be effective stimulators in the AMLR.[23-29] To better define the nature of the stimulating cell, the authors further fractionated the autologous non-T population by 2, 1 hr adherences to plastic into an adherent (95% esterase-positive, 90% phagocytic, referred to as Mφ) and a nonadherent population (85% Ig-positive, referred to as B cells). Each population was then tested at two ratios of responder to stimulator cells (2:1, 1:1) for its ability to induce proliferation among autologous T cells. In these experiments, reactivities were measured daily starting at day 4 and ending at day 11 of culture. The results of five such experiments are presented in Table 1 and are expressed as maximal reactivities. Note that although B cells are more effective stimulators in the AMLR, Mφ also induce substantial proliferation. The relatively low stimulatory capacity of Mφ may reflect suppression of measured blastogenesis either through the liberation of a soluble suppressive material or through secretion of cold thymidine rather than any intrinsic deficiency in their stimulatory capacity. It should be emphasized that maximal proliferation induced by the B population did not occur on the same day of culture as that induced by Mφ (data not shown). Thus, analysis of proliferation at only a single time point would be misleading.

Neither the B nor the Mφ population used as stimulators for these experiments are entirely pure. It is possible, therefore, that stimulation by each is mediated by a common cell type that contaminates both populations. To determine if Mφ represent one of the stimulating cells, a panel of Mφ-specific mAbs was generated. One of these antibodies (κ, μ) identifies a 120,000 dalton determinant displayed on the surface of 37 ± 3% of the Mφ from several HLA-DR disparate individuals. The specificity of this antibody, as determined by indirect immunofluorescence and microcytotoxicity, is demonstrated in Table 2. Three points concerning this data deserve emphasis. First, the Mac-120 antibody is specific for Mφ and does not bind to T cells, B cells, null cells, neutrophils, a human histiocytic, or a human promyelocyte cell line. Second, the Mac-120 reagent does not, in the assays used, react with all Mφ. Similar analysis of Mφ using the fluorescence-activated cell sorter (FACS) has also demonstrated the existence of two distinct Mφ populations. One population, representing approximately 1/2 of adherent, peripheral blood Mφ stains brightly with the Mac-120 reagent. The remaining 1/2 of the Mφ display at least a ten-fold lower density of the Mac-120 determinant. The third

Table 2
POPULATIONS OF CELLS IDENTIFIED BY MAC-120 AND ANTI-HLA-DR

Population assayed	Mac-120		Anti-HLA-DR	
	Fl	Cytotox.	Fl	Cytotox.
Adherent Mφ	37 ± 2.8	23 ± 8.8	94 ± 3	100
Phagocytic Mφ	35 ± 2.9	ND	ND	ND
Normal T cells	0	1	0	3
Human T cell line (CEM)	0	0	0	0
Normal B cells	0	0	90	58
Human B cell line (HLA-DR-positive, GM 130)	0	3	93	92
Human histiocytic cell line	0	5	ND	ND
Normal neutrophils	2	ND	ND	ND
Human promyelocyte cell line (HL-60)	0	ND	ND	ND

Note: The indicated cell populations were assayed for their reactivity with Mac-120 and anti-HLA-DR in either direct immunofluorescence (Fl) or indirect cytotoxicity (cytotox.). Phagocytic Mφ refers to whole PBMC that had been allowed to ingest latex particles and then quantitated for the frequency of fluorescence-positive, phagocytic cells. Normal T cells refers to E rosette-positive, adherent cell-depleted populations (94% T cells, <1% esterase-positive). Normal B cells refers to E rosette-negative, adherent cell-depleted populations (95% Ig-bearing, <2% esterase-positive), which may also include null cells. Results represent the mean for 2 or mean ± SE for 6 to 12 determinations. ND indicates not done.

point to be emphasized is that, in the authors' hands, virtually all (>90%) of adherent peripheral blood Mφ bear easily detectable HLA-DR determinants. Thus, the Mac-120+ as well as the Mac-120− population display HLA-DR determinants. This point will be substantiated subsequently.

The Mac-120 antibody was then used to cytolytically remove stimulator cells from the autologous B and Mφ populations (Table 3). To control for the nonspecific effects of dead cells, the Mφ population was also treated with a concentration of a monoclonal antilymphocyte antibody (ALA) that lysed a percentage of cells (30 to 40%) comparable to that lysed by the Mac-120 antibody. In each case, Mφ remaining after cytolysis with Mac-120 demonstrated a marked decrease in their ability to stimulate proliferation among autologous T cells. In contrast, Mac-120 treatment of the B cell population did not decrease their stimulatory capacity. Mφ remaining after limited cytolysis with the ALA were as effective as the original Mφ population in their stimulatory capacity. Addition of Mφ cytolytically treated with Mac-120 back to an AMLR between either T and B cells or T and whole Mφ did not inhibit proliferation (data not presented). This indicates that the decreased stimulation noted with Mac-120 treated cells did not represent the induction of suppressive influences.

These cytotoxicity experiments indicate that stimulating cells existing among the B population can be distinguished from those existing among the Mφ population. Furthermore, they suggest that not all Mφ are equally capable of serving as stimulators in the AMLR.

To pursue this concept of heterogeneity existing among Mφ with regard to their role as stimulators in the AMLR, a panning technique was developed that allowed direct comparison of the stimulatory capacity of Mac-120+ and Mac-120− populations. Adherent peripheral blood Mφ were incubated on a bacteriologic petri dish that had been coated with Mac-120. Nonadherent cells were removed by pipetting and cytolytically

Table 3

EFFECT OF A Mφ SPECIFIC, mAb (MAC-120) ON STIMULATOR CELLS IN AUTOLOGOUS B AND Mφ POPULATIONS

	Stimulator population				
	B, antisera Rx		Mφ, antisera Rx		
Responder T	MIg	Mac-120	MIg	Mac-120	ALA
Exp. 1	63,395	60,608	20,455	1,842	22,728
	(17)	(16)	(5.4)	(0.48)	(6.0)
Exp. 2	33,525	31,290	8,940	3,124	10,115
	(15)	(14)	(4.0)	(1.4)	(4.5)
Exp. 3	17,568	20,496	6,637	897	ND
	(18)	(21)	(6.8)	(0.92)	
Exp. 4	ND	ND	73,388	15,982	ND
			(11.9)	(2.6)	

Note: B and Mφ were treated by indirect cytotoxicity with MIg, a Mφ-specific mAb (Mac-120), or an ALA. 50,000 and 100,000 viable cells from each population were then compared for their ability to stimulate 100,000 autologous T cells in an AMLR. The results represent the maximal CPM among cultures containing responder and stimulator cells or as the stimulation indexes (in parentheses) for four experiments. The ALA was used in suboptimal concentrations so that it lysed approximately the same percentage of Mφ as Mac-120. N.D. indicates not done.

treated with Mac-120 to remove any residual Mac-120 positive cells. The adherent population was removed with xylocaine. Both populations were analyzed by the FACS with Mac-120 as well as with an antisera specific for nonpolymorphic regions of HLA-DR. The results of these studies demonstrated that the Mac-120$^+$ population contained >85% Mac-120$^+$ cells while the Mac-120$^-$ population contained less than 10% Mac-120$^+$ cells. Both Mac-120$^+$ and Mac-120$^-$ cells contained >90% HLA-DR positive Mφ. More importantly, both populations displayed a comparable density of HLA-DR determinants on their surface. Thus, while both populations are clearly different with regard to the frequency of Mac-120$^+$ cells they are comparable with regard to their display of HLA-DR determinants.

Each population was then compared for its ability to stimulate in an AMLR and an allogeneic mixed lymphocyte reaction (Table 4; these experiments also utilized two ratios of responder to stimulator cells). Mac-120$^+$ cells are effective stimulators in the AMLR while Mac-120$^-$ cells are not. Both populations were equivalent in their ability to stimulate in an allogeneic mixed lymphocyte culture (MLC). Addition of Mac-120$^-$ cells to an AMLR between T cells and the Mac-120$^+$ population simply diluted and did not suppress reactivity (data not presented). Finally, addition of culture fluid that was obtained from human Mφ cultured in fetal calf serum and that contained IL-1 activity did not reconstitute the ability of Mac-120$^-$ cells to stimulate in the AMLR. (Data not shown). When considered together, these findings indicate that only a subpopulation of Mφ are effective stimulators in the AMLR. Furthermore, they indicate that the relative difference in Mac-120$^+$ and Mac-120$^-$ cells to serve as stimulator cells cannot be ascribed to quantitative differences in their display of HLA-DR determinants.

B. Heterogeneity Among Responder Cells

The results of the studies presented to this point are compatible with the following two hypotheses. First, more than one cell type is capable of serving as a stimulator cell in the AMLR, but both induce proliferation among the same clone of T cell. Second,

Table 4
RELATIVE ABILITY OF MAC-120$^+$ AND MAC-120$^-$ Mφ TO STIMULATE IN THE AMLR

Responder T	Stimulating population	
	Mac-120$^+$ Mφ	Mac-120$^-$ Mφ
Exp. 1 Autologous	27,031	4,596
	(5.1)	(0.9)
Allogeneic	38,313	64,822
	(5.4)	(9.1)
Exp. 2 Autologous	8,936	1,156
	(8.9)	(1.2)
Allogeneic	35,908	43,617
	(13.7)	(16.7)

Note: Mac-120$^+$ and Mac-120$^-$ Mφ obtained by panning were tested in two concentrations for their ability to induce proliferation among autologous and allogeneic T cells. Results are presented either as CPM or stimulation indexes (in parentheses) for two experiments.

Table 5
NEGATIVE SELECTION OF T CELLS RESPONSIVE TO AUTOLOGOUS B OR Mφ

Responder populations	Stimulators (max. CPM)	
	B	Mφ
Exp. 1 T + B (BURD, no light)	16,342	5,462
T + B (BURD, light)	1,936	6,991
Exp. 2 T + B (BURD, no light)	23,654	4,321
T + B (BURD, light)	2,116	3,968
Exp. 3 T + Mφ (BURD, no light)	7,397	4,350
T + Mφ (BURD, light)	7,310	1,840
Exp. 4 T + Mφ (BURD, no light)	6,360	1,719
T + Mφ (BURD, light)	7,330	619

Note: T cells that proliferated in response to autologous B cells or Mφ were specifically suicided with BURD and light and their subsequent response to autologous B cells and Mφ compared. Controls consisted of cultures with BURD but not exposed to light. Results represent the maximal CPM in cultures of responder and stimulator cells.

the AMLR represents the sum proliferation of distinct T cell clones responding to distinct stimulating cells. To decide between these two possibilities, a negative selection technique was utilized. T cells proliferating in response to either Mφ or B cells were "suicided" by exposure to BURD and light. The remaining cells were assayed for their response to autologous B and Mφ populations (Table 5). The results of these experiments indicate the existence of two distinct groups of responding T cells. That is to say, negative selection of T cells responsive to the B population abrogated their subsequent response to B cells but did not diminish proliferation to Mφ. Conversely, negative selection of T cells responding to Mφ abrogated subsequent reactivity to Mφ, but did not diminish the subsequent reactivity to the B population. It should be noted that in these experiments the reactivity of the negatively selected populations was tested

Table 6
mAb T-29 DETECTS THE Mφ-RESPONSIVE T POPULATION

	Stimulators (max. CPM)	
Responding populations	**B**	**Mφ**
Exp. 1 T + MIg + C'	35,270	2,777
T + T-29 + C'	35,237	904
Exp. 2 T + MIg + C'	48,562	6,636
T + T-29 + C'	34,276	1,445
Exp. 3 T + MIg + C'	23,431	4,803
T + T-29 + C'	22,659	1,163
Exp. 4 T + MIg + C'	11,589	2,895
T + T-29 + C'	14,557	887
Exp. 5 T + MIg + C'	19,484	12,311
T + T-29 + C'	18,312	925
Exp. 6 T + MIg + C'	ND	4,561
T + T-15 + C'	ND	4,873
T + T-33 + C'	ND	3,279

Note: T cells were treated with either the control reagent MIg or with the mAb T-29 and complement. The recovered cells were then tested at equivalent concentrations of viable cells for their proliferative response to autologous B cells or Mφ. Results represent the maximal CPM for 5 experiments. T-15 and T-33 were similarly used to lyse an equivalent percentage of T cells.

after three, five, seven, and nine days of culture to control for the possibility that priming was induced during the negative selection procedure. In each instance, results are presented as maximal reactivities.

To confirm the existence of distinct, responding T cells in the AMLR, the authors developed a mAb reactive to Mφ-responsive T cells. This reagent, a κ, γ_{2b} mAb was made by fusing spleen cells from mice immunized with T cell blasts generated in the AMLR and isolated by gradient fractionation. Although the ligand that serves as a target for the antibody has not been characterized, the antibody, termed T-29, reacts with 10 ± 2% of the peripheral blood T cells from HLA-DR disparate individuals. T-29 does not bind, as determined by immunofluorescence and microcytotoxicity, to Mφ, B cells, or null cells.

T cells were cytolytically treated with T-29, then tested for their proliferative response to autologous B cells and Mφ. As demonstrated in Table 6, cytolysis with T-29 resulted in a selective decrease in the response to Mφ. Reactivity to B cells was not diminished. Cytolytic treatment of T cells with two other mAbs (T-15, T-33) that lysed the same percentage of T cells as T-29 did not decrease the AMLR to Mφ. These studies, in conjunction with the BURD experiments indicate the existence of two distinct T cell populations responding to two distinct stimulator populations in the AMLR. One population of T cells proliferates in response to signals from cells in autologous B-enriched populations. Whether the stimulating cell in this population is an Ig-bearing B cell, a null cell, or some other cell type is not known. Another distinct population of T cells identified by the T-29 reagent is induced to proliferate by signals from a subpopulation of HLA-DR$^+$, Mac-120$^+$ Mφ.

C. Function of Mac-120$^+$ Mφ and T-29$^+$ T Cells

As discussed in the introduction, the function of T cells activated in the AMLR is controversial. The authors' data suggests that the apparent controversy may reflect the fact that the AMLR is comprised of distinct T cell populations. It is possible that these distinct T cell populations mediate different effector and regulatory functions.

Table 7
ANTIGEN REACTIVITY AMONG POPULATIONS DEPLETED
OF MAC-120$^+$ Mϕ

Responding populations	Antigen used to induce reactivity		
	C. albicans	PPD	Collagen
Exp. 1 MIg	6,732	8,954	ND
Mac-120	345	682	ND
Exp. 2 MIg	18,069	13,521	ND
Mac-120	2,280	101	ND
Exp. 3 MIg	ND	ND	43%
Mac-120	ND	ND	11%

Note: T cell populations partially depleted of adherent cells were treated by indirect cytotoxicity with either the control reagent, MIg, or Mac-120. 100,000 viable cells from each population were compared for their reactivity to *C. albicans*, purified protein derivative (PPD), or bovine collagen. For reactivity to *C. albicans* and PPD, proliferative assays were used with results expressed as ΔCPM. For reactivity to collagen, cells from patients with rheumatoid arthritis were assayed for the ability of collagen to induce production of the LIF. Results are presented as % inhibition of migration (>20% inhibition of migration = + reactivity).

Since a portion of the cells interacting in the AMLR (i.e., T cells and Mϕ) also interact in vivo to initiate reactivity to soluble antigens, the role of Mac-120$^+$ Mϕ and T-29$^+$ T cells in T-dependent reactivity to soluble antigens was investigated.

T-enriched, partially adherent cell-depleted populations were cytolytically treated with either Mac-120 or the control MIg to completely remove Mac-120$^+$ cells. The populations were then compared for their ability to respond to three soluble antigens as determined by blast transformation and the synthesis of the lymphokine, leukocyte inhibition factor (LIF). As demonstrated in Table 7, cytolysis with Mac-120 markedly diminished reactivity to antigen irrespective of the assay used. Although only maximal reactivities are presented, the responses noted using suboptimal and supraoptimal concentrations of antigen were also comparably reduced by Mac-120 treatment.

These results indicate that Mac-120$^-$ cells cannot support antigen-induced T cell activation, but do not directly demonstrate that Mac-120$^+$ cells can. To investigate this, the panning technique previously described was utilized to obtain highly enriched Mac-120$^+$ and Mac-120$^-$ cells. Various proportions of each population were then compared for their ability to reconstitute antigen-induced T cell proliferation among autologous T-enriched, adherent cell-depleted populations (Table 8). The results are expressed as reactivity compared to that seen in whole peripheral blood mononuclear cells (PBMC) (% of control). Note that the adherent cell-depleted population displayed reactivity to *Candida albicans,* which was only 8% of that seen in the PBMC. Addition of as few as 0.1% Mac-120$^+$ cells reconstituted reactivity to 60% of control. Reactivity was restored to normal by the addition of 1.0% Mac-120$^+$ Mϕ. In contrast, addition of up to 10% Mac-120$^-$ Mϕ did not result in substantial restoration of reactivity (<20% of control). Addition of 10% Mac-120$^-$ Mϕ to whole PBMC did not result in any decreased reactivity to *Candida albicans* (10472 maximal ΔCPM in PBMC vs. 16630 maximal ΔCPM in whole PBMC + 10% Mac-120$^-$ cells). Thus, Mac-120$^-$ cells fail to support antigen-induced T cell proliferation among Mϕ-depleted T cells and do not suppress reactivity among whole PBMC.

While these studies suggest a requirement for Mac-120$^+$ Mϕ in antigen-induced activation of T cells, they do not indicate the nature of this requirement. It is clear that

Table 8
RELATIVE ABILITY OF MAC-120⁺ AND MAC-120⁻ Mφ TO RECONSTITUTE ANTIGEN REACTIVITY AMONG T-ENRICHED, Mφ-DEPLETED CELLS

	Mφ Added (%)			
Source of Mφ	0	0.1	1.0	10.0
Mac-120⁺	8%	59 ± 5%	81 ± 9%	130 ± 8%
Mac-120⁻	8%	10 ± 2%	13 ± 4%	15 ± 3%

Note: T-enriched, Mφ-depleted cells were reconstituted with the indicated final concentration of Mac-120⁺ or Mac-120⁻ Mφ. The reactivity of the mixtures to *C. albicans* was then assayed with results presented as a % of control (CPM in T + Mφ/CPM in whole PBMC). The results represent the arithmetic mean ± S.E. for 3 experiments.

tivation of T cells, they do not indicate the nature of this requirement. It is clear that activation of T cells by antigen requires two signals from the Mφ. First, Mφ are required to present antigen in a manner suitable for recognition by relevant T cells. This requires that T cells "see" not only determinants inherent in conventional antigens but also Mφ glycoproteins that are coded for by genes in the Ir region of the MHC.[9,14,44-49] Second, Mφ are required to liberate a soluble material, IL-1, necessary for T cell activation to proceed.[49-52] In contrast to the antigen presenting function of Mφ, this process is not restricted by products of Ir genes.[53] The next series of experiments indicate that Mac-120⁺ Mφ are required for appropriate presentation of antigen to T cells.

Various cell mixtures and soluble materials were assayed for their ability to reconstitute reactivity among T-enriched populations that were partially depleted of adherent cells and cytolytically treated with either a control reagent (MIg) or Mac-120 (Table 9). Note that while 10% autologous Mφ could reconstitute reactivity among Mac-120-treated cells (Table 9B) 10% autologous Mφ depleted of Mac-120⁺ cells could not (Table 9C). This indicates that the diminished reactivity seen among Mac-120-treated populations represents a qualitative and not simply a quantitative deficiency of Mφ. The relative inability of Mac-120-treated cells to reconstitute reactivity did not represent a toxic effect of dead or dying cells since Mφ treated with a concentration of ALA sufficient to lyse 30% of the Mφ were effective in reconstituting reactivity (Table 9D). Mφ from an individual disparate at both HLA-DR loci were not effective in restoring reactivity (Table 9E). It should be noted that allogeneic Mφ increased antigen reactivity among MIg treated cells, arguing against the possibility that a negative allogeneic effect was responsible for the failure of allogeneic cells to reconstitute reactivity in the Mac-120-depleted population. Finally, antigen reactivity could not be reconstituted by soluble products obtained from autologous Mφ cultured for 24 hr in fetal calf serum (Table 9F). That these Mφ culture fluids contained IL-1-like activity was demonstrated by two findings. First, they reconstituted antigen (OA)-induced T cell proliferation among partially adherent cell depleted, lymph node T cells from mice primed with OA.[62] Second, the culture fluids augmented the proliferation observed in the partially adherent cell-depleted populations used in Table 9 (Table 9A vs. Table 9F). The increase in reactivity noted upon addition of allogeneic Mφ most likely represents the nongenetically restricted effects of IL-1 or an allogeneic effect.

These data indicate that Mac-120⁺ but not Mac-120⁻ populations contain those Mφ required for the genetically restricted presentation of antigen to reactive T cells. Since this population also contains those Mφ that serve as the most effective stimulators in

Table 9

**RECONSTITUTION OF ANTIGEN-INDUCED PROLIFERATION AMONG
MAC-120-TREATED POPULATIONS**

Responding Population		Reactivity to *C. albicans*		
Antisera Rx	Reconstituted with	1/4	1/12 (ΔCPM)	1/36
A MIg	0	3902	3828	3064
Mac-120	0	186	224	99
B MIg	Autologous Mφ	6785	4198	3352
Mac-120	Autologous Mφ	3363	3032	1435
C MIg	Mac-120 Rx autologous Mφ	8676	8214	4771
Mac-120	Mac-120 Rx autologous Mφ	383	225	106
D MIg	ALA Rx autologous Mφ	4258	4879	3740
Mac-120	ALA Rx autologous Mφ	4164	4577	3552
E MIg	Allogeneic Mφ	5138	8820	6892
Mac-120	Allogeneic Mφ	1285	634	694
F MIg	IL-1	7726	6389	4680
Mac-120	IL-1	152	124	87

Note: PBMC partially depleted of adherent cells were treated by indirect cytotoxicity with either MIg or Mac-120, reconstituted with 10% of the indicated viable cells or IL-1-containing culture fluids and then tested for their proliferative reactivity to three concentrations of *C. albicans*. The results are presented as ΔCPM obtained in triplicate cultures from a single individual. IL-1 refers to a 50% concentration of culture fluids obtained from autologous Mφ, that had been incubated at 37°C for 24 hr in 10% FCS. ALA Rx autologous Mφ refers to Mφ cytolytically treated with suboptimal concentrations of an ALA so that 50% of the Mφ was lysed. Allogeneic indicates an individual disparate at both HLA-D loci.

the AMLR, the relationship among T cells responsive to Mφ in the AMLR and those T cells required for reactivity to soluble antigen was investigated. For these studies, two approaches were used. First, Mφ-responsive T cells were negatively selected using BURD and light. Since these T cells have been previously demonstrated to be distinct from those that proliferated in response to stimulation with autologous B cells, negative selection of T cells responsive to B cells was used as a control. As demonstrated in Table 10, negative selection of the T cells responsive to Mφ completely abrogated antigen-induced T cell proliferation. In contrast, this antigen reactivity was not diminished among populations responsive to autologous B cells.

Since the population of T cells responsive to Mφ in the AMLR is contained among T cells identified by the mAb T-29, it is predictable that cytolysis with T-29 should also diminish antigen-induced T cell reactivity. This is supported by the data presented in Table 11. Cytolysis of T-enriched populations with T-29 markedly diminished antigen-induced T cell proliferation and LIF release. In contrast, cytolytic treatment of the T cells with a mAb capable of removing a percentage of cells comparable to that removed by T-29 did not diminish antigen reactivity.

The authors have previously published data suggesting that T cells proliferating in the AMLR are required to help in the pokeweed mitogen (PWM)-stimulated production of Ig by autologous B cells.[25] These experiments analyzed the helper function of T populations negatively selected (by BURD and light) for cells proliferating in response to autologous non-T cells (B + Mφ). To determine the relative contribution of the T-29[+], Mφ-responsive T cell population to this helper activity, the following experiments were performed. T cells were cytolytically treated with T-29, the mAb T-15 (which

Table 10
REACTIVITY OF NEGATIVELY SELECTED T CELLS TO AUTOLOGOUS Mφ AND ANTIGENS

Responding populations	Maximal reactivity (CPM)		
	Media	*Candida*	PPD
A. Negative selection of Mφ-responsive T			
Exp. 1 T + Mφ + BURD, no light	909	6,373	12,611
T + Mφ + BURD, light	866	1,078	964
Exp. 2 T + Mφ + BURD, no light	1,324	14,496	34,279
T + Mφ + BURD, light	4,012	4,763	6,285
B. Negative selection of "B"-responsive T			
Exp. 1 T + B + BURD, no light	3,462	12,736	24,097
T + B + BURD, light	3,901	16,867	22,301
Exp. 2 T + B + BURD, no light	1,642	7,370	ND
T + B + BURD, light	2,819	13,670	ND

Note: T cells were cultured with either autologous Mφ (A) or autologous B-enriched populations (B) and BURD added as previously described. One-half of the cultures were exposed to cool, white light. All cultures were washed and compared at comparable concentrations of viable cells for their reactivity to media only, as well as three concentrations of *C. albicans* and PPD. Reactivity was measured by the incorporation of ^{3}H-TdR into DNA and is expressed as maximal CPM. ND indicates not done.

Table 11
REQUIREMENT FOR T-29$^+$ T CELLS IN ANTIGEN-INDUCED PROLIFERATION AND LYMPHOKINE SYNTHESIS

Responding populations	Reactivity (CPM)		LIF production
	PPD	*Candida*	Migration inhibition (%)
Exp. 1 T + MIg + C′	25,966	9,956	21.6
T + T-29 + C′	16,782	112	4.4
T + T-33 + C′	ND	8,290	ND
Exp. 2 T + MIg + C′	335	686	ND
T + T-29 + C′	35	183	ND
Exp. 3 T + T-33 + C′	ND	27,637	ND
T + MIg + C′	ND	27,530	ND
Exp. 4 T + T-15 + C′	32,834	13,499	ND
T + MIg + C′	ND	13,659	22.0
T + T-29 + C′	16,684	2,684	0

Note: T cells were treated in an indirect cytotoxicity assay with either the control reagents MIg, T-15, and T-33 or with the mAb T-29. 100,000 viable cells from each population were then compared for their proliferative reactivity to three concentrations of PPD, *C. albicans* or for their ability to synthesize LIF in response to a 1/6 dilution of *C. albicans*. For the proliferative studies, the results are expressed as maximal CPM for each antigen and for the LIF assays, expressed as the % inhibition of leukocyte migration noted by comparing the activity of culture fluids from cells incubated with or without antigen. ND indicates not done.

Table 12
REGULATION OF Ig PRODUCTION BY T-29$^+$ T CELLS

Populations added to auto. B/Mφ	Ig-producing populations (ng/Ig/culture)			
	Exp. 1	Exp. 2	Exp. 3	Exp. 4
No added Ts	0	125	140	815
T + MIg + C′	1475	ND	1625	ND
T + T-15 + C′	ND	850	ND	4000
T + T-29 + C′	175	300	950	2625

Note: T cells were treated with either the control reagents MIg or T-15 or with the mAb T 29 and complement. These treated T populations were cultured at ratios of 6/1, 3/1, or 1/1 with a constant number of autologous B/Mφ. Results are expressed as the mean maximal nanograms Ig synthesized per cell mixture. ND indicates not done.

removes a percentage of T cells comparable to that removed with T-29) or with the control reagent MIg. These three populations were then compared for their ability to help autologous B + Mφ synthesize immunoglobulin in response to two concentrations of PWM) (Table 12) (for these experiments the non-T population was not fractionated). The amount of Ig synthesized and released into the culture medium was quantitated using a competitive-binding RIA that detected all Ig classes. Note that in the absence of any added T cells, the B + Mφ population synthesizes only meager amounts of Ig. Thus, this population is deficient in helper cell activity. When compared to the MIg or T-15-treated T cells, populations depleted of T-29$^+$ cells were relatively deficient in helper activity. However, populations containing T-29-treated cells and autologous B + Mφ did synthesize more Ig than B + Mφ alone. It could be demonstrated that this did not result from incomplete removal of the T-29$^+$ T cells (data not presented). On the basis of this data it is suggested that while T-29$^+$ T cells can provide help for Ig synthesis so can T-29$^-$ T cells.

These in vitro studies indicate that a portion of the cells interacting to produce the AMLR include T cells required for antigen reactivity and helper activity and antigen presenting Mφ. If these same cells, i.e., T-29$^+$ T cells and Mac-120$^+$ Mφ, are also required for comparable reactivities in vivo, one would predict that either population might be defective in individuals manifesting anergy and hypogammaglobulinemia. To test this prediction, four patients with common variable immunodeficiency (i.e., cutaneous anergy in response to skin testing with five recall antigens and hypogammaglobulinemia) were analyzed for qualitative and quantitative aspects of T cell reactivity (Table 13). It should be stated at the outset that no clinical situation has been identified in which there is a quantitative deficiency of Mac-120$^+$ Mφ, including the four patients studied here. While the frequency of total T cells in each patient was moderately reduced (50.5 ± 1.3 vs. $75 \pm 4\%$), there was a complete absence of T-29$^+$ T cells. This was accompanied by an absence of AMLR reactivity to autologous Mφ, absent in vitro proliferative reactivity to soluble antigen (*Candida albicans*) and a relative preservation of the reactivity to autologous B cells. When compared to normal T cells, T cells from the three patients studied demonstrated a marked reduction in helper activity that was comparable to that mediated by normal T cells depleted of the T-29 positive population (Table 14). Thus, the functions ascribed to the T-29$^+$ T cells on the basis of in vitro manipulations are substantiated by examining a selected patient population in which T-29$^+$ T cells are deficient in vivo.

Table 13

REACTIVITY OF T CELLS FROM ANERGIC PATIENTS TO AUTOLOGOUS STIMULATOR CELLS AND CONVENTIONAL ANTIGEN

	% Positive Cells		Reactivity to		
	Total T	T-29$^+$ T	B	Mϕ	*Candida*
A. Normals (15)	75	10	7.1	4.7	9599
Mean ± S.E.	±4	±2	±1.2	±1.1	±1120
B. Patients					
1	48	0	5.0	1.1	260
2	56	1	3.1	0.3	21
3	54	1	4.3	0.8	437
4	49	1	2.1	0.9	887
Mean ± S.E.	50.5	0.8	3.6	0.8	401
	±1.3	±0.3	±0.6	±0.2	±182

Note: PBMC from 15 normal individuals (A) and 4 anergic patients (B) with hypogammaglobulinemia were compared for the frequency of E rosette cells (i.e., total T), the frequency of T cells detected by immunofluorescence with the T cell-specific mAb T-29 (T-29$^+$ T), their proliferative reactivity to two concentrations of either autologous B-enriched cells or Mϕ, and their proliferative response to three concentrations of *C. albicans*. Reactivity to autologous B or Mϕ is presented as maximal S.I. Reactivity to *Candida* is presented as ΔCPM (maximal CPM in cells cultured with antigen; CPM in cells cultured with media only).

Table 14

IG SYNTHESIS BY PATIENTS WITH COMMON VARIABLE IMMUNODEFICIENCY

T populations added to normal PBMC	Ng of Ig synthesized/ culture
None	75
Normal	425
Normal depleted of T-29$^+$ T cells	150
Patient 1	125
Patient 2	137
Patient 3	180

Note: The indicated T cell populations were added to normal PBMC in a ratio of 3:1 and 1:1. The cultures were incubated with two concentrations of PWM for seven days and maximal Ig synthesized and released into the culture fluid assayed by RIA.

IV. DISCUSSION

"Self"-recognition is crucially required for the initiation and expression of immunity. This is exemplified by the demonstration that activation of antigen-reactive T cells requires that they see nominal determinants inherent in conventional antigen as well as "self"-Ia determinants displayed by Mϕ.[9-14,44-49] It has been postulated that the T cell recognition unit required for this interaction either consists of two distinct receptors, one that interacts with "self"-Ia and the other that recognizes conventional antigen,[54,56] or a single receptor that recognizes a new, modified "self"-determinant generated by interactions between conventional antigen and Mϕ membrane Ia determinants.[55,56] In either case, it has been predicted that interactions between reactive T cells and either antigen alone or "self"-Ia determinants alone are not sufficient to initiate T cell activation.[57-59] However, the data presented here demonstrate that in the absence of added soluble antigen, antigen-reactive, and helper T cells can be induced to proliferate by Mϕ. Moreover, only a subpopulation of Mϕ capable of functioning as antigen-presenting cells are capable of inducing this T cell proliferation. In other words, antigen-reactive T cells can be activated, in vitro, by antigen-presenting cells in the absence of added soluble antigen.

It would appear, therefore, that data generated by the authors contradicts proposed theories concerning the nature of the receptor displayed by antigen-reactive, helper T cells.[9-14,44-49,54-56] However, there are several caveats concerning these findings that must be considered. First, it has not been definitively established that the Mϕ determinant that induces proliferation among the T-29$^+$ T cell population is indeed Ia. Although it has been possible to blunt the AMLR with anti-Ia (or anti-HLA-DR) antibodies, including F(ab)$'_2$ fragments of the antibodies,[24,29,35] this is also consistent with the interpretation that the stimulating determinant is only closely associated with Ia on the Mϕ membrane. This conclusion is supported by the finding that we can consistently and effectively abrogate the T-Mϕ AMLR with the Mac-120 mAb. Thus, the nature of the Mϕ-dependent stimulus that induces proliferation in the AMLR has not been established. Second, it is possible that the T-Mϕ AMLR represents reactivity among only a subpopulation of antigen-reactive helper cells that display high-affinity receptors for self and thus can be activated in the absence of conventional antigen. This is consistent with the finding that the Mϕ-responsive, T-29$^+$ population represents only 10% of the peripheral T cell pool. This frequency falls short of that theoretically required to accommodate the entire repertoire of antigen-reactive T cells. Moreover, the requirement for T-29$^+$ T cells has been investigated in terms of their response to only three antigens (Candida albicans, PPD, and collagen). It is possible that the T-29$^-$ cells are required for the reactivity to other antigens. Third, the authors have only demonstrated that the T-29$^+$ T cells are required for antigen-reactivity and not that they are themselves antigen-reactive. Although positive selection experiments have recently been presented that suggest that this is indeed the case,[40] a definitive statement concerning the response of these T cells to soluble antigens can only be made after examining the reactivity of cloned, Mϕ-responsive T cell lines. Thus, at this point the implication of the findings for understanding the structure of the receptor displayed by antigen-reactive helper cells are not certain. More data concerning the points raised is needed.

It should also be emphasized that the Mϕ-responsive, T-29$^+$ T cells contain a portion of T cells required to help in the polyclonal synthesis of Ig. In several experiments not presented here, the authors have found that addition of increasing numbers of T-29$^+$ T cells to autologous PBMC results in graded increases in Ig production. In other words, it has not been possible to demonstrate that the T-29$^+$ population can mediate feedback suppression. When considered together, these findings suggest that the T-29$^+$ subset resembles the murine Ly-1$^+$, Qa-1$^-$ T cell subset. A recent report by Lattime et al.[29] demonstrates that the Mϕ-responsive T cell in the murine AMLR is indeed Ly-1$^+$, Qa-1$^-$.[29]

Several investigators have reported that the T cells responsive in the AMLR are distinct from those reactive to alloantigens.[30,60,61] Data has been published showing that depletion of autologous reactive T cells by either suicide with BURD and light or cytolytic treatment with T-29 does not diminish the allogeneic response.[25,41] These studies clearly demonstrate that substantial alloreactivity can occur among populations depleted of autologous reactive T cells. There have been no experiments that directly assay the reactivity of autologous reactive cells to alloantigens. Thus, a decision concerning the reactivity of cells responsive in the AMLR to alloantigens also awaits studies using established T cell clones.

The technique of somatic cell hybridization to produce mAbs has provided the immunologists with powerful probes useful for exploring interactions among immunocompetent cells that are required for immunologic homeostasis. We have taken advantage of this technique to probe the phenomena of the AMLR. While much work remains before the significance of this phenomena is established, studies conducted by the authors clearly show that at least a portion of the AMLR represents communication between immunologically relevant cells. These findings indicate that the AMLR should serve as a useful model to further explore immunologic communication between Mϕ and T cells.

ACKNOWLEDGMENTS

The expert technical assistance of Ms. Marianne Newton and Ms. Karen Chinn and the secretarial assistance of Ms. Marilynn Marsh is appreciated.

REFERENCES

1. **Ehrlich. P.,** On immunity with special reference to cell life, *Proc. Roy. Soc. London Ser. B.,* 66, 424, 1900.
2. **Burnet, F. M.,** *The Clonal Selection Theory of Acquired Immunity,* Vanderbilt University Press, Nashville, 1959.
3. **Zinkernagel, R. M. and Doherty, P. C.,** H-2 compatibility requirement for T cell-mediated lysis of target cells infected with lymphocytic choriomeningitis. Different cytotoxic T cell specificities are associated with structures coded in H-2K and H-2D, *J. Exp. Med.,* 141, 1427, 1975.
4. **Doherty, P. C. and Zinkernagle, R. M.,** H-2 compatibility is required for T cell mediated lysis of target cells infected with lymphocytic choriomeningitis virus, *J. Exp. Med.,* 141, 502, 1975.
5. **Zinkernagle, R. M. and Doherty, P. C.,** MHC-restricted cytotoxic T cells: studies on the biological role of polymorphic major transplantation antigens determining T-cell restriction-specificity, function, and responsiveness, *Adv. Immunol.,* 27, 51, 1979.
6. **Shearer, G. M. et al.,** Cell-mediated lympholysis of trinitrophenyl-modified autologous lymphocytes. Effector cell specificity to modified cell surface components controlled by the H-2K and H-2D serological regions of the murine major histocompatibility complex, *J. Exp. Med.,* 151, 1348, 1975.
7. **Shearer, G. M., Rehn, T. G., and Schmitt-Verhulst, A. M.,** Role of the murine major histocompatibility complex in the specificity of in vitro T cell mediated lympholysis against chemically modified autologous lymphocytes, *Transplant. Rev.,* 29, 222, 1976.
8. **Bevan, M. J.,** The major histocompatibility complex determines susceptibility to cytotoxic T cells directed against minor histocompatibility antigens, *J. Exp. Med.,* 142, 1349, 1975.
9. **Yano, A., Schwartz, R. H., and Paul, W. E.,** Antigen presentation in the murine T-lymphocyte proliferative response. I. Requirement for genetic identity at the major histocompatibility complex, *J. Exp. Med.,* 146, 828, 1977.
10. **Thomas, D. W., Yamashita, U., and Shevach, E. M.,** The role of Ia antigens in T cell activation, *Immunol. Rev.,* 35, 97, 1977.
11. **Sprent, J.,** Role of H-2 gene products in the function of T helper cells from normal and chimeric mice in vivo, *Immunol. Rev.,* 42, 108, 1978.
12. **Zinkernagel, R. M., Callahan, G. M., Althage, A., Cooper, S., Streilein, J. W., and Skein, J.,** The lymphoreticular system in triggering virus plus self-specific cytotoxic T cells: evidence for T help, *J. Exp. Med.,* 147, 897, 1978.
13. **Kappler, J. W. and Marrack, P.,** The role of H-2 linked genes in helper T function. IV. Importance of T cell genotype and host environment in I-region and Ir gene expression, *J. Exp. Med.,* 148, 1510, 1978.

14. **Longo, D. L. and Schwartz, R. H.,** T-cell specificity for H-2 and Ir gene phenotype correlates with the phenotype of thymic antigen-presenting cells, *Nature (London)*, 287, 44, 1980.

15. **Jerne, N. K.,** The immune system: a web of V-domains, *Harvey Lect.*, 70, 93, 1975.

16. **Cosenza, H. and Köhler, H.,** Specific suppression of the antibody response by antibodies to receptors, *Proc. Nat. Acad. Sci. U.S.A.*, 69, 2701, 1972.

17. **Sy, M. S., Bach, B. A., Dohi, V., Nisonoff, A., Benacerraf, B., and Greene, M. I.,** Antigen and receptor driven regulatory mechanisms. I. Induction of suppressor T cells with anti-idiotypic antibodies, *J. Exp. Med.*, 150, 1216, 1979.

18. **Sy. M. S., Brown, A. R., Benacerraf, B., and Greene, M. I.,** Antigen- and receptor-driven regulatory mechanisms. III. Induction of delayed-type hypersensitivity to azobenzenearsonate with anti-cross-reactive idiotypic antibodies, *J. Exp. Med.*, 151, 896, 1980.

19. **Trenkner, E. and Riblet, R.,** Induction of antiphosphorycholine antibody formation by anti-idiotypic antibodies, *J. Exp. med.*, 142, 1121, 1975.

20. **Bona, C. and Paul, W. E.,** Cellular basis of regulation of expression of idiotype. I. T-suppressor cells specific for MOPC 460 idiotype regulate the expression of cells secreting anti-TNP antibodies bearing 460 idiotype, *J. Exp. Med.*, 149, 592, 1979.

21. **Adorini, L., Harvey, M., and Sercarz, E. E.,** The fine specificity of regulatory and antigen-binding interactions in the anti-lysozyme response, *Eur. J. Immunol.*, 9, 906, 1979.

22. **Etheredge, E. E., Shors, A. R., Hoheuthaner, K. L., and Najarion, J. S.,** Mitomycin C inactivation of leukocytes in the mixed leukocyte culture, *Transplantation*, 15, 331, 1973.

23. **Opelz, G., Kiuchi, M., Takasugi, M., and Terasaki, P. I.,** Autologous stimulation of human lymphocyte subpopulations, *J. Exp. Med.*, 142, 1327, 1975.

24. **Gottlieb, A. B., Fir, S. M., Yee, D. T., Wange, C. Y., Halper, J. P., Kunkel, H. G.,** The nature of the simulating cells in human allogeneic and autologous MLC reactions; role of isolated IgM-bearing B cells, *J. Immunol.*, 123, 1497, 1979.

25. **Hausman, P. B. and Stobo, J. D.,** Specificity and function of a human autologous reactive T cell, *J. Exp. Med.*, 149, 1537, 1979.

26. **MacDermott, R. P. and Stacey, M. E.,** Further characterization of the human autologous mixed lymphocyte reaction (MLR), *J. Immunol.*, 126, 729, 1981.

27. **Kuntz, M. M., Innes, J. B., and Weksler, M. E.,** Lymphocyte proliferation induced by autologous or allogeneic non-T lymphocytes, *J. Exp. Med.*, 143, 1042, 1976.

28. **Nussenzweig, M. D. and Steinman, R. M.,** Contribution of dendritic cells to stimulation of the murine syngeneic mixed leukocyte reaction, *J. Exp. Med.*, 151, 1196, 1980.

29. **Lattime, E. C., Gottlieb, S. H., and Stutman, O.,** Lyt 1 cells respond to Ia-bearing macrophages in the murine syngeneic mixed lymphocyte reaction, *Eur. J. Immunol.*, 10, 723, 1980.

30. **Sakane, R. and Green, I.,** Specificity and suppressor function of human T cells responsive to autologous non-T cells, *J. Immunol.*, 123, 584, 1979.

31. **Tomonari, K.,** Cytotoxic T cells generated in the autologous mixed lymphocyte reaction. I. Primary autologous mixed lymphocyte reaction, *J. Immunol.*, 124, 1111, 1980.

32. **Smith, J. B. and Knowlton, R. P.,** Activation of suppressor T cells in human autologous mixed lymphocyte culture, *J. Immunol.*, 123, 419, 1979.

33. **Innes, J. B., Juntz, M. M., Kim, Y. T., and Weksler, M. E.,** Induction of suppressor activity in the autologous mixed lymphocyte reaction and in cultures with Concanavalin A, *J. Clin. Invest.*, 64, 1608, 1979.

34. **Yu, D. T. Y., Chiorazzi, N., and Kunkel, H. G.,** Helper factors derived from autologous mixed lymphocyte cultures, *Cell. Immunol.*, 50, 305, 1980.

35. **Lattime, E. C., Gillis, S., David, C., and Stutman, O.,** Interleukin 2, production in the syngeneic mixed lymphocyte reaction, *Eur. J. Immunol.*, 11, 67, 1981.

36. **Smith, J. B.,** Stimulation of autologous and allogeneic human T cells by B cells occurs through separate B cell antigen systems, *Cell. Immunol.*, 36, 203, 1978.

37. **Stobo, J. D., Paul, S., Van Scoy, R. E., and Hermans, P. E.,** Suppressor thymus-derived lymphocytes in fungal infection, *J. Clin. Invest.*, 57, 319, 1976.

38. **Stobo, J. D. and Loehnen, C. P.,** Proliferative reactivity of T cells to autologous, cell-associated antigens, *Arthritis Rheum.*, 21, 210 (Suppl.), 1978.

39. **Raff, H. V., Picker, L. J., and Stobo, J. D.,** Macrophage heterogeneity in man: a subpopulation of HLA-DR bearing Mφ required for antigen induced T cell activation also contains stimulators for autologous reactive T cells, *J. Exp. Med.*, 152, 581, 1980.

40. **Hausman, P. B., Stites, D. P., and Stobo, J. D.,** Antigen-reactive T cells can be activated by autologous macrophages in the absence of added antigen, *J. Exp. Med.*, 153, 476, 1981.

41. **Hausman, P. B., Raff, H. V., Gilbert, R. C., Picker, L. J., and Stobo, J. D.,** T cells and macrophages involved in the autologous mixed lymphocyte reaction are required for the response to conventional antigens, *J. Immunol.*, 125, 1374, 1980.

42. **Wysocki, L. J. and Sato, V. L.,** "Panning" for lymphocytes: a method for cell selection, *Proc. Natl. Acad. Sci. U.S.A.,* 75, 2844, 1978.
43. **Rosenthal, A. S. and Shevach, E. M.,** The function of macrophages in antigen recognition by guinea pig T lymphocytes, *J. Exp. Med.,* 138, 1194, 1973.
44. **Shevach, E. M., Paul, W. E., and Green, D.,** Histocompatability-linked immune response gene function in guinea pigs. Specific inhibition of antigen-induced lymphocyte proliferation by alloantigen, *J. Exp. Med.,* 136, 1207, 1972.
45. **Shevach, E. M., Green, I., and Paul, W. E.,** Alloantiserum induced inhibition of immune response gene product function. II. Genetic analysis of target antigens, *J. Exp. Med.,* 139, 679, 1974.
46. **Shevach, E. M.,** The function of macrophages in antigen recognition by guinea pig T lymphocytes. III. Genetic analysis of the antigens mediating macrophage-T lymphocyte interaction, *J. Immunol.,* 116, 1482, 1976.
47. **Alpert, S. D., Jonsen, M. E., Broff, M. D., Schneeberger, E., and Geha, R.,** Macrophage T-cell interaction in man: handling of tetanus toxoid antigen by human monocytes, *J. Clin. Immunol.,* 1, 21, 1981.
48. **Schwartz, R. H., Yano, A., and Paul, W. E.,** Interaction between antigen-presenting cells and primed T lymphocytes: an assessment of Ir gene expression in the antigen-presenting cell, *Immunol. Rev.,* 40, 153, 1978.
49. **Unanue, E. R.,** The regulation of lymphocyte functions by the macrophage, *Immunol. Rev.,* 40, 227, 1978.
50. **Farrar, W. L., Mizel, S. B., and Farrar, J. J.,** Participation of lymphocyte activating factor (Interleukin 1) in the induction of cytotoxic T cell responses, *J. Immunol.,* 124, 1371, 1980.
51. **Smith, K. A., Lachman, L. B., Oppenheim, J. J., and Favata, M. F.,** The functional relationship of the interleukins, *J. Exp. Med.,* 151, 1551, 1980.
52. **Mizel, S. B. and Farrar, J. F.,** Revised nomenclature for antigen-nonspecific T-cell proliferation and helper factors, *Cell. Immunol.,* 48, 433, 1979.
53. **Farr, A. G., Dort, M. E., and Unanue, E. R.,** Secretion of mediators following T lymphocyte-macrophage interaction is regulated by the major histocompatibility complex, *Proc. Natl. Acad. Sci. U.S.A.,* 74, 3542, 1977.
54. **Von Boehmer, H., Haas, W., and Jerne, N. K.,** Major histocompatibility complex-linked immune-responsiveness is acquired by lymphocytes of low responder mice differentiating in thymus of high-responder mice, *Proc. Natl. Acad. Sci. U.S.A.,* 75, 2439, 1978.
55. **Zinkernagle, R. and Doherty, P.,** Immunological surveillance against altered self components by sensitised T lymphocytes in lymphocytic choriomeningitis, *Nature (London),* 251, 547, 1974.
56. **Janeway, C. E. and Jason, J. M.,** How T lymphocytes recognize antigen, *CRC Critical Reviews in Immunology,* 1, 2, 133, 1980.
57. **Lalande, M. E., McCutcheon, M. J., and Miller, R. G.,** Quantitative studies on the precursors of cytotoxic lymphocytes. VI. Second signal requirements of specifically activated precursor isolated 12h after stimulation, *J. Exp. Med.,* 151, 12, 1980.
58. **Larsson, E. L., Iscove, N. N., and Coutinho, A.,** Two distinct factors are required for induction of T-cell growth, *Nature (London),* 283, 664, 1980.
59. **Smith, K. A., Gilbridge, K. J., and Favata, M. F.,** Lymphocyte activating factor promotes T-cell growth factor production by cloned murine lymphoma cells, *Nature (London),* 287, 853, 1980.
60. **Tomonari, K., Wakisaka, A., and Aizawa, M.,** Self-recognition by autologous mixed lymphocyte reaction-primed cells, *J. Immunol.,* 125, 1596, 1980.
61. **Smith, J. B. and Knowlton, R. P.,** Autologous mixed lymphocyte culture responder T cells are in the Concanvailon-A reactive subpopulation and separate from alloreactive cells, *Immunol. Immunopathol.,* in press.
62. **Rosenwasser, L., Raff, H., and Stobo, J.,** Unpublished observations.

Chapter 4

mAbs TO HUMAN LYMPHOCYTE SURFACE ANTIGENS

Gideon Goldstein, John Lifter, and Robert Mittler

TABLE OF CONTENTS

I.   Introduction 72

II. Approaches to Generate mAbs 73

III. Human T Cell Antigens Defined by mAbs 73
     A.   Pan T Cell Antibodies 73
     B.   Helper/Inducer Subset 73
     C.   Suppressor/Cytotoxic Subset 76
     D.   Thymocyte-Specific Antibodies 77
     E.   Nonlineage-Specific Antibodies 77

IV. Regulatory Interactions Between T Cell Subsets as Defined by mAbs 78

V.   Analysis of Lymphocyte Differentiation and Maturation in
     Lymphoid Tissues Using mAbs 80

VI. Potential Applications of mAbs to T Cells 81
     A.   Basic and Applied Research Applications 81
     B.   Clinical and Diagnostic Applications 83
     C.   Therapeutic Applications 83

References 84

I. INTRODUCTION

Lymphocytes, the major cellular component of the immune system, have been classified into thymus–dependent T cells and thymus–independent B cells. These two main types of cells are important in the immune system because they mediate the recognition of antigens, both self and foreign. Lymphocytes also function as regulators of the immune response and this regulation is mediated by discrete interacting subclasses of T cells. One approach to clarifying the cellular and molecular bases of these regulatory interactions has been to establish the functional contribution of these T cell subpopulations to various kinds of immune responses. This type of analysis has enhanced our understanding of the developmental pathways of lymphocyte ontogeny as well as the molecular basis of the regulatory and effector activities of these different T cell subclasses.

Currently, the most effective technique for identifying and separating functionally distinct subclasses of T cells has come from studies of cell surface components. Following on from early work with alloantigens in mice,[1–3] the delineation of human T cell subsets in man has involved sheep red cell binding, Ig FcR binding, autoantibodies, and heteroantisera.[4–6] Direct application to man of the mouse work with alloantisera was attempted with adsorbed heteroantisera generated by immunizations of rabbits or goats with human lymphocytes. These techniques did not prove to be practical for widespread use because of considerable batch variations, frequent low titers, and the extensive tissue absorptions required to obtain specificity.[7,8] These shortcomings can now be overcome with the use of cell fusion techniques for the production of mAbs. Using this methodology, hybridoma–secreted mAbs, each with a single specificity, can be used to identify cell surface antigens whose existence was previously unknown. It appears now that potent and unlimited amounts of monospecific antibodies can be produced to identify and enumerate functional subsets of T lymphocytes.

This paper will review information concerning the generation and functional characterization of the OKT line of reagents, the molecular characterization of the antigens recognizing these mAbs, the distribution and specificity of these reagents with both cells and tissues and, finally, discuss the potential clinical and research applications of mAbs to T cells. A number of other pertinent mAbs and their relationship to the OKT series will also be discussed.

II. APPROACHES TO GENERATE mAbs

Recently described methods of somatic cell hybridization have resulted in the production of stabilized clones of antibody–secreting hybridomas.[9–12] This technology has led us as well as others to generate mAbs to human T cell differentiation antigens. The procedures of immunization, cell fusion, and clone selection for producing anti-T cell antibodies vary from laboratory to laboratory. Briefly, the OKT antibodies were generated in a mouse hybridoma system by immunizing mice with human E rosette–purified peripheral lymphocytes, thymocytes, T cell lines, or leukemic T cells.[13–21] Anti–pan T cell antibodies were obtained from cell fusions prepared from mice immunized with normal lymphocytes, T cell lines, and leukemic T cells, whereas anti–T cell subset antibodies were derived from mice immunized with normal lymphocytes and thymocytes. Screening of these hybridoma cultures for particular specificities, e.g., pan T, thymic, peripheral T, E rosette receptor, leukemic, etc., was assessed by first incubating the hybridoma–containing culture supernate with a panel of T cells, thymocytes, and B cells. This was followed by indirect immunofluorescent staining and flow cytometric analysis.[22-24] Hybridomas of interest were cloned and recloned and selected hybridomas were passed by peritoneal passage to produce ascitic fluid in mice.

III. HUMAN T CELL ANTIGENS DEFINED BY mAbs

In order to differentiate between mAbs with similar cell reactivities, it is imperative to analyze the cell distribution patterns of the specific antibodies and, at a molecular level, the antigens with which the antibodies are reacting. In this section the authors describe both the cellular distribution and molecular characteristics of the antigens recognized by a panel of T cell reactive antibodies.

A. Pan T Cell Antibodies

mAbs OKT1, OKT3, OKT11, and OKT11A were obtained by fusion of P3X63Ag8U1 myeloma cells with spleen cells from BALB/cJ mice previously immunized with purified human peripheral blood T cells.[22] Each of the four antibodies reacts with greater than 95% of peripheral blood T cells, and while OKT1 and OKT3 react with less than 10% of the thymocyte population, OKT11 and OKT11A are reactive with the vast majority of lymphocytes. In contrast, all are completely unreactive with B cells, null cells, granulocytes, and monocytes. OKT11 and OKT11A cross–react with Rhesus monkey T cells, whereas OKT1 and OKT3 do not. The reactivity patterns of these reagents suggest that they define mature T cell differentiation antigens.[19] Removal of cells bearing these antigens deletes all T cell functions.[25] Furthermore, T cell acute lymphoblastic leukemia cells (immature) are unreactive with OKT1 and OKT3, whereas T cell chronic lymphocytic leukemia cells and the T cells in mycosis fungoides are reactive with these antibodies.[19,26]

mAbs OKT1, OKT3, and OKT11 recognize different molecules on T cells as judged by SDS–PAGE of ^{125}I–labeled immunoprecipitates of membrane extracts. OKT1 precipitates a 67,000 dalton molecule that migrates as a single band under reducing and nonreducing conditions. Under identical conditions OKT3 antigen runs as a single band having a molecular weight of 21,000 daltons.[27] OKT11 precipitates a molecule with an apparent molecular weight of 45,000 daltons. OKT11A is currently being analyzed.

In addition to their distinct electrophoretic profiles, OKT3, OKT11, OKT11A, and OKT1 can be distinguished from each other by functional differences of the antigens with which they react. Recent studies by Van Wauwe et al.[28] demonstrated that subnanomolar concentrations of OKT3 exert a powerful mitogenic stimulus to peripheral blood T cells. Comparison of OKT3 mitogenic activity with phytohemagglutinin (PHA) and concanavalin A (Con A) on a weight to weight basis indicated that OKT3 stimulation was 20–fold more potent than PHA and 500-fold more potent than Con A. Chang et al.[29] confirmed and extended this observation by demonstrating that the OKT3 antibody inhibited the generation of cytotoxic effector cells in MLC and also inhibited target cell lysis mediated by allogeneic cytotoxic T cells. It was postulated that OKT3 reacts with the antigen–recognition structure on T cells and that OKT3, like anti–Id antibodies or antigen, combines with and subsequently perturbs the antigen receptor. This induces a mitogenic stimulus. Furthermore, OKT3 antibody, like the anti–Id antibody,[31,32] also inhibits T cell functions.

OKT3 induces T lymphocytes to secrete γ (immune) interferon (IF) similar to lectins.[33,34] IF secretion by T cells in response to OKT3 stimulation is dependent upon T cell mitogenesis. Addition of human plasma, which abrogates the mitogenic potential of OKT3, also inhibits IF secretion. Likewise, the substitution of F(ab')₂ or Fab fragments (poorly mitogenic) for OKT3 results in the loss of IF production. Exploration of the cellular requirements for γ IF production by T cells via OKT3 stimulation showed that monocytes were required for mitogenesis, an observation previously reported by Van Wauwe et al.[35]

Furthermore, it was shown that either the helper/inducer (OKT4+) subset or the suppressor/cytotoxic (OKT8+) subset in the presence of monocytes gave a mitogenic response to OKT3. However, only the OKT4+ subset in the presence of OKT3 and monocytes resulted in IF secretion.[34] Thus, it appears likely that the source of γ IF is the OKT4+ subset of peripheral blood lymphocytes.

In contrast with OKT3, both OKT1 and OKT11 (OKT11A) failed to induce mitogenesis in T cells and they did not interfere with the generation of cytotoxic effector cells. However OKT11A, previously shown to recognize the SRBC receptor on peripheral blood T cells,[21] significantly suppressed T cell proliferation induced by OKT3, purified protein derivative, tetanus toxoid, and allogeneic non–T cells.[36] ^{125}I–labeled OKT11A binding experiments indicated that an average of 2×10^4 antibody molecules are bound per cell. Thus OKT11A recognizes a sparsely represented cell surface determinant that is associated with the triggering of mitogenic responsiveness and the regulation of E rosette formation. Based on these observations it was suggested that the E rosette receptor of T cells is involved in the regulation of immune functions.

In addition to the pan T cell antibodies described above, several other laboratories have described similar reagents generally possessing a broader reactivity profile. Wang et al.[37] identified a protein complex of 69,000 and 71,000 daltons precipitated from membrane extracts of human T cells by a mAb termed anti–Leu–1. This antibody was found to be reactive with 80 to 95% of SRBC–rosetting cells from normal donors. Furthermore, anti–Leu–1 was reactive with greater than 95% of human thymocytes and a population of Ig+ cells from several patients with chronic lymphocytic leukemia, but is not expressed on normal B cells or Epstein–Barr virus–transformed peripheral blood B cells. Ledbetter et al.[38] have shown that anti–Leu–1 precipitates a 67,000 dalton polypeptide as well as a smaller molecule that, by internal labeling with [35S] methionine and pulse–chase studies, appears to be a precursor of the larger form. Based on these findings they suggested that Leu–1 is in fact the homologue to the Lyt–1 antigen in the mouse.[38] Like Lyt–1, Leu–1 is present in greater amounts on the helper/inducer subset than on the suppressor/cytotoxic subset and both antigens follow parallel distributions during T cell maturation.

Kamoun et al.[39] described a mAb designated 9.6 that identifies a 50,000 dalton surface protein that appears to be present on all E rosette forming cells and thymocytes. Blocking and lysostripping experiments indicated that the 9.6 antibody reacts with the SRBC receptor or with a closely associated structure. Cells preincubated with the 9.6 antibody and allowed to cap (determined by fluorescein staining with an anti- mouse reagent) were unable to form rosettes with SRBC. When 9.6 was replaced with mAb 10.2, which precipitates a 65 to 67,000 dalton surface protein expressed by 85 to 95% of peripheral E+ cells and thymocytes, no diminution of rosetting was observed despite the fact that 10.2 capped equally well.[40] Two additional antibodies, termed T101[41] and 17F12[42] identified an antigen of approximately 65,000 daltons that appears to define the same antigen as the 10.2 antibody.

Howard et al.[43] have identified a mAb termed anti–Leu–5. This antibody blocks rosette formation between T cells and SRBC. In this respect anti–Leu–5 is similar to OKT11, OKT11A, and 9.6. Like 9.6, anti–Leu–5 precipitates a single polypeptide with an apparent molecular weight of 40 to 50,000 daltons. In addition, 9.6 competes with anti–Leu–5 as judged by direct immunofluorescent staining with fluorescein–conjugated anti–Leu–5. Unlike OKT11 and OKT11A, anti–Leu–5 appears on null cells as well as on all thymocytes and peripheral T lymphocytes. Leu–5 appears to be a differentiation antigen in so far as its density on the cell surface decreases as the thymocyte matures to a peripheral T cell. Thus, subcapsular thymocytes have the highest density of Leu–5 followed by cortical thymocytes, medullary thymocytes, the suppressor/cytotoxic subset of peripheral T cells and lastly, the helper/inducer subset of peripheral T lymphocytes. In this respect anti-Leu–5 and OKT11A are dissimilar. Using a dual laser Cytofluorograf®, two color fluorescent analysis of peripheral T cells stained with rhodamine–conjugated OKT11A and fluorescein–conjugated OKT8 or OKT4 demonstrated that the OKT8[+] suppressor/cytotoxic population contained low densities of OKT11A. In contrast, the OKT4[+] helper/inducer subset contained a population of cells that had a high density of OKT11A.[44] Therefore, while it appears that OKT11A and anti-Leu–5 recognize determinants on the same population of cells, they are apparently separate antigens that probably have distinct biological functions.

Haynes et al.[45] described a mAb, designated 3A1, that appears to be a pan T cell antibody. 3A1 defines a T cell–specific antigen present on all T acute lymphoblastic leukemia or lymphoma cell lines and is absent on all Sezary T cells, normal B cells, and myeloid, monocytic and nonhematopoietic cell lines tested. On normal human lymphoid cells, 3A1 stains 85% of E rosette–positive PBMC while monocytes and B lymphocytes were 3A1[-]. 3A1 appears on 10 to 30% of spleen cells, 5 to 10% of bone marrow (BM) cells and 100% of adolescent thymocytes. SDS–PAGE of 3A1 immunoprecipitates revealed that the antigen is a 40,000 dalton single polypeptide that binds to lentil–lectin and Con A columns.[46] Lymphocyte function did not appear to be hampered in the presence of 3A1 antibody since 3A1 failed to inhibit rosetting, IgG or IgM FcR, or complement binding. Furthermore, 3A1 failed to block mitogen–induced blast transformation or in vitro T cell–dependent PWM–driven B cell differentiation. Functionally, the 3A1[+] population appears to be heterogeneous. 3A1[+] cells responded maximally to PHA and Con A, whereas the 3A1[-] population responded to PHA to a lesser extent and minimally to Con A. 3A1[+] cells in a 1:1 ratio with B cells provided maximal help for PWM–driven B cell differentiation. However, at increased ratios of 4:1 suppression of B cell differentiation was observed, suggesting the presence of suppressor cells. In addition, Con A stimulated 3A1[+] cells suppressed PWM–driven B cell differentiation to the same extent as the peripheral blood T cell population.[45]

Lastly, Beverley and Callard[47] have generated a mAb termed UCTH1. This antibody is similar in specificity to OKT3 as judged by both its mitogenic effect upon peripheral T cells and tissue distribution. Indirect fluorescent staining of E rosetted peripheral lymphocytes with UCTH1 and subsequent FACS analysis revealed two populations of cells as is the case with OKT3. The major population was UCTH1[+] (approximately 90% of the cells), whereas the remaining 10% was UCTH1[-]. Furthermore, the latter population failed to stain with OKT3. UCTH1[+] and UCTH1[-] populations sorted by FACS and cultured in the presence of either Con A, Protein A, or PHA clearly demonstrated that only the UCTH1[+] population could respond to the two lectins while the UCTH1[-] population responded weakly to protein A, a T–dependent B cell mitogen. Functionally, both helper and suppressor functions are contained within the UCTH1[+] population, as demonstrated by their ability to provide help in the generation of specific antibody responses to influenza virus, as well as their ability to suppress this response when allogeneic UCTH1[+] were added to responding PBMC.

B. Helper/Inducer Subset

OKT4, a mAb produced by fusion of P3X63Ag8U1 myeloma cells with CAF_1 spleen cells taken from a mouse immunized with purified human peripheral T cells,[15,16] was found to react with 55 to 60% of the peripheral T cell population and 80% or thymocytes by indirect immunofluorescence. Immunoprecipitation and SDS–PAGE demonstrated that OKT4 recognizes a single 60 to 62,000 dalton glycoprotein.[48,49] In the Ortho laboratories however, OKT4 antigen migrates as a 54,000 dalton glycoprotein.[50] OKT4 does not react with B cells, null cells, granulocytes, or monocytes.

The OKT4$^-$ population of T cells is equivalent to the TH$_2^+$ subset (defined by a selected and adsorbed heteroantiserum) that had been previously shown to contain suppressor/cytotoxic cells.[18] Both the OKT4$^+$ and OKT4$^-$ cell populations separated by fluorescent–activated cell sorting contain functionally discrete subsets. Both populations proliferate in response to Con A, PHA, and alloantigen, although the response to these stimulators is greater in the OKT4$^+$ subset than in the latter. OKT4$^+$ cells alone respond to soluble antigen while OKT4$^-$ cells alone are cytotoxic following allogeneic stimulation of unfractionated T cells. However, maximal development of the cytotoxic response requires both OKT4$^+$ and OKT4$^-$ populations during sensitization. These observations suggested that the OKT4$^+$ subset represents a helper population, whereas the OKT4$^-$ subset contains cytotoxic effector cells.

Further studies by Reinherz et al.[51] provided direct evidence that the OKT4$^+$ subset helped B lymphocyte differentiation in a PWM–driven system. Both B cell proliferation and intracytoplasmic Ig synthesis were facilitated by OKT4$^+$ but not OKT4$^-$ cells. Specifically, when isolated populations of T cells, T cell subsets, B cells, and T–B combinations were cultured in the presence of PWM for seven days, only the OKT4$^+$ population provided the required inductive signal(s) necessary to help autologous B cells proliferate and differentiate into plasma cells. These studies confirmed and extended the observations by Moretta et al.[6] demonstrating that the differentiation of B cells into plasma cells by PWM requires T cell help.

Recently, the authors developed several additional clones of antibody–secreting hybrids designated OKT4A, 4B, 4C, and 4D. Like OKT4, they react with 55 to 60% of peripheral T cells and 80% of thymocytes. By double staining, it was shown that they are all present on the same subset of cells. Immunoprecipitation and SDS–PAGE under reducing conditions revealed that OKT4A and OKT4B precipitate single glycoproteins of 54,000 daltons. However, OKT4C and OKT4D precipitate a polypeptide with a mol wt of 46,000 daltons.[50]

Bach et al.[52] discovered two patients whose staining patterns suggested that they possessed a rare polymorphism of the OKT4 antigen. Specifically, one patient's helper/inducer subset was recognized by OKT4A, 4B, 4C, and 4D antibodies (and not by OKT4) and the other was only recognized by OKT4C and 4D antibodies (and not by OKT4, 4A, and 4B). It is not clear from these studies whether epitope variation on a single molecule was occurring or whether deletions or changes in distinct differentiation antigens in the cell surface of human inducer T cells were detected.

In addition to OKT4 and OKT4A–D, Evans et al.[53] described two mAbs designated anti-Leu–3a and anti-Leu–3b that recognize distinct epitopes of the same cell population. Similarly to OKT4, Leu–3 reacts with 78 to 89% of thymocytes, 47 to 78% of peripheral E rosette–positive cells, precipitates an antigen with a molecular weight of 55,000 daltons, and may be the homologue of Lyt–3 in the mouse.[38] Whether or not anti-Leu–3a or 3b are identical to one of the OKT4, 4A–4D antibodies is unclear at this time.

C. Suppressor/Cytotoxic Subset

mAbs defining the suppressor/cytotoxic subset of peripheral blood T cells were generated by fusing P3X63Ag8U1 myeloma cells with spleen cells from a CAF$_1$ mouse immunized with human thymocytes.[10,11] Three stabilized clones were developed and designated OKT5, OKT8, and OKT8A. These antibodies have subclass differences (OKT5 is IgG$_1$, OKT8 is IgG$_{2a}$, and OKT8A is IgG$_2$) and preliminary evidence suggests that these antibodies recognize the same molecule. Two lines of evidence indicate that this is indeed the case. First, SDS–PAGE of immunoprecipitates from each of the antibodies yields a complex under reducing conditions with apparent molecular weights of 30,000 and 32,000 daltons.[48,50] Second, OKT8 and OKT8A compete with one another as measured by direct immunofluorescence staining and flow microfluorometric analysis.

OKT8 reacts with 80% of human thymocytes and 20 to 35% of peripheral T cells. As with the other OKT antibodies previously mentioned, OKT8 do not react with B cells, null cells, granulocytes, or monocytes. OKT8 activity on peripheral blood T cells is restricted to the previously defined TH_2^+ subpopulation. In functional studies, the OKT8 subset proliferates well in response to Con A and to alloantigens, but poorly to PHA, whereas the OKT4$^+$ subset responds vigorously to PHA.[51] In addition, cytotoxic effector cells generated by MLC are contained within the OKT8 subset.[18] Activation of OKT8$^+$ cells with Con A induces suppressor cells capable of dampening the generation of cytotoxic T lymphocytes (CTL) in MLC. Furthermore, like the TH_2^+ subpopulation, the OKT8$^+$ subset does not respond to soluble antigen.

D. Thymocyte–Specific Antibodies

OKT6[19] and NA1/34[55] are mAbs produced by lymphocyte hybrids derived from fusions of B cells from CAF$_1$ or BALB/cJ mice immunized with human thymocytes. Both OKT6 and NA1/34 react with approximately 70 to 85% of the thymocyte population and are unreactive with bone marrow (BM) cells and PBMC.[55] Both antibodies precipitate a 49,000 dalton glycoprotein[56,57] referred to as human thymocyte antigen (HTA–1). Associated with HTA–1 is a 12,000 dalton protein having a slightly slower electrophoretic mobility than β_2 microglobulin but nevertheless serologically cross–reactive with it.[55] The difference in gel mobility may be a result of a slight modification of β_2 microglobulin, a second related gene product, or a β_2 microglobulin polymorphism, as has been recently observed in the mouse. While neither OKT6 nor NA1/34 are expressed on lymphocytes outside the thymic compartment in normal individuals, several T cell acute lymphoblastic leukemias have been described that are reactive with OKT6 and NA1/34 and are therefore HTA–1$^+$.[19,58,59] Langerhans' cells in the skin are also reactive.[60] It has been suggested by McMichael et al.[56] that HTA–1 is analogous to the murine thymus leukemia (TL) antigen.

Finally, recent studies on normal thymocytes using antibodies NA1/34 and W6/32 (anti–HLA framework) suggested that the two antigens precipitated by these antibodies were reciprocally expressed.[56]

E. Nonlineage–Specific Antibodies

OKT9 is a mAb produced by a cloned hybridoma formed between spleen cells from CAF$_1$ mice immunized with T (thymic) acute lymphoblastic leukemia cells (T–ALL) and P3X63Ag8U1 myeloma cells.[20] Immunoprecipitation studies reveal that OKT9 reacts with a 90,000 dalton molecule under reducing conditions. It appears to be a disulfide–bonded dimer since it is 180,000 daltons under nonreducing conditions. Other mAbs have also been identified that precipitate an antigen of similar molecular weight and function.[61,62]

The OKT9 antibody reacts with a wide variety of leukemia and tumor cell lines (cALL, T-ALL, erythroid, myeloid, B-lymphoma, melanoma, etc.), leukemia cells taken directly from patients (T-ALL, non-T-ALL, AML), fetal thymus and liver, normal adult BM (myeloblasts, normoblasts, BFU-E, CFU-E), and activated lymphocytes (peripheral T cells and pediatric thymocytes).[20,58,63–65] All metabolically or mitogenically activated cell types studied have been shown to express this antigen. Synthesis of the antigen can be induced either to appear by mitogenic stimulation of normal resting lymphocytes (PHA, Con A, ionomycin + TPA for T cells; PWM for B cells), or to disappear by activating the maturation of leukemic cell lines (HL-60, HPB-ALL).[66,67]

Binding experiments, antigenic analyses, and cell distribution patterns have demonstrated that OKT9 recognizes the transferrin receptor.[20] It was determined that OKT9 and transferrin probably bind to different sites on the same molecule since OKT9 did not inhibit the binding of radiolabeled transferrin. The presence of transferrin receptors on the described cell types probably reflects the metabolic demands that are associated with cell proliferation and suggests that the OKT9 antibody may be used to identify activated and/or proliferating cells.

OKT10 is a mAb produced by lymphocyte hybrids derived from fusions of spleen cells from BALB/cJ mice immunized with human thymocytes.[22] Immunoprecipitation studies reveal that OKT10 precipitates a 45,000 dalton glycoprotein (reducing conditions) that appears to be an integral membrane protein.[67] OKT10 primarily reacts with early hematopoietic stem cells and various derivatives of these precursors. Specifically, these cells include thymocytes, and in the BM TdT$^+$ (terminal deoxynucleotidyl transferase) cells, B lymphocytes, as well as myeloblasts, promyelocytes, and some myelocytes.[68] The OKT10 antigen is also present on B cell lines as well as T cell lines. While OKT10 is neither a specific marker for T-lineage cells nor a marker restricted to a particular stage of T cell maturation, there appears to be a preferential reactivity for immature (thymic) T cells and their corresponding leukemias (T-ALL). Nevertheless, the majority of acute myeloid leukemias (AML) are also positive as are greater than 90% of common ALL (including the pre-B subclass) and some mature B-ALL.[65,66] Lastly, upon activation of resting T lymphocytes, this antigen has been shown to appear both in vivo[69] and in vitro, the latter following Con A stimulation.[67]

OKIa1 is a mAb produced from lymphocyte hybrids derived from fusions of spleen cells from BALB/cJ mice immunized with human peripheral E rosette-positive lymphocytes.[51] OKIa1 is reactive with the polypeptide framework of the Ia antigen which has been shown to be basically indistinguishable from that previously defined by heteroantisera, alloantisera, and mAbs to Ia-like molecules in man, guinea pigs, and mice.[70] Immunoprecipitation studies reveal that OKIa1 is reactive with a glycoprotein membrane complex composed of 29,000 and 34,000 dalton subunits.[48] OKIa1 reacts with the vast majority of B cells and macrophages (Mφ) (>90%) plus a subset of null cells (≈20%). No detectable resting T cells are OKIa1$^+$. Further analysis reveals that activated human T cells express Ia antigens.[51,71] Following mitogen activation with PHA or Con A and alloactivation in MLC, 20% and 70% of T cells, respectively, express the Ia antigen. On the other hand, only the inducer T cell population (OKT4$^+$) which proliferates maximally to soluble antigen, expresses Ia antigens after activation by tetanus toxoid.[15] Finally, the OKIa1 antibody has been shown to be present on T cells in certain disease states such as infectious disease, autoimmune disease, immunodeficiency diseases, and in certain leukemias, for example, ALL, AML, and chronic lymphatic leukemia.[70,72,73]

IV. REGULATORY INTERACTIONS BETWEEN T CELL SUBSETS AS DEFINED BY mAbs

OKT1* and OKT3 mAbs have been shown to identify greater than 95% of circulating peripheral human T cells. Treatment of purified peripheral T cells with antibody and

---

*OKT1 is an IgG$_1$ that does not fix complement. Cytotoxicity assays with OKT1 require use of a complement fixing α-mouse Ig as a second antibody.

complement abolishes all known T cell functions such as T cell proliferation with mitogens or allogeneic stimulation, T cell-mediated help during PWM-driven antibody responses in vitro, T cell-mediated suppression and the generation of CTL in response to allogeneic targets in MLC. Within the OKT1/OKT3 population two phenotypically and functionally distinct subpopulations reside. These subpopulations are detected by mAbs OKT4 and OKT8. OKT4 identifies 50 to 60% of normal human peripheral T cells and OKT8 identifies 30 to 40% of the T cell population. These two mutually exclusive subsets together represent greater than 95% of the human T cell pool and it remains uncertain whether peripheral cells lacking both OKT4 and OKT8 are truly T cells. Previous studies have shown that the OKT4[+] population contains cells capable of inducing both B cell differentiation and helping the development of alloreactive CTL precursors although it does not contain the precursors of these cells.[13,15] The OKT8[+] population on the other hand contains alloreactive precursor and effector CTL as well as suppressor cells.[18,74] Thus, the two subsets are functionally identified as helper/inducer and suppressor/cytotoxic subsets, respectively.

Considerable interaction occurs between these two subsets, as is demonstrated by the following observations. The OKT4[+] subset has been shown to contain both radiosensitive and radioresistant populations.[75,76] Irradiation of the OKT4[+] population and subsequent co-culture of these cells with nonirradiated OKT8[+] cells and B cells failed to suppress plaque-forming cells (PFC) in a PWM-driven system. In contrast, addition of nonirradiated OKT4[+] cells to this system resulted in marked suppression of PFC. Furthermore, when graded numbers of nonirradiated OKT4[+] cells were added to PWM-driven B cell cultures, the number of PFC generated did not follow a linear relationship with respect to added cells. The addition of moderate numbers of those cells resulted in a plateau effect and, subsequently, with the addition of further cells a diminution of the PFC response was obtained. In contrast to this observation, when irradiated OKT4[+] cells were added in graded numbers to the B cell cultures, a linear dose response curve was generated with respect to PFC.

Taken together, the above observations suggest that radiosensitive cells within the OKT4[+] subset are required for the generation of suppressor function by interacting with the OKT8[+] population. In addition, these data suggest that there may reside within the radiosensitive OKT4[+] population a novel suppressor cell bearing the OKT3[+],4[+],8[-] phenotype. This hypothesis is further supported by the observations of Thomas et al.[77] that small numbers of activated OKT4[+] cells (which retain the OKT4[+] phenotype following PWM activation) were able to suppress B cell differentiation by fresh OKT4[+] cells. In a recent report, Uchiyama et al.[78,79] described somewhat similar findings. These investigators described a mAb (anti-Tac) that reacts only with a subpopulation of mature PWM-activated T cells. When both the Tac[+] and Tac[-] populations were functionally analyzed for helper/inducer and suppressor/cytotoxic functions it was found that the Tac[+] population contained radioresistant help and radiosensitive suppression as well as CTL activity against allogeneic targets. In contrast, the Tac[-] population contained only radiosensitive helper cells. In addition to the OKT8[+] subset functioning as suppressors of B cell differentiation and Ig production, they also serve as CTL in the in vitro generation of hapten-altered (TNP) self-reactive human cytotoxic T lymphocytes. Studies directed toward a better comprehension of the role of T-T interaction in the generation of these killer cells have concluded that while the cytotoxic effector function is contained within the OKT8[+] subset, optimal cytotoxic responses to altered self-antigens required the presence of both OKT4[+] and OKT8[+] cells.[74] These observations suggest that cooperation between these subsets is essential for maximal amplification of killing. The following observations support this concept: OKT4[+] cells and not OKT8[+] cells generate helper factors during a mixed lymphocyte reaction and these amplify TNP-altered self-reactive CTL responses, and helper factors bypass the need for OKT4–OKT8 interaction in the CTL response. These observations as a whole demonstrate the importance of functional T-T interactions in the immunoregulation of both T and B cell differentiation.

Recently, Biddison et al.[80] further extended these findings by demonstrating that helper T lymphocytes are involved in the generation of human CTL responses to influenza virus. These investigators found that although influenza-immune CTL precursors and effectors are OKT3$^+$, OKT4$^-$, and OKT8$^+$, the generation of maximal CTL responses requires a helper T cell. Helper T cells can be obtained from either the OKT4$^+$ or OKT4$^-$ populations, but more potent help was generated by the OKT4$^+$ subset.

These findings further emphasize the importance of T-T interaction in regulation of the immune system. It is possible that the above studies represent a very preliminary picture of these regulatory circuits. It is hoped that further mAbs will help to dissect the complexities of normal immunoregulatory circuits and help elucidate their derangements in disease.

V. ANALYSIS OF LYMPHOCYTE DIFFERENTIATION AND MATURATION IN LYMPHOID TISSUES USING mAbs

mAbs have now been generated that recognize differentiation antigens that appear (or disappear) at precise stages of cell maturation. With the availability of such reagents, a number of laboratories have begun to study the ontogeny of T lymphocytes and their microanatomical locations within lymphoid tissues. Using this technology, the following analysis of T cell maturation and tissue distribution has been formulated.

To begin with, the BM contains two distinct lymphocyte populations related to T cells: lymphocytes of peripheral T cell phenotype and putative T lymphocyte precursors. The cells in the former population enter the BM from the blood following maturation (acquisition of T cell antigens) in the thymus. These cells express differentiation antigens that are exclusive to the T lymphoid lineage (OKT3, OKT4, OKT8, OKT11) that are absent on the proposed T lymphocyte precursors. In contrast, the cells in the latter population acquire differentiation antigens (OKT10, TdT) in the BM that are not lineage-specific, since OKT10 reacts with both early hematopoietic stem cells (BM, TdT$^+$ cells, myeloblasts, promyelocytes, and some myelocytes) and various derivatives of these precursors (thymocytes and B lymphocytes) and TdT is found in BM precursors of T lymphocytes and probably B lymphocytes.[68,81]

In the thymus, the earliest TdT$^+$ blasts (putative thymic precursors) bear a strong resemblance to the BM precursors (OKT10$^+$), yet, phenotypic differences suggest major differentiation steps between the two cell types.[59] Specifically, thymic blasts acquire differentiation antigens (not present on BM TdT$^+$ cells) within the thymus. These antigens are lost in an orderly fashion at various developmental stages in a continuous pattern from the cortex to the medulla.[82] The cortical thymocytes bear thymocyte-specific antigens (TdT$^+$,OKT6$^+$,10$^+$,4$^+$,5$^+$,8$^+$,11$^+$), while the medullary cell pattern approximates the staining pattern of peripheral T cells (OKT11$^+$,1$^+$,3$^+$,4$^+$,5$^+$,8$^+$). The latter population segregates into distinct OKT4$^+$ and OKT5/OKT8$^+$ subsets.[19] Noteworthy are 10 to 15% of thymocytes showing intermediate phenotypes between cortical and medullary thymocytes.[83]

Upon leaving the thymus, the T cell populations enter the peripheral blood and migrate to lymphohematopoietic organs and the gut. OKT4$^+$ cells are found to predominate in the peripheral blood (55 to 60% of peripheral T cell population), intestinal lamina propria and paracortical T cell areas in the lymph nodes and tonsils. There is a close association between the OKT4$^+$ cells and OKIa1$^+$ interdigitating reticular cells in the lymph nodes and tonsils and OKIa1$^+$ macrophages in the lamina propria, possibly suggesting that Ia-like antigens play a role in the local regulation of inducer T cell activity.[82,84,85] OKT8$^+$ cells are present in the peripheral blood (20% of the peripheral T cell population) and constitute the larger part of the T cell population in normal human BM and gut epithelium.[82] Some OKT8$^+$ cells are seen in the paracortical areas of the tonsils and lymph nodes, yet unlike OKT4$^+$ cells, are not found to be associated with OKIa1$^+$ reticular cells. Lastly, T lymphocytes (OKT3$^+$) can be found within the white pulp of the spleen (approximately 30% of mononuclear cells) with equal proportions of OKT4$^+$ and OKT8$^+$ cells (16 to 17%). OKT10$^+$ cells have also been detected in the spleen (19% of mononuclear cells).

VI. POTENTIAL APPLICATIONS OF mAbs TO T CELLS

A. Basic and Applied Research Applications

As described in sections IV and V, the anti-T cell mAbs are providing a great deal of information on the physiological and anatomical interrelationships among the cells of the immune system. At the present time the authors believe that only the OKT3, OKT4 and OKT5/OKT8 antibodies are uniquely found on T lineage cells, although the nonlineage-specific mAbs provide valuable information on the state of maturation and function when used in conjunction with these lineage-specific reagents. While it is certain that other mAbs specific for T lineage antigens will be isolated, much will be learned when researchers, continuing the work described in Sections IV and V, use combinations of mAbs in double labeling and/or multiple depletion experiments.

Another area of increasing interest is the use of the anti-T cell mAbs in the evaluation of clinical disease. To date, most attempts to monitor and diagnose disease have focused on quantitating the T lymphocyte subpopulations in peripheral blood. When used in combination with the white cell differential count, the anti-T cell mAbs provide a knowledge of the absolute numbers of T lymphocytes as well as the number of lymphocytes belonging to each of the T cell subpopulations. In these studies the ratio of helper/inducer to suppressor/cytotoxic cells, the OKT4/OKT8 ratio, has been particularly interesting since it provides a measure of the intersubpopulation balance within the immune system. Changes in this ratio may be due to changes in the proportions of T cells within each subpopulation and/or changes in the absolute number of cells within a subpopulation(s).

The anti-T cell mAbs are providing new information on the etiology of disease. Six major groups of diseases are currently being studied with these reagents:

1. Lymphoid and nonlymphoid malignancies
2. Infectious diseases
3. Autoimmune diseases
4. Allergic diseases
5. Immunodeficiencies
6. Transplantation patients

Classification of a leukemia into a T cell or non-T cell (i.e., B cell, monocytic) malignancy can clearly be done with these reagents. More interestingly, the stage of differentiation of a leukemia may be determined. Leukemias derived from early thymocytes express surface antigens of an immature thymic phenotype (OKT10 and/or OKT9), whereas malignancies derived from a more mature thymocyte express surface antigens found on peripheral T lymphocytes (OKT3, OKT4, OKT8).[19] Adult chronic

T cell leukemias (including mycosis fungoides) express mature subset phenotypes.[26,86] Further investigations may allow physicians to prescribe a specific therapy most appropriate for the maturational stage of the leukemia. Studies in nonlymphoid malignancies are at an early stage but preliminary indications are that each type will be associated with a characteristic pattern of immunoregulatory disturbance and that excess suppressor cells (low OKT4/OKT8 ratio) are most commonly seen with metastatic disease.[87]

Within the field of infectious disease, interesting data is being obtained about T lymphocyte subpopulations during viral infection. In both infectious mononucleosis and cytomegalovirus infection there is a large increase in suppressor/cytotoxic (OKT8$^+$) lymphocytes that is accompanied by a decrease in the OKT4/OKT8 ratio. In infectious mononucleosis many of the lymphocytes also display the DR antigen (OKIa1$^+$) and OKT9 and OKT10 antigens. These phenotypes are indicative of physiological activation and suggest that the newly mature suppressor/cytotoxic lymphocytes may be regulating the B cell activation associated with this disease.[69,88] In cytomegalovirus mononucleosis the reduced OKT4/OKT8 ratio is accompanied by a reduced responsiveness of lymphocytes to Con A as demonstrated by in vitro assays.[89] This suppressed immunological state may be responsible for the protracted course of the illness and the increased risk of bacterial and fungal superinfections. In both diseases, clinical recovery is associated with a return of the OKT4/OKT8 ratio to more normal levels.

The subset changes that occur during hepatitis B infection are similar, though milder in degree to those of infectious mononucleosis. The reduced OKT4/OKT8 ratio in chronic hepatitis B infection is due to a decrease in the absolute number of OKT4$^+$ lymphocytes with normal absolute numbers of OKT8$^+$ cells.[90] In acute hepatitis the reduced ratio is due to an increase in the OKT8$^+$ lymphocytes. The ratio returns to more normal values after disappearance of the hepatitis B antigen and appearance of antibody to the B antigen in the blood. In contrast, hepatitis A virus infection causes an increase in the OKT4/OKT8 ratio and is characterized by rapid clinical recovery.

These studies of infectious disease are beginning to suggest that microorganisms may be able to induce an increase in the suppressive state in the host organism, permitting unchecked proliferation of the parasitic microbe and a prolonged course of disease.

The size of the T cell population and further division of these lymphocytes into the OKT4$^+$ and OKT8$^+$ subpopulations is also being studied in many autoimmune diseases including rheumatoid arthritis,[91] systemic lupus erythematosus,[92] multiple sclerosis,[93] Sjogren's disease,[94] thyroid disease, and myasthenia gravis.[95] These diseases are generally characterized by an increase in the OKT4/OKT8 ratio but may also be associated with defects in the interrelationships among the T lymphocyte subpopulations. These changes in the lymphocyte subpopulations are associated with reduced or impaired suppressor activity and may be accompanied by the development of autoantibodies. In the case of rheumatoid arthritis and multiple sclerosis, remission of the disease appears to be associated with a return of the OKT4/OKT8 ratio to more normal values.

Studies of patients with allergies, specifically atopic dermatitis, suggested an association between active atopic dermatitis and reduced suppressor/cytotoxic cells, resulting in an elevated OKT4/OKT8 ratio. In accordance with these findings a proportion of patients with hay fever due to ragweed pollen also revealed an increase in the OKT4/OKT8 ratio.[96]

Patients with acquired hypogammaglobulinemia often present with a lowered OKT4/OKT8 ratio that is representative of either reduced helper activity (due to a reduction in the number of OKT4$^+$ cells) or elevated suppressor activity (due to an increase in the number of OKT8$^+$ cells).[97,98] Characteristic of this disease, many of the OKT8$^+$ T cells are shown to be activated (OKIa1$^+$) and preliminary in vitro experiments have shown that depletion of these cells restores helper activity, as demonstrated by the production of Ig after stimulation with PWM.

B. Clinical and Diagnostic Applications

Anti-T cell mAbs may find clinical use in the diagnosis or classification of disease and monitoring therapy or disease course. It is possible to use these reagents to examine peripheral blood, exudates, and tissue sections, although most work has been done with the mononuclear cells isolated from peripheral blood. At the present time most analyses utilize an indirect immunofluorescent technique although methods which employ enzyme or colloidal gold-labeled reagents are becoming more widespread.[99,100] Additionally, the development of rapidly automated analytical methods gives the promise of making this type of analysis more widely available in clinical medicine.[23]

While the similarities of T cell subpopulation changes that occur in diverse diseases may suggest that a diagnosis based solely on the lymphocyte counts will be unlikely, when the overall immune profile is considered, many interesting and significant diagnostic associations are evident. Simple changes in the OKT4/OKT8 ratio may be highly informative and diagnostically significant when there is some preexisting knowledge of the disease or more likely the class of disease. For example, infectious mononucleosis is characterized by a large increase in OKT8+ lymphocytes but is distinguished from other diseases by the fact that many of these suppressor cells express the DR antigen (OKIa1+) as a sign of activation.[69] In the case of renal transplant recipients, the OKT4/OKT8 ratio allows the clinician to distinguish between kidney damage caused by the activation of latent viruses (lowered ratio) from that caused by rejection (increased ratio) allowing the most appropriate therapy to be instituted.[89]

Success in monitoring therapy with the anti-T cell mAbs is being demonstrated in the area of renal transplantation. The risk of organ rejection can be correlated with the OKT4/OKT8 ratio, with values greater than normal predictive of an "at risk" situation.[101] Interestingly, values lower than normal are predictive of a controlled rejection process but also indicative of a susceptibility to infection. In this situation the most appropriate therapy may be to continue the reduction in immunosuppressive drugs in order for the patient's immune system to recover sufficiently to control the infection.[89]

Patients with rheumatoid arthritis will also benefit from a regime that includes monitoring of the subpopulations and the OKT4/OKT8 ratio. Response to therapy and the beginning of clinical remission has been associated with a normalization of the ratio in certain patients who presented with an elevated ratio.[91]

The mAb OKT9, coupled to a suitable radioisotope, may prove to be a useful reagent for in vivo diagnostic imaging and allow for the localization of clusters of dividing cells such as tumors. In order for the antibody to have access to all regions of the body, it may be necessary to cleave the molecule into the smaller Fab or $F(ab')_2$ fragments. The specificity of the mAb and the high-specific activity of the radioisotope will in all likelihood allow imaging to be accomplished with small amounts of material.

C. Therapeutic Applications

The anti-T cell mAbs are potentially highly specific therapeutic agents that can be produced to the standards of purity and consistency required of a pharmaceutical agent and may serve as general or subpopulation-specific immunosuppressive agents. It is already apparent that OKT3 can function as an immunosuppressive drug and be of value in the management of transplant rejection or graft-vs.-host disease.[101–103] OKT3 exerts a direct immunosuppressive effect on the in vitro development and effecting of T cell-mediated killing[29] and may, for this reason, function in vivo as both an immediate pharmaceutical immunosuppressive agent in addition to its subsequent effect in deleting OKT3[+] cells.

It is interesting to note that those diseases characterized by an altered OKT4/OKT8 ratio may be best treated with an anti-T cell mAb specific for only one T cell subpopulation. Using one of these reagents as a drug may allow the physician the opportunity to selectively delete a subpopulation, either in vivo or perhaps in vitro, which may serve as an effective therapeutic agent if it can be demonstrated that the clinical situation is affected by the imbalance in the T cell subpopulations.

mAbs used as therapeutic agents may function in vivo in concert with the complement system or may increase opsonization of the cells carrying the unique antigen. It may also be possible to conjugate a toxin or chemotherapeutic drug to the antibody and use the specificity of the reagent to concentrate a lethal dose in a target tissue.

Currently, mAbs are being developed for the treatment of leukemia, graft-vs.-host disease associated with BM transplantation, and acute rejection of renal transplants.

Leukemia-reactive mAbs could be used to treat patients directly in vivo or to remove, in vitro, leukemia cells from a sample of a patient's BM prior to whole body irradiation followed by infusion of the leukemia-depleted stem cells into the patient. Recently, the efficacy of such serotherapy in the treatment of ALL has been tested in patients using mAbs.[104,105] Preliminary studies using J-5, a mAb specific for a common ALL antigen (CALLA) and L17F12, a mAb reactive with the majority of human T lymphocytes and thymocytes,[42] showed the antibodies rapidly bound to leukemic cells. This resulted in marked reductions of circulating lymphocytes. Unfortunately this response was transient and attributable in part to antigenic modulation of leukemic cells. These studies represent only a beginning in this type of therapy and with proper dosage scheduling and in vitro monitoring, it is possible that these obstacles can be overcome.

The elimination of graft-vs.-host disease in recipients of donor BM transplants may also be an appropriate therapeutic application for anti-T cell mAbs. OKT3 is currently being used to inactivate and remove immunocompetent T cells from donor BM. The marrow is subsequently used to reconstitute the immune system in children suffering from severe combined immunodeficiency disease or in leukemia patients who have been treated with whole body irradiation and intensive chemotherapy.[102,103] In preliminary studies, successful engraftment of donor cells in the recipient's BM has been demonstrated and the severity of the graft-vs.-host disease appears to be reduced.

Whether the successful management of the disease in all cases will respond to the in vitro treatment of donor BM with OKT3 prior to transplant or will require continued in vivo immunosuppression by injection of OKT3 into the recipient is the topic of current clinical investigations.

The most successful therapeutic application of the anti-T cell mAbs has been in the management of acute rejection of renal transplants. OKT3, in doses of 5 mg or less per day, has been shown to be an effective immunosuppressive agent that has contributed to the reversal of acute rejection episodes.[101] Expanded clinical studies are presently underway to study further the therapeutic potential of this agent.

REFERENCES

1. **Cantor, H. and Boyse, E. A.,** Functional subclasses of T lymphocytes bearing different Ly antigens. I. Generation of functionally distinct T-cell subclasses in a differentiative process independent of antigen, *J. Exp. Med.,* 141, 1376, 1975.

2. **Jandinski, J., Cantor, H., Tadakuma, T., Peavy, D. L., and Pierce, C. W.,** Separation of helper T cells from suppressor T cells expressing different Ly components. I. Polyclonal activation: suppression and helper activities are inherent properties of distinct T-cell subclasses, *J. Exp. Med.,* 143, 1382, 1976.

3. **McKenzie, I. F. C. and Potter, T.,** Murine lymphocytes surface antigens, *Adv. Immunol.,* 27, 181, 1979.

4. **Evans, R. L., Lazarus, H., Penta, A. C., and Schlossman, S. F.,** Two functionally distinct subpopulations of human T cells that collaborate in the generation of cytotoxic cells responsible for cell-mediated lympholysis, *J. Immunol.,* 129, 1423, 1978.

5. **Jondal, M., Holm, G., and Wigzell, H.,** Surface markers on human T and B lymphocytes. I. A large population of lymphocytes forming nonimmune rosettes with sheep red blood cells, *J. Exp. Med.,* 136, 207, 1972.

6. **Moretta, L., Webb, S. R., Grossi, C. E., Lydyard, P. M., and Cooper, M. D.,** Functional analysis of two human T cell subpopulations: help and suppression of B cell responses by T cells bearing receptor of IgM or IgG, *J. Exp. Med.,* 146, 184, 1977.

7. **Strelkauskas, A. J., Schauf, V., Wilson, B. S., Chess, L., and Schlossman, S. F.,** Isolation and characterization of naturally occurring subclasses of human peripheral blood cells with regulatory functions, *J. Immunol.,* 123, 83, 1979.

8. **Moretta, L., Ferrarini, M., Mingari, M. C., Moretta, A., and Webb, S. R.,** Subpopulations of human T cells identified by receptors for immunoglobulin and mitogen responsiveness, *J. Immunol.,* 117, 2171, 1976.

9. **Köhler, G. and Milstein, C.,** Continuous cultures of fused cells secreting antibody of predefined specificity, *Nature (London),* 256, 495, 1975.

10. **Trucco, M. M., Stocker, J. W., and Ceppelini, R.,** Monoclonal antibodies against human lymphocyte antigens, *Nature (London),* 273, 666, 1978.

11. **Koprowski, H., Steplewski, Z., Herlyn, D., and Herlyn, M.,** Study of antibodies against human melanoma produced by somatic cell hybrids, *Proc. Natl. Acad. Sci. U.S.A.,* 75, 3405, 1978.

12. **Williams, A. F., Galfre, G., and Milstein, C.,** Analysis of cell surfaces by xenogeneic myeloma-hybrid antibodies: differentiation antigens of rat lymphocytes, *Cell,* 12, 663, 1977.

13. **Reinherz, E. L., Kung, P. C., Goldstein, G., and Schlossman, S. F.,** A monoclonal antibody with selective reactivity with functionally mature human thymocytes and all peripheral human T cells, *J. Immunol.,* 123, 1312, 1979.

14. **Kung, P. C., Goldstein, G., Reinherz, E. L., and Schlossman, S. F.,** Monoclonal antibodies defining distinctive human T cell surface antigens, *Science,* 206, 347, 1979.

15. **Reinherz, E. L., Kung, P. C., Goldstein, G., and Schlossman, S. F.,** Separation of functional subsets of human T cells by a monoclonal antibody, *Proc. Natl. Acad. Sci. U.S.A.,* 76, 4061, 1979.

16. **Reinherz, E. L., Kung, P. C., Goldstein, G., and Schlossman, S. F.,** Further characterization of the human inducer T cell subset defined by monoclonal antibody, *J. Immunol.,* 123, 2894, 1979.

17. **Reinherz, E. L., Kung, P. C., Breard, J. M., Goldstein, G., and Schlossman, S. F.,** T cell requirements for generation of helper factor(s) in man: analysis of the subsets involved, *J. Immunol.,* 124, 1883, 1980.

18. **Reinherz, E. L., Kung, P. C., Goldstein, G., and Schlossman, S. F.,** A monoclonal antibody reactive with the human cytotoxic/suppressor T cell subset previously defined by a heteroantiserum termed TH_2, *J. Immunol.,* 124, 1301, 1980.

19. **Reinherz, E. L., Kung, P. C., Goldstein, G., Levey, R. H., and Schlossman, S. F.,** Discrete stages of human intrathymic differentiation: analysis of normal thymocytes and leukemic lymphoblasts of T-cell lineage, *Proc. Natl. Acad. Sci. U.S.A.,* 77, 1588, 1980.

20. **Sutherland, R., Delia, D., Schneider, C., Newman, R., Kemshead, J., and Greaves, M.,** Ubiquitous cell surface glycoprotein on tumour cells is proliferation-associated receptor for transferrin, *Proc. Natl. Acad. Sci. U.S.A.,* 78, 4515, 1981.

21. **Verbi, W., Greaves, M. F., Koubek, K., Janossy, G., Stein, H., Kung, P., and Goldstein, G.,** OKT11 and OKT11A: monoclonal antibodies with pan T reactivity which block sheep erythrocyte "receptors" on T cells, *Eur. J. Immunol.,* in press.

22. **Kung, P. C., Talle, M. A., DeMaria, M. E., Butler, M. S., Lifter, J., and Goldstein, G.,** Strategies for generating monoclonal antibodies defining human T-lymphocyte differentiation antigens, *Transplant. Proc.,* 12 (Suppl. 1), 141, 1980.

23. **Hoffman, R. A., Kung, P. C., Hansen, W. P., and Goldstein, G.,** Simple and rapid measurement of human T lymphocytes and their subclasses in peripheral blood, *Proc. Natl. Acad. Sci. U.S.A.,* 77, 4914, 1980.

24. **Kung, P. C., Talle, M. A., DeMaria, M., Ziminski, N., Look, R., Lifter, J., and Goldstein, G.,** Creating a useful panel of anti-T cell monoclonal antibodies, *Int. J. Immunopharmacol.,* 3, 175, 1981.

25. **Kung, P. C. and Goldstein, G.,** Human T cell differentiation antigens detected by monoclonal antibodies, in *Monoclonal Antibodies and T Cell Hybridomas,* Hammerling, U., Hammerling, G. J., and Kearney, J., Eds., Elsevier, Amsterdam, in press.

26. **Kung, P. C., Berger, C. L., Goldstein, G., LoGerfo, P., and Edelson, R. L.,** Cutaneous T cell lymphoma: characterization by monoclonal antibodies, *Blood,* 57, 261, 1981.

27. **van Agthoven, A., Terhorst, C., Reinherz, E. L., and Schlossman, S. F.,** Characterization of T cell surface glycoproteins T1 and T3 present on all human peripheral T lymphocytes and functionally mature thymocytes, *Eur. J. Immunol.,* 11, 18, 1981.

28. **Van Wauwe, J. P., De Mey, J. R., and Goossens, J. G.,** OKT3: a monoclonal anti-human T lymphocyte antibody with potent mitogenic properties, *J. Immunol.,* 124, 2708, 1980.

29. **Chang, T. W., Kung, P. C., Gingras, S. P., and Goldstein, G.,** Does OKT3 monoclonal antibody react with an antigen-recognition structure on human T cells? *Proc. Natl. Acad. Sci. U.S.A.,* 78, 1805, 1981.

30. **Chang, T. W. and Gingras, S. P.,** OKT3 monoclonal antibody inhibits cytotoxic T lymphocyte mediated cell lysis, *Int. J. Immunopharmacol.,* 3, 183, 1981.

31. **Eichmann, K.,** Expression of function of idiotypes of lymphocytes, *Adv. Immunol.,* 26, 195, 1978.

32. **Binz, H.,** Local graft-versus-host reaction in mice specifically inhibited by anti-receptor antibodies, *Scand. J. Immunol.,* 4, 79, 1975.

33. **Pang, R. H. L., Yip, Y. K., and Vilcek, J.,** Immune interferon induction by a monoclonal antibody specific for human T cells, *Cell. Immunol.,* 64, 304, 1981.

34. **Chang, T. W., Testa, D., Kung, P. C., Perry, L., Dreskin, H. J., and Goldstein, G.,** Cellular origin and interactions involved in γ-interferon production induced by OKT3 monoclonal antibody, *J. Immunol.,* 128, 585, 1982.

35. **Van Wauwe, J. and Goossens, J.,** Mitogenic actions of Orthoclone OKT3 on human peripheral blood lymphocytes: effects of monocytes and serum components, *Int. J. Immunopharmacol.,* 3, 203, 1981.

36. **Van Wauwe, J., Goossens, J., DeCock, W., Kung, P., and Goldstein, G.,** Suppression of human T-cell mitogenesis and E-rosette formation by the monoclonal antibody OKT11A, *Immunology,* in press.

37. **Wang, C. Y., Good, R. A., Ammirati, P., Dymbort, G., and Evans, R. L.,** Identification of a p69,71 complex expressed on human T cells sharing determinants with B-type chronic lymphatic leukemia cells, *J. Exp. Med.,* 151, 1539, 1980.

38. **Ledbetter, J. A., Evans, R. L., Lipinski, M., Cunningham-Rundles, C., Good, R. A., and Herzenberg, L. A.,** Evolutionary conservation of surface molecules that distinguish T lymphocyte helper/inducer and cytotoxic/suppressor subpopulations in mouse and man, *J. Exp. Med.,* 153, 310, 1981.

39. **Kamoun, M., Martin, P. J., Hansen, J. A., Brown, M. A., Siadek, A. W., and Nowinski, R. A.,** Identification of a human T lymphocyte surface protein associated with the E-rosette receptor, *J. Exp. Med.,* 153, 207, 1981.

40. **Haynes, B. F.,** Human T cell antigens as defined by monoclonal antibodies, *Immunol. Rev.,* 57, 1, 1981.

41. **Royston, I., Majda, J. A., Baird, S. M., Meserve, B. L., and Griffiths, J. C.,** Human T cell antigens defined by monoclonal antibodies: the 65,000 dalton antigen of T cells (T65) is also found on the chronic lymphocytic leukemia cells bearing surface immunoglobulin, *J. Immunol.,* 125, 725, 1980.

42. **Engleman, E. G., Warnke, R., Fox, R. I., Dilley, J., Benike, C. J., and Levy, R.,** Studies of a human T lymphocyte antigen recognized by a monoclonal antibody, *Proc. Natl. Acad. Sci. U.S.A.,* 78, 1791, 1981.

43. **Howard, F. D., Ledbetter, J. A., Wong, J., Bieber, C. P., Stinson, E. B., and Herzenberg, L. A.,** A human T lymphocyte differentiation marker defined by monoclonal antibodies that block E-rosette formation, *J. Immunol.,* 126, 2117, 1981.

44. **Yip, S.,** Personal communication, 1981.

45. **Haynes, B. F., Eisenbarth, G. S., and Fauci, A. S.,** Human lymphocyte antigens: production of a monoclonal antibody that defines functional thymus-derived lymphocyte subsets, *Proc. Natl. Acad. Sci. U.S.A.,* 76, 5829, 1979.

46. **Haynes, B. F., Mann, D. L., Hemler, M. E., Schroer, J. A., Shelhamer, J. H., Eisenbarth, G. S., Strominger, J. L., Thomas, C. A., Mostowski, H. S., and Fauci, A. S.,** Characterization of a monoclonal antibody that defines an immunoregulatory T cell subset for immunoglobulin synthesis in humans, *Proc. Natl. Acad. Sci. U.S.A.,* 77, 2914, 1980.

47. **Beverley, P. C. L. and Callard, R. E.,** Distinctive functional characteristics of human "T" lymphocytes defined by E rosetting or a monoclonal anti-T cell antibody, *Eur. J. Immunol.,* 11, 329, 1981.

48. **Terhorst, C., van Agthoven, A., Reinherz, E. L., and Schlossman, S. F.,** Biochemical analysis of human T lymphocyte differentiation antigens T4 and T5, *Science,* 209, 520, 1980.
49. **Bach, J. F.,** Unpublished data, 1981.
50. **Rao, P.,** Unpublished data, 1981.
51. **Reinherz, E. L., Kung, P. C., Pesando, J. M., Ritz, J., Goldstein, G., and Schlossman, S. F.,** Ia determinants on human T-cell subsets defined by monoclonal antibody, *J. Exp. Med.,* 150, 1472, 1979.
52. **Bach, M. -A., Phan-Dinh-Tuy, F., Bach, J. F., Wallach, D., Biddison, W. E., Sharrow, S. O., Goldstein, G., and Kung, P. C.,** Unusual phenotypes of human inducer T cells as measured by OKT4 and related monoclonal antibodies, *J. Immunol.,* 127, 980, 1981.
53. **Evans, R. L., Wall, D. W., Platsoucas, C. D., Siegal, F. P., Fikrig, S. M., Testa, C. M., and Good, R. A.,** Thymus-dependent membrane antigens in man: inhibition of cell mediated lympholysis by monoclonal antibodies to TH₂ antigen, *Proc. Natl. Acad. Sci. U.S.A.,* 78, 544, 1981.
54. **Kung, P. C. and Goldstein, G.,** Functional and developmental compartments of human T lymphocytes, *Vox Sang.,* 39, 121, 1980.
55. **Cotner, T., Mashimo, H., Kung, P. C., Goldstein, G., and Strominger, J. L.,** Human T cell surface antigens bearing a structural relationship to HLA antigens, *Proc. Natl. Acad. Sci. U.S.A.,* 78, 3859, 1981.
56. **McMichael, A. J., Pilch, J. R., Galfre, G., Mason, D. Y., Fabre, J. W., and Milstein, C.,** A human thymocyte antigen defined by a hybrid myeloma monoclonal antibody, *Eur. J. Immunol.,* 9, 205, 1979.
57. **Ziegler, A. and Milstein, D.,** A small polypeptide different from β₂-microglobulin associated with a human cell surface antigen, *Nature (London),* 279, 243, 1979.
58. **Haynes, B. F., Metzgar, R. S., Minna, J. D., and Bunn, P. A.,** Phenotypic characterization of cutaneous T-cell lymphoma. Use of monoclonal antibodies to compare with other malignant T cells, *N. Engl. J. Med.,* 304, 1319, 1981.
59. **Bradstock, K. F., Janossy, G., Pizzolo, G., Hoffbrand, A. V., McMichael, A., Pilch, J. R., Milstein, C., Beverley, P., and Bollum, F. J.,** Subpopulations of normal and leukemic human thymocytes: an analysis with the use of monoclonal antibodies, *J. Natl. Cancer Inst.,* 65, 33, 1980.
60. **Fithian, E., Kung, P., Goldstein, G., Rubenfeld, M., Fenoglio, C., and Edelson, R.,** Reactivity of Langerhans' cells with hybridoma antibody, *Proc. Natl. Acad. Sci. U.S.A.,* 78, 2541, 1981.
61. **Bramwell, M. E., and Harris, A.,** An abnormal membrane glycoprotein associated with malignancy in a wide range of different tumors, *Proc. R. Soc. London Ser. B.,* 201, 87, 1978.
62. **Omary, M. B., Trowbridge, I. S., and Minowada, J.,** Human cell surface glycoprotein with unusual properties, *Nature (London),* 286, 888, 1980.
63. **Delia, D., Newman, R., Greaves, M. F., Goldstein, G., and Kung, P.,** Induction of differentiation in T-ALL cell lines with phorbol ester (TPA), in *Proceedings of the Leukemia Marker Conference,* Knapp, W., Ed., Academic Press, New York, 1981, 293.
64. **Kersey, J. H., LeBien, T. W., Gajl-Peczalska, K., Nesbit, M., Jansen, J., Kung, P., Goldstein, G., Sather, H., Coccia, P., Siegel, S., Bleyer, A., and Hammond, D.,** Acute lymphoblastic leukemia/lymphoma: cell markers define phenotypic heterogeneity, in *Proceedings of the Leukemia Marker Conference,* Knapp, W., Ed., Academic Press, New York, in press.
65. **Greaves, M. F., Verbi, W., Rao, J., Kung, P., and Goldstein, G.,** Monoclonal antibodies probes for leukemic heterogeneity and haematopoietic differentiation, in *Proc. of the Leukemia Marker Conference,* Knapp, W., Ed., Academic Press, New York, 3, 283, 1981.
66. **Greaves, M., Delia, D., Sutherland, R., Rao, J., Verbi, W., Kemshead, J., Robinson, J., Hariri, G., Goldstein, G., and Kung, P.,** Expression of the OKT monoclonal antibody defined antigenic determinants in malignancy, *Int. J. Immunopharmacol.,* in press.
67. **Terhorst, C., van Agthoven, A., LeClair, K., Snow, P., Reinherz, E. L., and Schlossman, S. F.,** Biochemical studies of the human thymocyte cell-surface antigens T6, T9 and T10, *Cell,* 23, 771, 1981.
68. **Janossy, G., Tidman, N., Papageorgiou, E. S., Kung, P. C., and Goldstein, G.,** Distribution of T lymphocyte subsets in the human bone marrow and thymus: an analysis with monoclonal antibodies, *J. Immunol.,* 126, 1608, 1981.
69. **De Waele, M., Thielemans, C., and Van Camp, B. K. G.,** Characterization of immunoregulatory T cells in EBV-induced mononucleosis by monoclonal antibodies, *N. Engl. J. Med.,* 304, 460, 1981.
70. **Schlossman, S. F., Chess, L., Humphreys, R. E., and Strominger, J. L.,** Distribution of Ia-like molecules on the surface of normal and leukemic cells, *Proc. Natl. Acad. Sci. U.S.A.,* 73, 1288, 1976.
71. **Evans, R. L., Faldetta, T. J., Humphreys, R. E., Pratt, D. M., Yunis, E. J., and Schlossman, S. F.,** Peripheral human T cells sensitized in mixed leukocyte culture synthesize and express Ia-like antigens, *J. Exp. Med.,* 148, 1440, 1978.

72. **Reinherz, E. L., Nadler, L. M., Rosenthal, D. S., Moloney, W. C., and Schlossman, S. F.,** T cell subset characterization of human T-CLL, *Blood,* 53, 1066, 1979.

73. **Reinherz, E. L., Parkman, R., Rappeport, J., Rosen, F. S., and Schlossman, S. F.,** Aberrations of suppressor T cells in human graft-versus-host disease, *N. Engl. J. Med.,* 300, 1061, 1979.

74. **Friedman, S. M., Hunter, S. B., Irigoyen, O. H., Kung, P. C., Goldstein, G., and Chess, L.,** Functional analysis of human T cell subsets defined by monoclonal antibodies. II. Collaborative T-T interactions in the generation of TNP-altered-self-reactive cytotoxic T lymphocytes, *J. Immunol.,* 126, 1702, 1981.

75. **Thomas, Y., Sosman, J., Irogoyen, O., Friedman, S. M., Kung, P. C., Goldstein, G., and Chess, L.,** Functional analysis of human T cell subsets defined by monoclonal antibodies. I. Collaborative T-T interactions in the immunoregulation of B cell differentiation, *J. Immunol.,* 125, 2402, 1980.

76. **Thomas, Y., Sosman, J., Irigoyen, O., Rogozinski, L., Friedman, S. M., and Chess, L.,** Interactions among human T cell subsets, *Int. J. Immunopharmacol.,* 3, 193, 1981.

77. **Thomas, Y., Rogozinski, L., Irigoyen, O., Friedman, S. M., Kung, P. C., Goldstein, G., and Chess, L.,** Functional analysis of human T cell subsets defined by monoclonal antibodies. IV. Induction of suppressor cells within the OKT4$^+$ population, *J. Exp. Med.,* 150, 459, 1981.

78. **Uchiyama, T., Broder, S., and Waldmann, T. A.,** A monoclonal antibody (anti-Tac) reactive with activated and functionally mature human T cells. I. Production of anti-Tac monoclonal antibody and distribution of Tac ($^+$) cells, *J. Immunol.,* 126, 1393, 1981.

79. **Uchiyama, T., Nelson, D. L., Fleisher, T. A., and Waldmann, T. A.,** A monoclonal antibody (anti-Tac) reactive with activated and functionally mature human T cells. II. Expression of Tac antigen on activated cytotoxic killer T cells, suppressor cells, and on one of two types of helper cells, *J. Immunol.,* 126, 1398, 1981.

80. **Biddison, W. E., Sharrow, S. O., and Shearer, G. M.,** T cell subpopulations required for the human cytotoxic T lymphocyte response to influenza virus: evidence for T cell help, *J. Immunol.,* 127, 487, 1981.

81. **Crawford, D. H., Francis, G. E., Wing, M. A., Edwards, A. J., Janossy, G., Hoffbrand, A. V., Prentice, H. G., Secher, D., McConnell, I., Kung, P. C., and Goldstein, G.,** Reactivity of monoclonal antibodies with human myeloid precursor cells, *Br. J. Haematol.,* 49, 209, 1981.

82. **Janossy, G., Tidman, N., Selby, W. S., Thomas, J. A., Granger, S., Kung, P. C., and Goldstein, G.,** Human T lymphocytes of inducer and suppressor type occupy different microenvironments, *Nature (London),* 288, 81, 1980.

83. **Tidman, N., Janossy, G., Bodger, M., Granger, S., Kung, P. C., and Goldstein, G.,** Delineation of human thymocyte differentiation pathways utilizing double-staining techniques with monoclonal antibodies, *Clin. Exp. Immunol.,* 45, 457, 1981.

84. **Bhan, A. K., Reinherz, E. L., Poppema, S., McCluskey, R. T., and Schlossman, S. F.,** Location of T cell and major histocompatibility complex antigens in the human thymus, *J. Exp. Med.,* 152, 771, 1980.

85. **Poppema, S., Bhan, A. K., Reinherz, E. L., McCluskey, R. T., and Schlossman, S. F.,** Distribution of T cell subsets in human lymph nodes, *J. Exp. Med.,* 153, 30, 1981.

86. **Berger, C. L., Warburton, D., Raafat, J., LoGerfo, P., and Edelson, R. L.,** Cutaneous T-cell lymphoma: neoplasm of T cells with helper activity, *Blood,* 53, 642, 1979.

87. **Ginns, L. C., Goldenheim, P. D., Miller, L. G., Burton, R. C., Gillick, L., Colvin, R. B., Goldstein, G., Kung, P. C., Hurwitz, C., and Kazemi, H.,** T-lymphocyte subsets in smoking and lung cancer analysis by monoclonal antibodies, *N. Engl. J. Med.,* submitted.

88. **Reinherz, E. L., O'Brien, C., Rosenthal, P., and Schlossman, S. F.,** The cellular basis for viral-induced immunodeficiency: analysis by monoclonal antibodies, *J. Immunol.,* 125, 1269, 1980.

89. **Carney, W. P., Rubin, R. H., Hoffman, R. A., Hansen, W. P., Healey, K., and Hirsch, M. S.,** Analysis of T lymphocyte subsets in cytomegalovirus mononucleosis, *J. Immunol.,* 126, 2114, 1981.

90. **Thomas, H. C., Brown, D., Routhier, G., Janossy, G., King, P. C., Goldstein, G., and Sherlock, S.,** Inducer and suppressor T-cells in HBV induced liver disease, *Hepatology,* in press.

91. **Veys, E. M., Hermans, P., Schindler, J., Kung, P. C., Goldstein, G., Symoens, J., and Van Wauwe, J.,** Evaluation of T cell subsets with monoclonal antibodies in patients with rheumatoid arthritis, *J. Rheumatol.,* in press.

92. **Morimoto, C., Reinherz, E. L., Schlossman, S. F., Schur, P. H., Mills, J. A., and Steinberg, A. D.,** Alterations in immunoregulatory T cell subsets in active systemic lupus erythematosus, *J. Clin. Invest.,* 66, 1171, 1980.

93. **Reinherz, E. L., Weiner, H. L., Hauser, S. L., Cohen, J. A., Distaso, J. A., and Schlossman, S. F.,** Loss of suppressor T cells in active multiple sclerosis. Analysis with monoclonal antibodies, *N. Engl. J. Med.,* 303, 125, 1980.

94. **Fox, R. I., Carstens, S. A., Sabharwal, N., Robinson, C. A., Howell, F., Kung, P., and Vaughan, J. H.,** Alterations of lymphocyte subsets in Sjogren's syndrome, *Arthritis Rheum.,* submitted.

95. **Berrih, S., Gaud, C., Bach, M. -A., Le Brigard, H., Binet, J. P., and Bach, J. F.,** Evaluation of T cell subsets in myasthenia gravis using anti-T cell monoclonal antibodies, *Clin. Exp. Immunol.,* 45, 1, 1981.

96. **Alexander, J. F., Ishizaka, K., Norman, P. S., Kagey-Sobotka, A., and Lichtenstein, L. M.,** Peripheral blood helper and suppressor lymphocytes in ragweed hay fever, *Am. Acad. Allerg.,* in press.

97. **Reinherz, E. L., Geha, R., Wohl, M. E., Morimoto, C., Rosen, F. S., and Schlossman, S. F.,** Immunodeficiency associated with loss of T4$^+$ inducer T-cell function, *N. Engl. J. Med.,* 304, 811, 1981.

98. **Rubinstein, A., Sicklick, M., Mchra, V., Rosen, F. S., and Levey, R. H.,** Antihelper cell autoantibody in acquired agammaglobulinemia, *J. Clin. Invest.,* 67, 42, 1981.

99. **DeWaele, M., De Mey, J., Moeremans, M., and Van Camp, B. K. G.,** The Immuno-gold staining method: an immunocytochemical procedure for leucocyte characterization by monoclonal antibodies, in *Proceedings of the Leukemia Marker Conference,* Knapp, W., Ed., Academic Press, New York, in press.

100. **Pepys, E. O., Tennent, G. A., and Pepys, M. B.,** Enumeration of T and B lymphocytes in whole peripheral blood: absence of a null cell population, *Clin. Exp. Immunol.,* 46, 229, 1981.

101. **Cosimi, A. B., Colvin, R. B., Burton, R. C., Rubin, R. H., Goldstein, G., Kung, P. C., Hansen, W. P., Delmonico, F. L., and Russell, P. S.,** Use of monoclonal antibodies to T-cell subsets for immunologic monitoring and treatment in recipients of renal allograft, *N. Engl. J. Med.,* 305, 308, 1981.

102. **Atkinson, K., Hansen, J. A., Storb, R., Goehle, S., Goldstein, G., and Thomas, E. D.,** Human T cell subpopulations identified by monoclonal antibodies after human marrow transplantation. I. Helper-inducer and cytotoxic-suppressor subsets, *Blood,* submitted.

103. **de Bruin, H., Astaldi, A., Leupers, T., van de Griend, R. J., Dooren, L. J., Schellekens, P. T. A., Tanke, H. J., Roos, M., and Vossen, J. M.,** T lymphocyte characteristics in bone marrow-transplanted patients. II. Analysis with monoclonal antibodies, *J. Immunol.,* 127, 244, 1981.

104. **Miller, R. A., Maloney, D. G., McKillop, J., and Levy, R.,** In vivo effects of murine hybridoma monoclonal antibody in a patient with T-cell leukemia, *Blood,* 58, 78, 1981.

105. **Ritz, J., Pesando, J. M., Sallan, S. E., Clavell, L. A., Notis-McConarty, J., Rosenthal, P., and Schlossman, S. F.,** Serotherapy of acute lymphoblastic leukemia with monoclonal antibody, *Blood,* 58, 141, 1981.

106. **Ritz, J., Pesando, J. M., Notis-McConarty, J., Lazarus, H., and Schlossman, S. F.,** A monoclonal antibody to human acute lymphoblastic leukemia antigen, *Nature (London),* 283, 583, 1980.

Chapter 5

APPLICATIONS OF HYBRIDOMA TECHNOLOGY TO AUTOIMMUNITY*

Joyce Rauch,** Robert S. Schwartz, and B. David Stollar

TABLE OF CONTENTS

I.   Introduction 92

II.   Spontaneously Occurring Monoclonal Autoantibodies 92

III.   Monoclonal Autoantibodies in Experimental Autoimmune Disease 95

IV.   Hybridoma Autoantibodies as Tools in the Identification and
       Characterization of the Relevant Antigens and Antibodies in
       Experimental Autoimmune Disease 96
       A.   Experimental Myasthenia Gravis 96
       B.   Experimental Models of Systemic Lupus Erythematosus 97
             1.   Antierythrocyte and Antithymocyte Antibodies 97
             2.   Antinucleic Acid Antibodies 98
             3.   Anti–Sm Antibodies 102
       C.   Experimentally Induced Antibodies Related to Graves' Disease ...104

V.   Idiotypic Analysis of Hybridoma Autoantibodies 104

VI.   Antiidiotypic Antibodies as Immunotherapeutic Agents 105

VIII. Conclusions 106

References 107

*Supported by NIH Grant AM27232.
**Joyce Rauch is a Fellow of the Medical Research Council of Canada.

develop SLE have been subjected to extensive analyses. Although there are common pathogenetic features among them, no common etiologic factor has been identified.[67] The murine lupus syndrome may therefore result from many different abnormalities that ultimately cause the B cell hyperactivity and the immune complex lesions that characterize the disease. Moreover, different abnormalities appear to cause the production of different autoantibodies, even within the same autoimmune strain. In the MRL/1 mouse, for instance, the anti–DNA response is related to polyclonal B cell activation, whereas anti–Sm antibody production does not correlate with B cell hyperactivity.[70] Thus, an examination of different classes of autoantibodies from the same animal will be necessary to define the specific immunological and genetic mechanisms that cause their production.

IV. HYBRIDOMA AUTOANTIBODIES AS TOOLS IN THE IDENTIFICATION AND CHARACTERIZATION OF THE RELEVANT ANTIGENS AND ANTIBODIES IN EXPERIMENTAL AUTOIMMUNE DISEASE

A. Experimental Myasthenia Gravis

Myasthenia gravis has been the focus of intense research over the past two decades. This disease results from an immune–mediated disruption of AChR in the postsynaptic membrane of striated muscle.[73] The myasthenic individual produces antibodies against several antigenic determinants on the surface of the AChR molecule. Some of these antibodies interact with complement, and thereby lyse the postsynaptic membrane, whereas others cross–link the receptors and thereby perturb the membrane. One of the enigmas of myasthenia gravis is the lack of correlation between the level of anti–AChR antibody in the serum and the clinical severity of the disease. Perhaps in the spectrum of antibodies only some are pathogenetic.

The electric organ of the torpedo eel, *Torpedo californica,* contains high concentrations of AChR suitable for purification. Animals immunized with *Torpedo* AChR develop experimental MG, a condition that mimics human myasthenia gravis. α–Bungarotoxin, a snake venom toxin, binds specifically and with high affinity, to the acetylcholine interaction site on the receptor molecule. It thus provides an excellent ligand for detecting and analyzing antibodies to AChR. Gomez et al.[74] prepared 11 stable cloned hybridoma cell lines that secrete antibodies against purified *Torpedo* AChR. These hybridomas were produced by fusing spleen cells from a rat that had been immunized with *Torpedo* AChR with a mouse myeloma cell line. The binding of six of these antibodies to AChR was inhibited by α–bungarotoxin.

Moshly–Rosen and colleagues[75] also studied monoclonal hybridoma antibodies against AChR. An immunochemical analysis of these antibodies was performed with the AChR used for immunization and with two AChR derivatives: a trypsin–digested fragment that retains the pharmacologic myasthenic activity of intact AChR, and a reduced and methylated derivative that lacks this activity. The results demonstrated that the mAbs bind to antigenic determinants that are exposed on membrane–bound AChR receptors. Moreover, some of the antibodies recognize antigenic determinants on the trypsinized receptor, but not the denatured receptor. Moshly–Rosen et al.[75] proposed that the myasthenic potential of the receptor molecule resides within a group of determinants that are present on trypsinized AChR, and that antibodies directed against these determinants may have pathological effects. By contrast, the antibodies that recognize determinants on the denatured receptor are probably not associated with myasthenic activity, and may even have preventive or therapeutic activity.

The pathogenicity of anti–AChR antibodies has been demonstrated in vivo by passive develop SLE have been subjected to extensive analyses. Although there are common pathogenetic features among them, no common etiologic factor has been identified.[67] The murine lupus syndrome may therefore result from many different abnormalities that ultimately cause the B cell hyperactivity and the immune complex lesions that characterize the disease. Moreover, different abnormalities appear to cause the production of different autoantibodies, even within the same autoimmune strain. In the MRL/1 mouse, for instance, the anti–DNA response is related to polyclonal B cell activation, whereas anti–Sm antibody production does not correlate with B cell hyperactivity.[70] Thus, an examination of different classes of autoantibodies from the same animal will be necessary to define the specific immunological and genetic mechanisms that cause their production.

IV. HYBRIDOMA AUTOANTIBODIES AS TOOLS IN THE IDENTIFICATION AND CHARACTERIZATION OF THE RELEVANT ANTIGENS AND ANTIBODIES IN EXPERIMENTAL AUTOIMMUNE DISEASE

A. Experimental Myasthenia Gravis

Myasthenia gravis has been the focus of intense research over the past two decades. This disease results from an immune–medicated disruption of AChR in the postsynaptic membrane of striated muscle.[73] The myasthenic individual produces antibodies against several antigenic determinants on the surface of the AChR molecule. Some of these antibodies interact with complement, and thereby lyse the postsynaptic membrane, whereas others cross–link the receptors and thereby perturb the membrane. One of the enigmas of myasthenia gravis is the lack of correlation between the level of anti–AChR antibody in the serum and the clinical severity of the disease. Perhaps in the spectrum of antibodies only some are pathogenetic.

The electric organ of the torpedo eel, *Torpedo californica*, contains high concentrations of AChR suitable for purification. Animals immunized with *Torpedo* AChR develop experimental MG, a condition that mimics human myasthenia gravis. α–Bungarotoxin, a snake venom toxin, binds specifically and with high affinity, to the acetylcholine interaction site on the receptor molecule. It thus provides an excellent ligand for detecting and analyzing antibodies to AChR. Gomez et al.[74] prepared 11 stable cloned hybridoma cell lines that secrete antibodies against purified *Torpedo* AChR. These hybridomas were produced by fusing spleen cells from a rat that had been immunized with *Torpedo* AChR with a mouse myeloma cell line. The binding of six of these antibodies to AChR was inhibited by α–bungarotoxin.

Moshly–Rosen and colleagues[75] also studied monoclonal hybridoma antibodies against AChR. An immunochemical analysis of these antibodies was performed with the AChR used for immunization and with two AChR derivatives: a trypsin–digested fragment that retains the pharmacologic myasthenic activity of intact AChR, and a reduced and methylated derivative that lacks this activity. The results demonstrated that the mAbs bind to antigenic determinants that are exposed on membrane–bound AChR receptors. Moreover, some of the antibodies recognize antigenic determinants on the trypsinized receptor, but not the denatured receptor. Moshly–Rosen et al.[75] proposed that the myasthenic potential of the receptor molecule resides within a group of determinants that are present on trypsinized AChR, and that antibodies directed against these determinants may have pathological effects. By contrast, the antibodies that recognize determinants on the denatured receptor are probably not associated with myasthenic activity, and may even have preventive or therapeutic activity.

The pathogenicity of anti–AChR antibodies has been demonstrated in vivo by passive share Id. An early example is that of monoclonal cold agglutinins,[56] which are divided into four distinct groups on the basis of cross-Id specificities. Moreover, cold agglutinins with anti–I specificity were found to have Id specificities distinct from those with anti–Pr specificity.[57] These observations found support in the demonstration that the amino acid sequences of the V regions of anti–I and anti–Pr antibodies differ.[58] By contrast, rabbit antisera against the H chains of two IgM monoclonal anti–I antibodies identified a V_H marker that is present on both anti–I and anti–i cold agglutinins.[59] Interestingly, this marker was also present on 8% (3/38) of myeloma and Waldenstrom macroglobulinemia proteins that lacked cold agglutinin activity. Cross-Id specificity also exists among monoclonal rheumatoid factors.[60,61] Two groups of these Id, termed Po and Wa, exist among monoclonal rheumatoid factors[62] and a third Id family defines the monoclonal rheumatoid factor that reacts with DNA–histone.[46] Po molecules from unrelated individuals have identical amino acid sequences in four of their six complementarity determining regions. By contrast, the idiotypic determinant of the Wa group seems related either to light chain framework structures or the J segments of these molecules.[63]

The presence of a shared V-region marker among Ig from different individuals suggests that the serologically defined structure has a genetic origin. Evidence in inbred mice[64] and in families of rabbits[65] supports this view. The study of a human family demonstrated cross–reactive Id on the rheumatoid factors of four of the patient's first–degree relatives, spanning three generations, irrespective of their HLA type.[66] Although the proband's rheumatoid factor was not monoclonal, the results suggest that the Id was inherited in this family.

In summary, studies of spontaneously occurring monoclonal autoantibodies have provided abundant precedents for investigations of hybridoma–produced autoantibodies. The ability of these proteins to define submolecular epitopes, and thus to bind structures that are shared by different antigens, is an important feature that we will see again with hybridoma autoantibodies. Finally, these earlier experiments showed the advantages of monoclonal autoantibodies in the analysis of Id and their potentialities for structural and genetic studies of autoantibodies.

III. MONOCLONAL AUTOANTIBODIES IN EXPERIMENTAL AUTOIMMUNE DISEASE

The heterogeneous mixtures of autoantibodies present in serum have been subjected to immunochemical and functional analyses,[67–72] and although these efforts have provided information on the nature of autoantibodies as a whole, technical limitations prevented an understanding of the molecular diversity of the autoantibody repertoire. Hybridoma technology, by contrast, affords the means to "pluck out" individual, spontaneously occurring autoantibodies from the autoimmune individual, to produce them in large quantitites, and to subject them to rigorous biochemical, immunochemical, and functional analyses.

Presently, each experimental system has similar objectives in the production of monoclonal autoantibodies. This is not to oversimplify the situation, nor to underestimate the importance of any individual study, but to suggest that common rationales and purposes unite this work. The most obvious use of monoclonal autoantibodies is to focus on specificity. This goal is important because the origins of autoimmune diseases will be known, not from studies of nonspecific phenomena, but from the application of techniques that reveal specific lesions.[1] Specificity is particularly relevant to studies of the systemic lupus erythematosus (SLE)–like diseases of mice. Several mouse strains (NZB, B/W, MRL/Mp-1pr (MRL/1), MRL/Mp-+/+ (MRL/++), and BXSB) that

Table 2
MONOCLONAL Ig WITH POLYSPECIFIC BINDING REACTIONS

Species	Specificities	Ref.
Human	IgG, DNP, DNA	47
Human	IgG,DNP	44, 45
Human	Nucleic acid, DNP	48
Human	IgG, cardiolipin	49
Human	IgG, DNA–histone	46
Human	DNA, DNP, heparin	50
Rabbit	Menadione, DNP	42
Rabbit	IgG, peptidoglycan	38
Mouse	Menadione, DNP	39, 40
Mouse	DNA, DNP	43

DNA to its native form. Hapten inhibition experiments indicated that purines, pyrimidines, and dinitrophenyl derivatives can inhibit DNA binding by these myeloma proteins over a wide range of concentrations.

These kinds of polyspecific reactions have also been observed with monoclonal human Ig. For instance, monoclonal rheumatoid factors that can also bind to DNP[44,45] and DNA–histone[46] have been found. One mAb reacts with three molecules: IgG, DNP, and DNA.[47] A human myeloma protein reacts similarly to the above–mentioned mouse myeloma proteins[43] in that it binds both to DNP and DNA,[48] and an IgMλ molecule that reacts with cardiolipin also binds to an acrylic plastic.[49] This latter activity was responsible for the antibody's false–positive rheumatoid factor activity, which was traced to the acrylic powder employed in the test. Cardiolipin and the plastic particle may share a chemical group that serves as a determinant for this molecule. One unusual monoclonal IgM binds to DNA, DNP, and heparin.[50]

Absorption and elution experiments with polyclonal antinuclear antibodies and rheumatoid factors have revealed that they, too, can have polyspecific serological activity. Certain antinuclear antibodies can react not only with cell nuclei, but also with surface membranes of human leukocytes.[51] Rheumatoid factor anti–IgG antibodies can also react with nucleosomes[52] or with cell nuclei.[53,54]

Michaelides and Eisen[39] referred to the multiple–binding reactions of monoclonal Ig as "strange". They seem strange, however, only because of expectations about specificity in antigen–antibody reactions. In order to understand these "strange" reactions the frame of reference must be shifted from the molecular to the submolecular. The demonstration that two apparently unrelated antigens, menadione and DNP, share a common submolecular structure serves as an example. Michaelides and Eisen[39] argued convincingly that this common structure can react with the combining region of a single antibody molecule. Their view coincides with that of Landsteiner,[55] who explained almost 50 years earlier that the action of antibodies extended to structures chemically similar to those of the homologous antigen. Later in this review further examples of this principle will be shown, as revealed by hybridoma–produced monoclonal autoantibodies. The discussion of these kinds of polyspecific autoantibodies, with particular emphasis on their medical implications will then be continued. Before leaving the subject of spontaneously produced mAbs, another of their attributes, cross–idiotypic specificity, will be dealt with briefly.

mAbs are ideal immunogens for the production of anti–Id sera because of the ease of purification of homogeneous Id. Soon after the unique serological determinants on antibody molecules were discovered, it was noted that Ig from different individuals can

Chapter 5

APPLICATIONS OF HYBRIDOMA TECHNOLOGY TO AUTOIMMUNITY*

Joyce Rauch, ** Robert S. Schwartz, and B. David Stollar**

TABLE OF CONTENTS

I.   Introduction 92

II.   Spontaneously Occurring Monoclonal Autoantibodies 92

III.   Monoclonal Autoantibodies in Experimental Autoimmune Disease 95

IV.   Hybridoma Autoantibodies as Tools in the Identification and
        Characterization of the Relevant Antigens and Antibodies in
        Experimental Autoimmune Disease 96
        A.   Experimental Myasthenia Gravis 96
        B.   Experimental Models of Systemic Lupus Erythematosus 97
                1.   Antierythrocyte and Antithymocyte Antibodies 97
                2.   Antinucleic Acid Antibodies 98
                3.   Anti–Sm Antibodies 102
        C.   Experimentally Induced Antibodies Related to Graves' Disease   ...104

V.   Idiotypic Analysis of Hybridoma Autoantibodies 104

VI.   Antiidiotypic Antibodies as Immunotherapeutic Agents 105

VIII.   Conclusions 106

References 107

*Supported by NIH Grant AM27232.
**Joyce Rauch is a Fellow of the Medical Research Council of Canada.

transfer of myasthenia gravis serum antibodies from human to mouse[76] and from rat to rat.[77] Lennon and Lambert[78] and Richman et al.[79] independently demonstrated that passive myasthenia gravis can also be produced by a monoclonal hybridoma antibody against AChR. Lennon and Lambert[78] found that two hybridoma antibodies bind to antigenic determinants that are remote from the binding site for cholinergic ligands. Nevertheless, they impaired neuromuscular transmission. It thus appears unnecessary for an anti–AChR antibody to inhibit the binding of neurotransmitter with the receptor site for an impairment of neuromuscular transmission. Richman et al.[79] had similar results. Two of their monoclonal anti–AChR antibodies, when injected i.v. into normal rats, induced an acute myasthenic syndrome. The binding of one of these antibodies to AChR was only partially blocked by α–bungarotoxin, and the binding of the other was actually increased by the venom. The failure of four other hybridoma anti–AChR antibodies to produce disease may have been due to their lack of cross–reactivity with mammalian AChR, or a requirement for binding to a specific portion of the AChR molecule. Another consideration in work of this type is the subclass of the antibody, and hence its effector function. Despite their preliminary nature, these results imply that a single antibody–producing clone may be sufficient to cause the lesions of myasthenia gravis.

Anti–AChR mAbs are useful probes of the molecular structure of the AChR *Torpedo* AChR consists of four subunits: α, β, γ, δ, in the ratio of 2:1:1:1. AChR from other species have a similar pattern. Tzartos and Lindstrom[80] have produced 17 cell lines that produce antibodies against *Torpedo* AChR and its subunits, as well as mAbs against muscle from electric eel and fetal calf. By analyzing these antibodies with whole receptor, separated subunits, the individual subunit fragments, Tzartos and Lindstrom could map the regions on the receptor to which particular antibodies bind. Their findings show that some of these antibodies are species–specific, but about half of them cross–react with receptors of other species. Many of the cross–reacting antibodies bind to the α-subunit that Lindstrom refers to as the Main Immunogenic Region. It is not the ACh binding site. There is evidence that this region is highly conserved between species. The use of hybridoma monoclonal anti–AChR antibodies to probe the fine structure of the AChR and, at the same time, to determine their pathogenicity could define precisely the mechanism that causes myasthenia gravis.

B. Experimental Models of Systemic Lupus Erythematosus

1. Antierythrocyte and Antithymocyte Antibodies

Thus far, antibodies that are induced by heterologous immunization, but which nevertheless function as autoantibodies have been discussed. Hybridomas that produce autoantibodies without prior immunization should now be considered. They are representative of spontaneously occurring autoantibodies. The first such autoantibodies were described by Bussard and Pages,[81,82] who fused peritoneal cells from unimmunized NZB mice with mouse plasmacytoma cells. Bussard[83] had previously shown that peritoneal cells from unstimulated NZB mice produce antibodies that react with bromelin–treated isologous erythrocytes. Similarly, the hybridomas also produce antibodies against bromelin–treated mouse red blood cell antibodies.[81] DeHeer, Pages, and Bussard[84] found that the IgM antierythrocyte autoantibodies produced by their hybridomas bind to the HB autoantigen, a cryptic erythrocyte autoantigen that is exposed by proteolysis with bromelin.[85,86] Autoantibodies against this antigen occur spontaneously in aging mice of all strains, including NZB mice, and they are probably of no pathogenetic significance. By contrast, autoantibodies directed against an exposed (i.e., bromelin–independent) erythrocyte antigen are unique to NZB mice and probably cause the hemolytic anemia of that strain.[86] DeHeer et al.[84] did not find hybridomas that secrete such autoantibodies, presumably because their screening procedure employed only bromelin–treated erythrocytes.

Klotz et al.[87] have recently described two IgG hybridoma antibodies that have serological reactivities that are characteristic of the NZB antierythrocyte autoantibody. The hybridoma antibodies react with antigen exposed on the surface of mouse erythrocytes and do not cross–react with erythrocytes of other species. Three thymocyte–specific hybridoma antibodies from NZB/NZW F_1 mice were also reported by this group. Two of these antibodies were IgA2a and the third was an IgM.

2. Antinucleic Acid Antibodies

Production of antibodies to nucleic acids (especially to DNA) is characteristic of SLE.[68] The mechanism responsible for their formation is unknown. They may result from immunization by nucleic acid antigens,[88–91] or they may arise spontaneously from clones of cells that are unique to autoimmune individuals. Alternatively, clones with a potential for the spontaneous secretion of autoantibodies may exist in all individuals, but the immunoregulatory mechanisms that control them may be absent or impaired in autoimmune individuals.[92] Hybridoma technology provides the means to test these proposals and to answer basic questions concerning the nature, heterogeneity, distribution, and regulation of clones of antibody–producing cells in SLE.

Eilat et al.[93] fused spleen cells from an unimmunized NZB/NZW F_1 mouse with MPC–11 myeloma cells. One of the hybrid clones they obtained produced an IgG_3 that binds ribosomal RNA with high affinity. This antibody does not bind significantly to DNA, tRNA, or synthetic single and double–stranded polynucleotides. In a later report, Eilat and co-workers[94] suggested that this hybridoma autoantibody recognizes a trinucleotide sequence of single–stranded RNA that consists of guanine, cytosine, and uracil residues. Preliminary experiments with pooled sera from NZB/NZW F_1 mice showed antigen–binding patterns similar to those of the mAb. The monoclonal autoantibody may therefore be representative of other RNA–binding autoantibodies of NZB/NZW F_1 mice.

The production of hybridomas that secrete anti–DNA antibodies was first described by Andrzejewski et al.[95] The clones were derived from the fusion of spleen cells from unimmunized MRL/1 mice with the MPC–11 or SP2/O–Ag–14 plasmacytoma cell lines. The antigenic specificities of four anti–DNA hybridoma antibodies were studied by a competitive RIA using native (double–stranded) DNA, denatured (single–stranded) DNA, a mixture of oligonucleotides from a DNA digest, and a mixture of four mononucleotides. These experiments showed that each autoantibody has a distinct specificity.

Andrzejewski and coworkers[96] continued this work with tests of many nucleic acid antigens and synthetic polynucleotides for their ability to inhibit the binding of monoclonal autoantibodies to single–stranded DNA. Each antibody was found to have a unique antigen–binding profile, and in all cases there was binding to several different nucleic acid antigens (Figure 1). The most reasonable explanation for the apparent multiplicity of the binding reactions is the presence of cross–reacting epitopes among the various ligands. One implication of these findings is that the heterogeneity among anti–DNA antibodies in SLE may reflect diversity, not only among autoreactive clones, but also among the serological reactions of individual antibodies.

The antigen–binding analyses of Andrzejewski et al.[96] demonstrated that some of the hybridoma autoantibodies have marked specificity for nucleic acid bases. Others, by contrast, react with several different polynucleotides and therefore recognize a common structure in these molecules, such as the sugar–phosphate backbone. The sugar–phosphate backbone of nucleic acids consists of phosphate groups in phosphodiester–linkage separated by three carbon atoms of adjacent sugar molecules. Other biological molecules

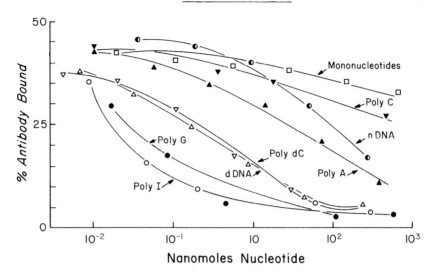

FIGURE 1. Solid–phase competitive RIA of hybridoma H104, selected originally as an anti–DNA antibody.

also contain phosphodiester–linked phosphate groups that are separated by three carbon atoms. These molecules include phospholipids, with cardiolipin (diphosphatidyl glycerol) as a typical example (Figure 2). The resemblance between the two different classes of molecules in this regard provided the rationale for a test of the ability of phospholipids to inhibit the binding of anti–DNA mAbs to DNA.[97] Some, but not all, of the antibodies reacted strongly with several phospholipids, and in a few cases the phospholipids were stronger competitors than DNA itself (Figure 3).

These results prompted additional experiments. It was found that cardiolipin can inhibit the antinuclear antibody reaction of a monoclonal anti–DNA autoantibody, that an anti–DNA antibody can prolong the activated partial thromboplastin test in a manner characteristic of a lupus anticoagulant (presumably by binding to the phospholipid that the test requires), and that phospholipids, as well as polynucleotides, specifically inhibit idiotype–anti–idiotype reactions of anti–DNA antibodies[97] (Figure 4). These diverse reactions of a monoclonal Ig indicate the ability of the autoantibody to bind to structures that contain phosphate esters (Figure 5). They recall the previously discussed polyspecific serological reactions of spontaneous monoclonal autoantibodies, and of induced mAbs. The results suggest that the identification of certain lupus autoantibodies as anti–DNA antibodies may indicate the fortuitous choice of DNA as the test antigen. They imply, moreover, that some of the diversity of autoantibody reactions in SLE may result from the presence of a relatively simple antigenic structure in a variety of biological molecules. Finally, the presence of readily detectable cardiolipin–binding antibodies in the sera of MRL/1 mice[123] suggests that such polyspecific antibodies may constitute an important fraction of the autoantibody population in these animals.

Hahn et al.[98] have used hybridomas to study a different aspect of anti–DNA antibodies. They produced hybridoma anti–DNA antibodies by the fusion of spleen cells from NZB/NZW F$_1$ mice, MRL/1, and BSXB mice with mouse myeloma cells. The isoelectric points of 10 of these hybridoma antibodies range from pH 5 to 9. Two of the antibodies have antigen inhibition patterns similar to those of serum anti–DNA an-

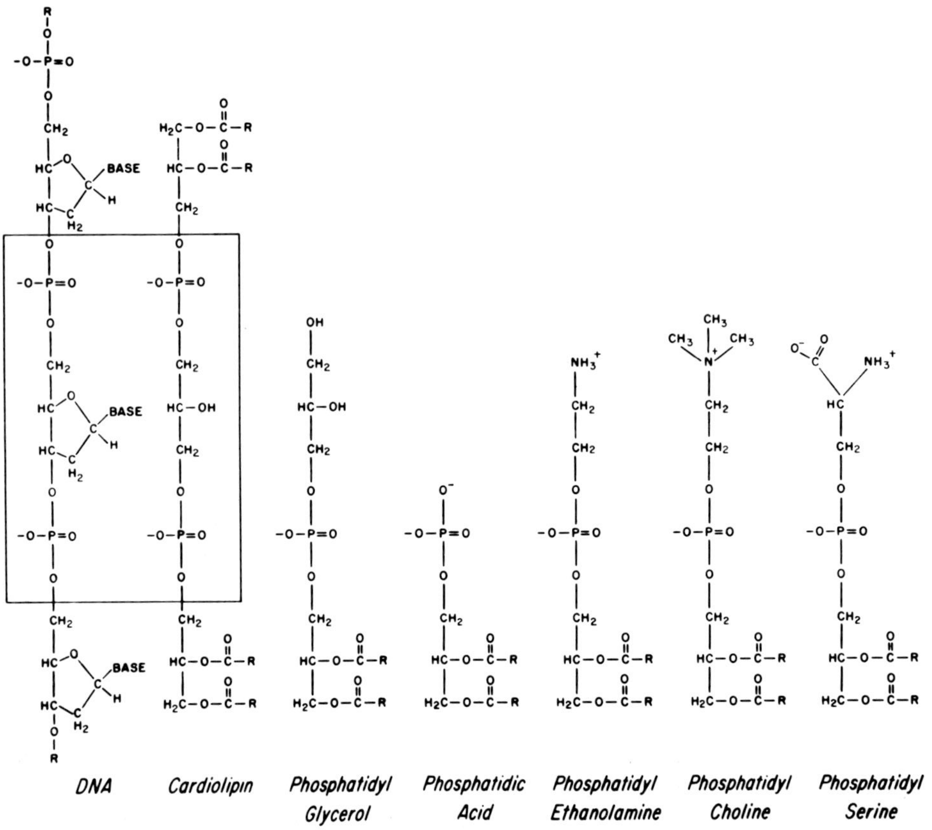

FIGURE 2. Chemical formulas of DNA and phospholipids. (From Lafer, E. M., Rauch, J., Andrzejewski, C., Jr., Mudd, D., Furie, B., Schwartz, R. S., and Stollar, B. D., *J. Exp. Med.*, 153, 897, 1981. With permission.

tibodies. These two antibodies are inhibited by both native and single–stranded DNA, but not by single–stranded RNA or poly(I)·poly(C). Ebling and Hahn[99] showed that sera from autoimmune mice contain IgG anti-native DNA antibodies with pI values ranging from pH 5.5 to 9.0, and that antibodies with high pIs (8.0 to 8.5) are more frequent than those with low pIs. Glomerular eluates of MRL/1 and NZB/NZW F_1 mice contain a restricted number of DNA–binding bands, all of which focus at pH 8.0 to 9.0. This result suggests that anti–DNA antibodies with isoelectric points of pH 8 to 9 may be more nephritogenic than other subpopulations. Thus, an analysis of hybridoma anti–DNA antibodies with similar DNA–binding characteristics, but with different isoelectric points, may reveal the relative pathogenicity of different subpopulations of auto-antibodies.

Tron and colleagues[100] have isolated 25 anti–DNA–secreting clones from fusions between spleen cells from NZB/NZW F_1 mice and mouse plasmacytoma cells. One of these antibodies was analyzed by a competitive RIA. It binds strongly to both native and single–stranded DNA. Reactivity with native DNA also occurs in the *Crithidia luciliae* assay. This type of reactivity to both native and denatured DNA has been demonstrated in many SLE sera.

Marion and Briles[101] also obtained hybridomas from spleen cells of NZB/NZW F_1 mice. They found that the number of hybridomas obtained from each fusion paralleled serum anti–DNA titers. As expected, older mice, with the highest serum anti–DNA

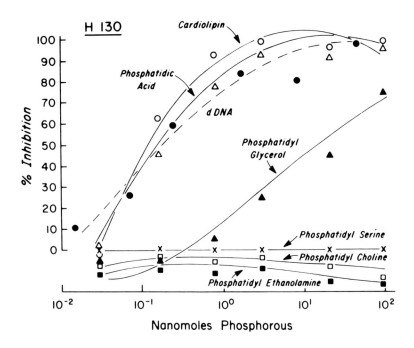

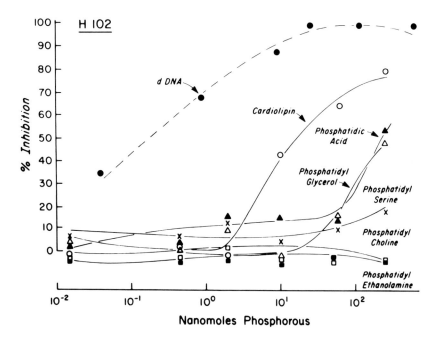

FIGURE 3A. Solid-phase competitive RIA of two mAbs, H130 and H102, selected originally on the basis of their binding to DNA. (From Lafer, E. M., Rauch, J., Andrzejewski, C., Jr., Mudd, D., Furie, B., Schwartz, R. S., and Stollar, B. D., *J. Exp. Med.*, 153, 897, 1981. With permission.)

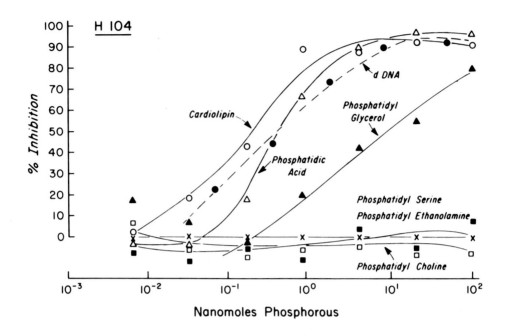

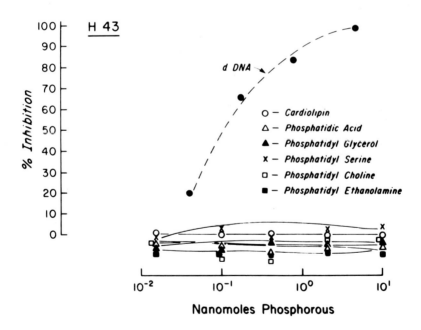

FIGURE 3B. Solid-phase competitive RIA of two mAbs, H104 and H43, selected originally on the basis of their binding to DNA. (From Lafer, E. M., Rauch, J., Andrzejewski, C., Jr., Mudd, D., Furie, B., Schwartz, R. S., and Stollar, B. D., *J. Exp. Med.*, 153, 007, 1981. With permission.)

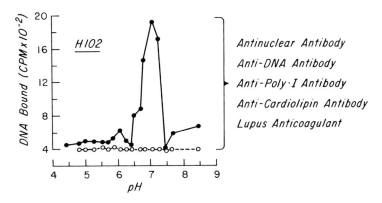

*Multiple Serological Manifestations
of a Monoclonal Lupus Autoantibody*

FIGURE 4. Polyspecific activities of a lupus autoantibody. The isolectric focusing patterns of the antibody are typical of a monoclonal Ig. ●-----● DNA–binding of eluates from the focusing gel; o–o–o, DNA–binding of the same eluates after incubation with cardiolipin.

titers, gave the greatest number of anti–DNA hybridomas. There was also a direct correlation in a given mouse, between the isotype distribution of serum anti–DNA antibodies and the isotype representation of hybridoma anti–DNA antibodies. As a group, the hybridoma antibodies were heterogeneous, both by isoelectric focusing and with regard to specificity for native and single–stranded DNA and Poly(I)·poly(C). These results are simlar to those obtained by other groups mentioned earlier.

Pisetsky et al.[124] analyzed the binding specificity of an anti–DNA antibody secreted by an MRL/l–derived hybridoma and found a preference for denatured DNA, but binding to native DNA also occurred. This antibody reacted with ribohomopolymers and deoxyribohomopolymers, but its ability to bind these ligands was influenced by their base composition. Poly(dT) produced the strongest inhibition of all the homopolymers tested, and the antibody bound maximally to a polynucleotide of >18 nucleotides. The authors believe that a bivalent mode of interaction stabilizes this antibody, or that both of its combining sites must occupy epitopes on the same DNA molecule.

3. Anti–Sm Antibodies

Antibodies to the Sm antigen are present in about 2/3 of SLE patients,[102] and they are highly specific for this disease.[103,104] They are also produced by MRL/l and MRL/ ++ mice.[72] Lerner and colleagues[105] have constructed MRL/l–derived hybridomas that produce monoclonal autoantibodies that are specific for either Sm, DNA, or RNA. These antibodies were examined by immunoprecipitation, PAGE, and immunofluorescence techniques. The anti–Sm antibody gave an immunoprecipitation pattern that is identical with that of a human anti–Sm antibody. They also demonstrated that on all five of the small RNAs that are immunoprecipitated by anti–Sm sera are also precipitated by the monoclonal anti–Sm antibody. Immunofluorescence patterns with mouse monoclonal anti–Sm and human serum anti–Sm antibodies were also identical. The anti–Sm mAb has been used to establish a quantitative RIA for anti–Sm antibody, which could replace the less sensitive and less accurate techniques in current use. Although anti–Sm antibodies seem limited to SLE, their levels in serum do not correlate with clinical activity. Lerner et al.[105] suggest that inadequacies of the currently available assays account for the lack of sensitivity that such a correlation requires.

C. Experimentally Induced Antibodies Related to Graves' Disease

A hybridoma that produces an antibody of quite a different nature than those discussed thus far was described by Yavin et al.[106] They fused spleen cells from mice that had been immunized with solubilized preparations of thyrotropin receptor. mAbs that bind to thyroid membranes were produced. Thyrotropin (TSH) specifically inhibits the binding of these antibodies, a result that indicates that they are antireceptor antibodies. They do not, however, stimulate adenylate cyclase activity in thyroid cells. By contrast, autoantibodies that both inhibit TSH binding and stimulate adenylate cyclase activity seem implicated in the pathogenesis of Graves' disease.[107,108] Recent studies indicate that the TSH receptor consists of two components: a glycoprotein and a ganglioside.[109,110] The mAbs described by Yavin and coworkers[106] bind to the glycoprotein portion of the receptor, and thus identify its TSH–binding component. The inability of these antibodies to stimulate adenylate cyclase activity is consistent with the hypothesis that interaction with the glycoprotein component alone is insufficient to transmit the TSH "message" to the cyclase system. Thus, the TSH receptor may require both the ganglioside and the glycoprotein for complete expression of its function.

V. IDIOTYPIC ANALYSIS OF HYBRIDOMA AUTOANTIBODIES

A second line of research with monoclonal autoantibodies involves analysis of their Id cross–reactivities. An accounting of the specificity of autoantibodies requires not only definitions of their ligand–binding specificities, but also estimates of their Id diversity. Cross–reacting idiotypes shared by autoantibodies would suggest the existence of related clones, or families of antibodies. Precedents for the presence of cross–reacting Id in spontaneously produced monoclonal autoantibodies have been discussed above. In the murine model of MG, Schwartz et al.[111] demonstrated cross–reactive Id on experimentally induced antibodies to the AChR. These cross–reactivities were also found with induced anti–AChR antibodies from various mouse strains, as well as from rats, rabbits, and monkeys.

Nisonoff and Lamoyi[112] have argued that this type of extensive cross–reactivity could signal that the anti–Id antibodies share an epitope with the original antigen (in the case of Schwartz et al.,[111] the original antigen would be AcChR and the anti–Id antibody would share a determinant with AcChR). They point out that such cross–reactions could be misinterpreted as having genetic implications, whereas they actually represent binding of serum antibody to a structure that resembles the original antigen. Their fascinating article should be read by all concerned with this field.

Id analysis of hybridoma monoclonal autoantibodies is still in its early stages and most of this work is ongoing and hitherto unpublished. In the Tufts laboratory, Andrzejewski and coworkers[96] produced anti–Id antibodies in rabbits against several anti–DNA hybridoma antibodies. These anti–Id antibodies were defined by their ability to inhibit the binding of the homologous anti–DNA antibody to DNA. Quantitative RIAs were established for each Id–anti–Id pair and they were used both to seek cross–reactive Id and to measure serum levels of Id. Id–anti–Id interactions were antiinhibitible, with the same order of antigen preference as in competitive DNA binding assays.[96] These analyses were done with two hybridomas, H102 and H43. Three of six hybridoma anti–DNA antibodies shared idiotypy to varying degrees with H102. The other idiotype, H43, was detected on only one of the six hybridoma autoantibodies. A third Id, currently under investigation, appears to share determinants with many other hybridoma autoantibodies.[123]

Despite their preliminary nature, these studies lead to some conclusions. The Id cross–reactions appear to stem from similarities in the antigen–binding regions of the

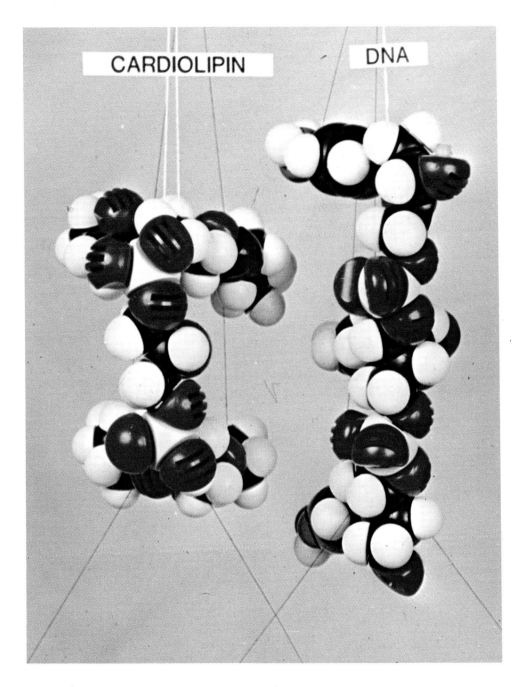

FIGURE 5. CPK space-filling atomic models of the polar region of cardiolipin (left) and a portion of a single strand of DNA backbone (right). A common surface feature, which is the probable basis for serological cross-reactivity, is a similar spacing between phosphate groups in the two structures. In cardiolipin (diaphosphatidyl glycerol) two phosphates are separated by the three carbon atoms of the central glycerol to which they are linked as phosphoesters. In DNA, the phosphates are separated by three carbon atoms of deoxyribose, and also occur in phosphoester linkage. This surface of cardiolipin projects from membranes or micelles and is repeated in many adjacent molecules on any one such structure. Micelles of phosphatidic acid, in which there is only one phosphate group per glycerol, show a weaker cross-reaction with the hybridoma antibodies that react with cardiolipin. The phosphatidic acid micelles would also present an array of repeating phosphate groups exposed to aqueous solvent. The backbone of DNA is a surface feature as well, and is accessible to antibody. The precise spacing of phosphate groups required for reaction with antibackbone antibodies may occur either on single strands in denatured DNA or in native DNA.

autoantibodies because anti–Id blocks the binding of the hybridoma antibodies to DNA. Furthermore, antigen (i.e., DNA and other polynucleotides) inhibits the Id–anti–Id interactions. Although each autoantibody tested has unique antigen–binding specificities, anti–Id antibodies can, in some cases, detect common determinants in their binding sites. Moreover, cross–reactive Id occur not only in hybridoma anti–DNA antibodies that are produced by clones derived from the same MRL/1 mouse, but also in antibodies produced by clones derived from different MRL/1 mice. This finding suggests that such cross–reactive Id may derive from families of germ line genes (see the cautionary note above). The Id cross–reactions, together with the multiple antigenic reactivities of individual hybridoma anti–DNA antibodies[96,97] discussed earlier, indicate that the repertoire of autoantibody–producing clones in SLE may be smaller than previously envisioned.

VI. ANTIIDIOTYPIC ANTIBODIES AS IMMUNOTHERAPEUTIC AGENTS

There are many important and exciting implications if there is Id restriction (or if there are predominant Id) in autoimmune diseases. Jerne[113] proposed that anti–Id reactions are powerful regulators of immune responses. According to this theory, the mechanism of specific immunoregulation consists of a system of Id in which each Id corresponds to a complementary anti–Id. The finding that T and B cells possess functionally active Id structures on their surfaces[114] fulfilled an important expectation of this theory. The presence of Id structures on suppressor T cells[114] provides an obvious mechanism for the specific down–regulation of Ir. Anti–Id antibodies are capable of suppressing,[115,116] or under certain conditions, initiating, antibody responses.[114] Wigzell et al.[117] have proposed that anti–Id reactions may be useful in the control of autoimmune disease. The feasibility of such treatment has however been questioned because of the apparent heterogeneity of autoantibodies. The recent evidence that some autoantibodies may be unexpectedly restricted, and the demonstration of Id cross–reactivities among hybridoma monoclonal autoantibodies, argue the practicability of anti–Id control of autoimmunity.

A recent review article[118] briefly summarized one such attempt. Anti–Id antibodies were raised in rats against three anti–AChr mAbs. Each was shown to cross-react with the other hybridoma antibodies. The anti–Id antibodies inhibited only a proportion of the serum anti–AChR antibodies in experimental autoimmune myasthenia gravis, and notwithstanding their production of anti–Id antibodies, the rats developed electrophysiological evidence of experimental myasthenia gravis when immunized with AChR. Nevertheless, a significant reduction of anti–AChR antibody was observed. This encouraging result suggests that an even greater decrease in antibody production might occur after treatment with a pool of anti–Id antibodies.

A more recent experiment by Zanetti and Bigazzi[119] concerns the in vivo effects of heterologous anti–Id antibodies on autoimmune thyroiditis. Repeated injections of anti–Id antibodies into sublethally X–irradiated Buffalo rats that spontaneously develop antoimmune thyroiditis, resulted in a significant diminution in the levels of serum autoantibodies to rat thyroglobulin and a concomitant decrease in Id–bearing cells in their spleens. This experiment did not use hybridoma monoclonal autoantibodies, but affinity–purified serum antibodies. Nevertheless, it is pertinent to the feasibility of anti–Id immunotherapy in established autoimmune disease. Inhibitory or suppressive effects of anti–Id antibodies have been observed in systems in which anti–Id treatment starts before or at the time of immunization.[114,115] In spontaneously occurring autoimmune diseases, however, autosensitization occurs long before any treatment can begin. Zanetti and Bigazzi[119] attempted to solve this problem by sublethal X–irradiation of the animal before administration of anti–Id antibodies. This type of nonspecific immunosuppression, combined with the use of selective and specific anti–Id reagents, may hold promise for the future of immunotherapeutic regulation of autoimmune disease.

VII. CONCLUSIONS

In a short time, studies of monoclonal autoantibodies have helped to sharpen the focus of fundamental questions about autoimmunity. Two major assumptions that underlie the studies of hybridoma–derived antibodies are that the mAbs obtained, and thus the clones being tested, are representative of the actual in vivo clonal populations, and that the specificities of monoclonal autoantibodies depend only on the gene products of the spleen cells used in fusion, and not on new combinations of chains from spleen cell and myeloma cell fusion partners. To help ensure the latter condition, fusions are now done when possible with myeloma cell lines that do not synthesize or secrete Ig chains. When Ig–secreting myeloma cells are used, it may be necessary to purify the relevant subpopulation of hybridoma products. Eilat and Laskov[120] have described such a procedure that required preparation of Fab fragments and affinity chromatography on an antigen-Sepharose column to remove all combinations with myeloma chains. An important recent development for the application of hybridoma technology to human disease is the availability of human myeloma cell lines for fusion.[121,122] Those available do secrete Ig, so the recombination of parental chains must still be considered until nonsynthesizing cell lines are developed. To test the other assumption, that hybridoma products are representative of in vivo autoantibody production, analyses of complex antibody populations in autoimmune sera will still have to be done parallel with analyses of mAbs. The information gained from the latter will guide a rational approach to studies of the serum populations.

One of the long–standing questions in autoimmunity, reemphasized by studies of monoclonal autoantibodies, has concerned the nature of the immunizing stimulus in these conditions. As noted earlier in this review, even though autoreactivity can be detected with a particular antigen, it is possible that this is a fortuitous result and the selected test reagent is in fact a cross–reacting antigen. The spontaneous occurrence of monoclonal Ig that combine with such apparently diverse structures as IgG and nucleosome subunits of chromatin serves as a reminder of this ambiguity. So does the finding that a single hybridoma product derived from an MRL/1 lupus mouse can react with denatured DNA, polyriboinosinate, cardiolipin, and a phospholipid involved in the thromboplastin generation assay. One might consider the latter Ig to be an anti–DNA antibody, but we cannot be certain that DNA stimulated its production. The question that may be asked is whether it will be possible, even by extensive analysis, to identify a unique immunogen for autoreactivity. One approach will be to immunize normal animals with suspected autoimmunogens and to determine whether mAbs from these animals show the same spectrum of cross–reactions as those derived from animals with spontaneous autoimmunity. It may turn out to be a general feature of monoclonal products that each antibody recognizes a restricted structure that recurs in many different molecules of apparently diverse nature and that likely immunogens can be identified even if some individual clonal products react strongly with several serologically tested antigens.

Experiments with autoimmune–derived hybridomas are also helping to focus questions concerning the genetic background of autoimmune disease. It has been known for some time that normal individuals have B cells capable of producing autoreactive Ig, and thus contain genes for autoreactive Ig. Are they, in fact, the clones that are expanded in autoimmune disease? Examination of these and other related questions are just beginning. The use of hybridomas to generate Id–anti–Id reagents and gene probes will provide powerful reagents for seeking the answers.

REFERENCES

1. **Miller, K. and Schwartz, R. S.,** Suppressor cells in autoimmune diseases, *Adv. Int. Med.,* 27, 281, 1982.
2. **Kritzman, J., Kunkel, H. G., McCarthy, J. et al.,** Studies of a Waldenstrom–type macroglobulin with rheumatoid factor properties, *J. Lab. Clin. Med.,* 57, 905, 1961.
3. **Drussin, L. M., Litwin, S. D., Armstrong, M. et al.,** Waldenstrom's macroglobulinemia in a patient with a chronic biologic false–positive serologic test for syphilis, *Am. J. Med.,* 56, 429, 1974.
4. **Christenson, W. N. and Dacie, J. V.,** Serum proteins in acquired haemolytic anemia (auto–antibody type), *Br. J. Haematol.,* 3, 153, 1957.
5. **Dellagi, K., Brouet, J.–C., Schenmetzler, C. et al.,** Chronic hemolytic anemia due to a monoclonal IgG cold agglutinin with anti–Pr specificity, *Blood,* 57, 189, 1981.
6. **Latov, N., Sherman, W. H., Nemni, R. et al.,** Plasma–cell dyscrasia and peripheral neuropathy with a monoclonal antibody to peripheral–nerve myelin, *N. Engl. J. Med.,* 303, 618, 1980.
7. **Bonomo, L., Dammacco, F., Tursi, A. et al.,** Waldenstrom's macroglobulinemia with anti-IgG activity: a series of five cases, *Clin. Exp. Immunol.,* 6, 531, 1970.
8. **Grey, H. M., Kohler, P. F., Terry, W. D. et al.,** Human monoclonal G–cryoglobulins with anti–γ–globulin activity, *J. Clin. Invest.,* 47, 1875, 1968.
9. **Heimer, P. and Nosenzo, C. J.,** Pseudoglobulin rheumatoid factors, *J. Immunol.,* 94, 502, 1965.
10. **Curtain, C. C., Baumgarten, A. and Pye, J.,** Coprecipitation of some cryomacroglobulins with immunoglobulins and their fragments, *Arch. Biochem.,* 112, 37, 1965.
11. **Brouet, J.-C., Clauvel, J.-P., Danon, F. et al.,** Biologic and clinical significance of cryoglobulins, *Am. J. Med.,* 57, 775, 1974.
12. **Gorevic, P. C., Kassab, H., Levo, Y. et al.,** Mixed cryoglobulinemia: clinical aspects and long-term follow-up of 40 patients, *Am. J. Med.,* 69, 287, 1980.
13. **Zinneman, H. H., Levi, D., and Seal, U. S.,** On the nature of cryoglobulins, *J. Immunol.,* 100, 594, 1968.
14. **Kosaka, M. and Solomon, A.,** Hyperviscosity syndrome associated with an idiopathic monoclonal IgA-rheumatoid factor, *Am. J. Med.,* 69, 145, 1980.
15. **Taylor, H. and Abraham, G. N.,** Characterization of a monoclonal IgA rheumatoid factor. II. Evidence for reactivity with a specific IgG Fc fragment determinant, *Clin. Exp. Immunol.,* 13, 529, 1973.
16. **Stone, M. J. and Metzger, H.,** Binding properties of a Waldenstrom's macroglobulin antibody, *J. Biol. Chem.,* 243, 5977, 1968.
17. **Harboe, M., Van Furth, R., Schubothe, H. et al.,** Exclusive occurrence of K chains in isolated cold haemagglutinins, *Scand. J. Haematol.,* 2, 259, 1965.
18. **Macris, N. T., Capra, J. D., Frankel, G. J. et al.,** A lambda light chain cold agglutinin-cryomacroglobulin occurring in Waldenstrom's macroglobulinemia, *Am. J. Med.,* 48, 524, 1970.
19. **Feizi, T.,** Lambda chains in cold agglutinins, *Science,* 156, 1111, 1967.
20. **Roelcke, D., Pruzanski, W., Ebert, W. et al.,** A new monoclonal cold agglutinin Sa recognizing terminal *N*-acetyl neuraminyl groups on the cell surface, *Blood,* 55, 677, 1980.
21. **Hakamori, S.,** Blood group ABH and Ii antigens of human erythrocytes: chemistry, polymorphism, and their developmental change, *Semin. Hematol.,* 17, 39, 1981.
22. **Fudenberg, H. H. and Kunkel, H. G.,** Physical properties of red cell agglutinins in acquired hemolytic anemia, *J. Exp. Med.,* 106, 689, 1957.
23. **Harboe, M. and Torsok, H.,** Protein abnormalities in the cold haemagglutination syndrome, *Scand. J. Haematol.,* 6, 416, 1969.
24. **Killander, A., Killander, J., Phillipson, L. et al.,** A monoclonal gammamacroglobulin complexing with lecithin, in *Nobel Symposium 3: Gamma Globulins,* Killander, J., Ed., Interscience, New York, 1967, 359.
25. **Gisler, R. and Pillot, J.,** Activite anticardiolipide liée a un complexe macroglobuline de Waldenstrom-IgG cryoprécipitant, *Immunochemistry,* 5, 543, 1968.
26. **Cooper, M. R., Cohen, H. J., Huntley, C. C. et al.,** A monoclonal IgM with antibody-like specificity for phospholipids in a patient with lymphoma, *Blood,* 43, 493, 1974.
27. **Risen, W., Rudikoff, S., Oriol, R. et al.,** An IgM Waldenstrom with specificity against phosphoryl-choline, *Biochemistry,* 14, 1052, 1975.
28. **Thiagarajan, P., Shapiro, S. S., and DeMarco, L.,** Monoclonal immunoglobulin Mλ coagulation inhibitor with phospholipid specificity, *J. Clin. Invest.,* 66, 397, 1980.
29. **Intrator, L., Andre, C., Chenal, C. et al.,** A monoclonal macroglobulin with antinuclear activity, *J. Clin. Pathol.,* 32, 450, 1979.
30. **Lindstrom, F. D., Hed, J., and Enestrom, S.,** Renal pathology of Waldenstrom's macroglobulinemia with monoclonal antiglomerular antibodies and nephrotic syndrome, *Clin. Exp. Immunol.,* 41, 196, 1980.

31. **Toh, B. H., Ceredig, R., Cornell, F. N. et al.,** Multiple myeloma and monoclonal IgA with anti-actin reactivity, *Clin. Exp. Immunol.,* 30, 379, 1977.

32. **Micouin, C., Rivat, C., Bensa, J. C. et al.,** A human immunoglobulin in a myeloma protein with anti-gastric parietal cell autoantigen activity, *Clin. Exp. Immunol.,* 27, 78, 1977.

33. **Hauptman, S. and Tomasi, T. B., Jr.,** A monoclonal IgM protein with antibody-like activity for human albumin, *J. Clin. Invest.,* 53, 932, 1973.

34. **Wager, O., Rasanen, J. A., Haltia, K. et al.,** M components with antibody activity. Anti-smooth muscle, anti-thyroglobulin and anti-streptolysin-O activity in fine M component sera, *Ann. Clin. Res.,* 3, 86, 1971.

35. **Florin-Christensen, A., Roux, M. E. B., and Arana, R. M.,** Cryoglobulins in acute and chronic liver diseases, *Clin. Exp. Immunol.* 16, 599, 1974.

36. **Cream, J. J.,** Peripheral vascular disease and annular erythema with selective IgA deficiency and mixed cryoglobulinemia, *Br. J. Dermatol.,* 85, 546, 1971.

37. **Miyagawa, S. and Sakamoto, K.,** Characterization of cryoprecipitates in pemphigus. Demonstration of pemphigus antibody using the IF technic, *J. Invest. Dermatol.,* 69, 673, 1977.

38. **Bokich, V. A., Chiao, J. W., Bernstein, D. et al.,** Homogeneous rabbit 7S anti–IgG with antibody specificity for peptidogylcan, *J. Exp. Med.,* 138, 1184, 1973.

39. **Michaelides, M. C. and Eisen, H. N.,** The strange cross–reaction of memadione (vitamin K_3) and 2,4 dinithophenyl ligands with a myeloma protein and some conventional antibodies, *J. Exp. Med.,* 140, 687, 1974.

40. **Rosenstein, R. W., Musson, R. A., Armstron, M. et al.,** Contact regions for dinithrophenyl and menodione haptens in an immunoglobulin binding more than 1 antigen, *Proc. Natl. Acad. Sci. U.S.A.,* 69, 877, 1972.

41. **Richards, F. F., Konigsberg, R. W., Rosenstein, R. W. et al.,** On the specificity of antibodies. Biochemical and biophysical evidence indicates the existence of polyfunctional antibody combining regions, *Science,* 187, 130, 1975.

42. **Johnston, M. F. M. and Eisen, H. N.,** Cross–reactions between 2, 4–dintrophenyl and menadione (vitamin K_3) and the general problem of antibody specificity, *J. Immunol.,* 117, 1189, 1976.

43. **Schubert, D., Jobe, A., and Cohn, M.,** Mouse myelomas producing precipitating antibody to nucleic acid bases and/or nitrophenyl derivatives. *Nature (London),* 220, 882, 1962.

44. **Hannestad, K.,** Monoclonal and polyclonal M rheumatoid factors with anti–di and anti–trinitrophenyl activity, *Clin. Exp. Immunol.,* 4, 55, 1969.

45. **Warner, N. L., Mackenzie, M. R., and Fudenberg, H. H.,** Anti–antibody activity of a monoclonal macroglobulin, *Proc. Natl. Acad. Sci. U.S.A.,* 68, 2846, 1971.

46. **Agnello, V., Arbetter, A., de Kasep, G. A., Powell, R., Tan, E. M., and Joslin, F.,** Evidence for a subset of rheumatoid factors that cross–react with DNA–histone and have a distinct cross–idiotype, *J. Exp. Med.,* 151, 1514, 1980.

47. **Hannestad, K.,** M rheumatoid factors reacting with nitrophenyl groups and denatured deoxyribo-nucleic acids, *Ann. N.Y. Acad. Sci.,* 168, 63, 169.

48. **Reisen, W. and Morell, A.,** A human myeloma protein with specificity against dinitrophenyl and nucleic acid derivatives, *Immunochemistry,* 9, 979, 1972.

49. **Merlini, G., Forsgren, A., Turesson, I., et al.,** An IgM monoclonal protein with multiple scrol ogical specificities, *Clin. Exp. Immunol.,* 37, 276, 1979.

50. **Tolleshaug, H. and Hannestad, K.,** Binding of ligands to a monoclonal IgM macroglobulin with multiple specificity, *Immunochemistry,* 12, 173, 1975.

51. **Rekvig, O. P. and Hannestad, K.,** Certain polyclonal antinuclear antibodies cross–react with the surface membrane of human lymphocytes and granulocytes, *Scand. J. Immunol.,* 6, 1041, 1977.

52. **Hannestad, K. and Stollar, B. D.,** Certain rheumatoid factors react with nucleosomes, *Nature (London),* 275, 671, 1978.

53. **Hannestad, K.,** Certain rheumatoid factors react with both IgG and an antigen associated with cell nuclei, *Scand. J. Immunol.,* 7, 127, 1978.

54. **Johnson, P. M.,** IgM–rheumatoid factors cross reactive with IgG and a cell nuclear antigen: apparent ''masking'' in original serum, *Scand. J. Immunol.,* 9, 461, 1979.

55. **Landsteiner, K.,** *The Specificity of Serological Reactions,* Dover Publications, New York, 1936, 54.

56. **Williams, R. C., Kunkel, H. G., and Capra, J. D.,** Cross idiotypic with C.A., *Science,* 161, 379, 1968.

57. **Feizi, T., Kunkel, H. G., and Roelke, D.,** Cross idiotypic specificity among cold agglutinins in relation to combining activity for blood group related antigens, *Clin. Exp. Immunol.,* 18, 283, 1974.

58. **Riesen, W. F., Majaniemi, I., Huser, H. et al.,** Variable region subgroups and specificity of cold agglutinins, *Scand. J. Immunol.,* 8, 145, 1978.

59. **Feizi, T., Lecomte, J., and Childs, R.,** An immunoglobulin heavy chain variable region (V_H) marker associated with cross–reactive idiotypes in man, *Clin. Exp. Immunol.*, 30, 233, 1977.
60. **Kunkel, H. G., Angello, V., Joslin, F. et al.,** Cross–idiotypic specificity among monoclonal IgM proteins with anti–globulin activity, *J. Exp. Med.*, 137, 331, 1973.
61. **Forre, O., Dobloug, J. H., Michaelson, T. E. et al.,** Evidence of similar idiotypic determinants on different rheumatoid factor populations, *Scand. J. Immunol.*, 9, 281, 1979.
62. **Carson, D. A. and Lawrence, S.** Idiotypes in rheumatoid sera, *Arthritis Rheum.*, 21, 550, 1978.
63. **Andrews, D. W. and Capra, J. D.,** Complete aminoacid sequence of variable domains from two monoclonal human anti–gamma globulins of the Wa cross–reactive idiotypic group, *Proc. Natl. Acad. Sci. U.S.A.*, 78, 3799, 1981.
64. **Makela, O. and Karjalainen, K.,** Inherited immunoglobulin idiotypes of the mouse, *Immunol. Rev.*, 34, 119, 1977.
65. **Eichmann, K. and Kindt, T. J.,** The inheritance of individual antigenic specificities of rabbit antibodies to streptococcal carbohydrates, *J. Exp. Med.*, 134, 532, 1971.
66. **Pasquali, J.–L., Fong, S., Tsoukas, C. et al.,** Inheritance of immunoglobulin M rheumatoid–factor idiotypes, *J. Clin. Invest.*, 66, 863, 1980.
67. **Theofilopoulos, A. N., McConahey, P. J., Izui, S., Eisenberg, R. A., Pereira, A. B., and Creighton, W. D.,** A comparative immunologic analysis of several murine strains with autoimmune manifestations, *Clin. Immunol. Immunopathol.*, 15, 258, 1980.
68. **Andrews, B. S., Eisenberg, R. A., Theofilopoulos, A. N., Izui, S., Wilson, C., McConahey, P. S., Murphy, E. D., Roths, J. B., and Dixon, F. J.,** Spontaneous murine lupus–like syndrome. Clinical and immunopathological manifestations of several strains, *J. Exp. Med.*, 148, 1198, 1978.
69. **Steward, M. W., Katz, F. E., and West, N. S.,** The Role of low affinity antibody in immune complex disease. The quantity of anti–DNA antibodies in NZB/W F_1 hybrid mice, *Clin. Exp. Immunol.*, 21, 121, 1975.
70. **Pisetsky, D. S., McCarty, G. A., and Peters, D. V.,** Mechanisms of autoantibody production in autoimmune MRL mice, *J. Exp. Med.*, 152, 1302, 1980.
71. **Lindstrom, J., Einarson, B., and Merlie, J.,** Immunization of rats with polypeptide chains from torpedo acetylcholine receptor causes an autoimmune response to receptors in rat muscle, *Proc. Natl. Acad. Sci. U.S.A.*, 75, 769, 1978.
72. **Eisenberg, R. A., Tan, E. M., and Dixon, F. J.,** Presence of anti–Sm reactivity in autoimmune mouse strains, *J. Exp. Med.*, 147, 582, 1978.
73. **Lewin, R.,** Myasthenia gravis under monoclonal scrutiny, *Science*, 211(2), 38, 1981.
74. **Gomez, C. M., Richman, D. P., Berman, P. W., Burres, S. A., Arnason, B. G. W., and Fitch, F. W.,** Monoclonal antibodies against purified nicotinic acetylcholine receptor, *Biochem. Biophys. Res. Commun.*, 88, 575, 1979.
75. **Moshly–Rosen, D., Fuchs, S., and Eshhar, Z.,** Monoclonal antibodies against defined determinants of acetylocholine receptor, *FEBS Lett.*, 106, 389, 1979.
76. **Toyka, K. V., Drachman, D. B., Griffin, D. E., Pestronk, A., Winkelstein, J. A., Fishbeck, K. H., and Kao, I.,** Myasthenia gravis. Study of humoral immune mechanisms by passive transfer to mice, *N. Eng. J. Med.*, 296, 125, 1977.
77. **Lindstrom, J., Engel, A. G., Seybold, M. E., Lennon, V. A., and Lambert, E. H.,** Pathological mechanisms in experimental autoimmune myasthenia gravis in rats with anti–acetylcholine receptor antibodies, *J. Exp. Med.*, 144, 739, 1976.
78. **Lennon, V. A. and Lamberg, E. H.,** Myasthenia gravis induced by monoclonal antibodies to acetylcholine receptors, *Nature (London)*, 285, 238, 1980.
79. **Richman, D. P., Gomez, C. M., Berman, P. W., Burres, S. A., Fitch, F. W., and Arnason, B. G. W.,** Monoclonal anti–acetylcholine receptor antibodies can cause experimental myasthenia, *Nature (London)*, 286, 738, 1980.
80. **Tzartos, S. J. and Lindstrom, J. M.,** Monoclonal antibodies used to probe acetylcholine receptor structure: localization of the main immunogenic region and detection of similarities between subunits, *Proc. Natl. Acad. Sci. U.S.A.*, 77, 755, 1980.
81. **Bussard, A. E. and Pages, J. M.,** Establishment of a permanent hybridoma producing a mouse autoantibody, *Prog. Clin. Biol. Res.*, 26, 167, 1978.
82. **Pages, J. M. and Bussard, A. E.,** Establishment and charaterization of a permanent murine hybridoma secreting monoclonal autoantibodies, *Cell. Immunol.*, 41, 188, 1978.
83. **Bussard, A. E.,** Antibody formation in nonimmune mouse peritoneal cells after incubation in gum containing antigen, *Science*, 153, 887, 1966.
84. **DeHeer, D. H., Pages, J. M., and Bussard, A. E.,** Specificity of anti–erythrocyte autoantibodies secreted by a NZB–derived hybridoma and NZB peritoneal cells, *Cell. Immunol.*, 49, 135, 1980.

85. **Linder, E. and Edgington, T. S.,** Antigenic specificity of anti–erythrocyte autoantibody responses by NZB mice: identification and partial characterization of two erythrocyte surface auto antigens, *J. Immunol.,* 108, 1615, 1972.

86. **DeHeer, D. H., Linder, E. J., and Edgington, T. S.,** Delineation of spontaneous erythrocyte autoantibody responses of NZB and other strains of mice, *J. Immunol.,* 120, 825, 1978.

87. **Klotz, J. L., Phillips, M. L., Miller, M. M., and Teplitz, R. L.,** Monoclonal autoantibody production by hybrid cell lines, *Clin. Immunol. Immunopathol.,* 18, 368, 1981.

88. **Talal, N.,** Immunologic and viral factors in the pathogenesis of systemic lupus erythematosus, *Arthritis Rheum.,* 13, 887, 1970.

89. **Lambert, P. H. and Dixon, F. J.,** Genesis of anti–nuclear antibody in NZB/W mice: role of genetic factors and of viral infections, *Clin. Exp. Immunol.,* 6, 829, 1970.

90. **Dubroff, L. M. and Reid, R. J., Jr.,** Hydralazine–pyrimidine interactions may explain hydralazine–induced lupus erythematosus, *Science,* 208, 404, 1980.

91. **Tan, E. M.,** Immunopathology and pathogenesis of cutaneous involvement in systemic lupus erythematosus, *J. Invest. Dermatol.,* 67, 360, 1976.

92. **Quimby, F. and Schwartz, R. S.,** The etiopathogenesis of systemic lupus erythematosus, *Pathobiol. Annu.,* 8, 35, 1978.

93. **Eilat, D., Asofsky, R., and Laskov, R.,** A hybridoma from an autoimmune NZB/NZW mouse producing monoclonal antibody to ribosomal—RNA, *J. Immunol.,* 124, 766, 1980.

94. **Eilat, D., Ben Sasson, S. A., and Laskov, R.,** A ribonucleic acid–specific antibody produced during autoimmune disease: evidence for nucleotide sequence specificity, *Eur. J. Immunol.,* 10, 841, 1980.

95. **Andrzejewski, C., Jr., Stollar, B. D., Lalor, T. M., and Schwartz, R. B.,** Hybridoma autoantibodies to DNA, *J. Immunol.,* 124, 1499, 1980.

96. **Andrzejewski, C., Jr., Rauch, J., Lafer, E. M., Stollar, B. D., and Schwartz, R. S.,** Antigen–binding diversity and idiotypic cross–reactions among hybridoma autoantibodies to DNA, *J. Immunol.,* 126, 226, 1981.

97. **Lafer, E. M., Rauch, J., Andrzejewski, C., Jr., Mudd, D., Furie, B., Schwartz, R. S., and Stollar, B. D.,** Polyspecific monoclonal lupus autoantibodies reactive with both polynucleotides and phospholipids, *J. Exp. Med.,* 153, 897, 1981.

98. **Hahn, B. H., Ebling, F., Freeman, S., Clevinger, B., and Davie, J.,** Production of monoclonal murine antibodies to DNA by somatic cell hybrids, *Arthritis Rheum.,* 23, 942, 1980.

99. **Ebling, F. and Hahn, B. H.,** Restricted subpopulations of DNA antibodies in kidneys of mice with systemic lupus. Comparison of antibodies in serum and renal eluates, *Arthritis Rheum.,* 23, 392, 1980.

100. **Tron, F., Charron, D., Bach, J.–F., and Talal, N.,** Establishment and characterization of a murine hybridoma secreting monoclonal anti–DNA autoantibody, *J. Immunol.,* 125, 2805, 1980.

101. **Marion, T. N. and Briles, D. E.,** Analysis of autoimmune anti–DNA antibody responses using somatic cell hybridization, in *Monoclonal Antibodies and T Cell Hybridomas,* Hammerling, G., Hammerling, U., and Kearney, J. F., Eds., Elsevier/North Holland, Amsterdam, 1981.

102. **Notman, D. D., Kurata, N., and Tan, E. M.,** Profiles of antinuclear antibodies in systemic rheumatic diseases, *Ann. Intern. Med.,* 83, 464, 1975.

103. **Sharp, G. C., Irvin, W. S., Mau, C. M., Holman, H. R., McDuffie, F. C., Hess, E. V., and Schmid, F. R.,** Association of antibodies to ribonucleoprotein and Sm antigens with mixed connective tissue disease, systemic lupus erythematosus, and other rheumatic diseases, *N. Engl. J. Med.,* 295, 1149, 1976.

104. **Nakamura, R. M., Peebles, C., and Tan, E. M.,** Microhemagglutination test for detection of antibodies and nuclear Sm and ribonucleoprotein antigens in systemic lupus erythematosus and related diseases, *Am. J. Clin. Pathol.,* 70, 800, 1978.

105. **Lerner, E. A., Lerner, M. R., Janeway, C. A., Jr., and Steitz, J. A.,** Monoclonal antibodies to nucleic acid–containing cellular constituents: probes for molecular biology and autoimmune disease, *Proc. Natl. Acad. Sci. U.S.A.,* 78, 2737, 1981.

106. **Yavin, E., Yavin, Z., Schneider, M. D., and Kohn, L. D.,** Monoclonal antibodies to the thyrotropin receptor: implications for receptor structure and the action of autoantibodies in Graves' disease, *Proc. Natl. Acad. Sci. U.S.A.,* 78, 3180, 1981.

107. **Smith, B. R. and Hall, R.,** Thyroid–stimulating immunoglobulins in Graves' disease, *Lancet,* 2, 427, 1974.

108. **Mehdi, S. W. and Nussey, S. S.,** A radio–ligand receptor assay for the long–acting thyroid stimulator. inhibition by the long–acting thyroid stimulator of the binding of radioiodinated thyroid–stimulating hormone to human thyroid membranes, *Biochem. J.,* 145, 105, 1975.

109. **Kohn, L. D., Consiglio, E., DeWolf, M. J. S., Grollman, E. F., Ledley, F. D., Lee, G., and Morris, N. P.,** Thyrotropin receptors and gangliosides, *Adv. Exp. Med. Biol.,* 125, 487, 1980.

110. **Kohn, L. D., Consiglio, E., Aloj, S. M., Beguinot, F., DeWolf, M. J. S., Yavin, E., Yavin, Z., Meldolesi, M. F., Shifrin, S., Gill, D. L., Vitti, P., Lee, G., Valente, W. A., and Grollman, E. F.,** The structure of the thyrotropin [TSH] receptor: potential role of gangliosides and relationship to receptor for interferon and bacterial toxin, in *International Cell Biology,* Schweiger, H. G., Ed., Lange and Springer, West Berlin, 1980, 696.

111. **Schwartz, M., Novick, D., Givol, D., and Fuchs, S.,** Induction of anti–idiotypic antibodies by immunization with syngeneic spleen cells educated with acetylcholine receptor, *Nature (London),* 273, 543, 1978.

112. **Nisonoff, A. and Lamoyi, E.,** Implications of the presence of an internal image of the antigen in anti–idiotypic antibodies; possible application to vaccine production (hypothesis), *Clin. Immunol. Immunopathol.,* 21, 397, 1981.

113. **Jerne, N. K.,** Towards a network theory of the immune system, *Ann. Immunol. (Paris),* 124C, 373, 1974.

114. **Eichmann, K.,** Expression and function of idiotypes in lymphocytes, *Adv. Immunol.,* 26, 195, 1978.

115. **Hart, D. A., Wang, A. L., Pawlak, L. L., and Nisonoff, A.,** Suppression of idiotypic specificities in adult mice by administration of antiidiotypic antibody, *J. Exp. Med.,* 135, 1293, 1972.

116. **Nisonoff, A., Ju, S. T., and Owen, F. L.,** Studies of structure and immunosuppression of cross–reactive idiotype in strain A mice, *Transplant. Rev.,* 34, 89, 1977.

117. **Wigzell, H., Binz, H., Frischknecht, H., Peterson, P., and Sege, K.,** Possible role of auto-idiotypic immunity in auto-immune disease, in *Genetic Control of Autoimmune Disease,* Rose, N. R., Bigazzi, P. E., and Warner, N. L., Eds., Elsevier/North–Holland, New York, 1978, 327.

118. **Vincent, A.,** Idiotype restriction in myasthenia gravis antibodies, *Nature (London),* 290, 293, 1981.

119. **Zanetti, M. and Bigazzi, P. E.,** Anti–idiotypic immunity and autoimmunity. I. *In vitro* and *in vivo* effects of anti–idiotypic antibodies to spontaneously occurring autoantibodies to rat thyroglobulin, *Eur. J. Immunol.,* 11, 187, 1981.

120. **Eilat, D. and Laskov, R.,** Production of anti–RNA antibody by hybridoma cells: purification from mixed immunoglobulin products, *Mol. Immunol.,* 18, 589, 1981.

121. **Olsson, L. and Kaplan, H. S.,** Human–human hybridomas producing monoclonal antibodies of pre-defined antigenic specificity, *Proc. Natl. Acad. Sci. U.S.A.,* 77, 5429, 1980.

122. **Croce, C. M., Linnenbach, A., Hall, W., Steplewski, Z., and Koprowski, H.,** Production of human hybridomas secreting antibodies to measles virus, *Nature (London),* 288, 488, 1980.

123. **Rauch, J.,** Manuscript in preparation.

124. **Pisetsky, D. S.,** Manuscript submitted.

Chapter 6

FUNCTIONAL T CELL HYBRIDOMAS PRODUCING NONSPECIFIC IMMUNOREGULATORY FACTORS

Amnon Altman, Robert D. Schreiber, and David H. Katz

TABLE OF CONTENTS

I.   Introduction 114

II.   Somatic Cell Hybrid Construction 115

III. Allogeneic Effect Factor (AEF) 115
      A.   Biological Effects of AEF 115
      B.   AEF Secretion by T Cell Hybridomas 116
            1.   Biological Activities of Hybridoma Supernatants 116
            2.   Inhibition of Biological Activity by Anti–*Ia* Antibodies 116

IV.   T Cell Growth Factor (TCGF) 118
      A.   Properties of TCGF 118
      B.   TCGF Production by T Cell Hybridomas 119
            1.   Cellular Characteristics of TCGF Production 119
            2.   Biochemical Analysis 121

V.   Mφ Activating Factor (MAF) 122
      A.   Properties of MAF 122
      B.   MAF Production by T Cell Hybridoma 124
            1.   Assays 124
            2.   Cellular Characteristics of MAF Production by
                  T Cell Hybridoma 125
            3.   Biochemical Analysis of T Cell Hybridoma MAF 125

VI.   Discussion and Concluding Remarks 127

Acknowledgments 128

References 128

I. INTRODUCTION

Ever since it was established that immune responses (Ir) involve complex interactions among T cells, B cells, and Mφ,[1] scientists have been searching for soluble factors that mediate such interactions by acting as communication signals between the cells producing them and other cells carrying the relevant acceptor sites for such factors. The impressive amount of effort invested in the search for such immunoregulatory mediators has resulted in the discovery of a number of soluble lymphokines produced by various cellular components of the immune system.[2] To illustrate the complexity of this situation, a multitude of soluble immunoregulatory factors can be generated by stimulation with specific heterologous antigens, alloantigens, or mitogens, either in vivo or in vitro. They are produced by T cells, B cells, or Mφ they suppress or help Ir, they are antigen–specific or nonspecific, they bear or lack antigenic determinants encoded by the MHC of the species, and they are either MHC–restricted or unrestricted in their action on target cells.

Analysis of the structure–function relationships among various lymphokines has been especially problematic in the case of the antigen–nonspecific factors. Depending on the biological assay system used for detecting their activity, these lymphokines have been given many different acronyms. Several facts impose serious limitations on the usefulness of the conventionally derived lymphokine preparations. First, assigning the production of these lymphokines to T cells has been indirect in that activated T cell–enriched populations were shown to produce these mediators. However, these cell populations contain other cell types and it is difficult to rule out Mφ (or other antigen–processing cells) since these are normally required for T cell activation. Secondly, the use of heterogeneous cell populations in many cases results in the production of different types of lymphokines in the same culture. Thus, examples exist to indicate that culture supernatants may contain mixtures of antigen–specific suppressor factors produced by different T suppressor cells,[3] antigen–specific and nonspecific factors,[4–6] and suppressor and helper factors.[7] Furthermore, it is known today that stimulation of antigen–primed T cells with specific antigen, a method that is routinely used for the preparation of antigen–specific factors,[8] also leads to the production of the antigen–nonspecific lymphokine, TCGF[9,10] (more recently termed Interleukin 2 (IL–2)[11]), as well as other nonspecific lymphokines.[12] Finally, the amounts of lymphokine available for structural studies from conventionally prepared culture supernatants are limited.

Because of these limitations, considerable efforts have been made recently to establish monoclonal lines of permanently growing T cells that are capable of secreting various lymphokines. The availability of such lines should overcome the problems mentioned above, particularly in terms of providing large quantities of a given lymphokine that allows detailed biochemical analyses. Two experimental approaches have been used to obtain lymphokine–secreting T cell lines. The first one has been to screen a large number of T cell leukemias for constitutive or facultative (i.e., following mitogen stimulation) lymphokine production. This has resulted in the identification of several lymphokine–secreting murine,[13–16,90] owl monkey,[17] or human[18,19] leukemic T cells.

The other approach has taken advantage of the technique of somatic cell hybridization as refined by Köhler and Milstein[20] for immunologically relevant cells. This technology, developed initially for the construction of hybrid cell lines of the B cell lineage, was subsequently extended to the construction of T cell hybridomas by fusion of either normal or activated T cells with established T lymphoma lines.[21–23] However, in early studies of this type these hybridomas failed to exhibit functional T cell properties of the normal T cell partner. More recently, several laboratories have been successful in constructing T cell hybridomas expressing T cell function of the nonlymphoma partner as manifested by the active secretion of soluble mediators capable of exerting immunoregulatory effects of antigen–specific[24–36] and nonspecific[37–42] nature, as well as class (IgE)–selective effects.[43]

The purpose of this communication is to summarize the authors' recent studies on murine T cell hybridomas secreting a number of antigen–nonspecific lymphokines and to briefly review other recent studies pertaining to the same issue.

II. SOMATIC CELL HYBRID CONSTRUCTION

In all reported studies concerning T cell hybrids secreting antigen–nonspecific lymphokines, the HAT–sensitive variant of the AKR–derived thymoma, BW5147, has been used as the malignant cell partner for fusion. The normal T cells used in these studies were either unstimulated cells from naive donors,[39] or T cell–enriched populations activated by heterologous antigens,[37,40,41] or alloantigens.[37,38,91] In one case, PHA–stimulated, IL–2–secreting LBRM–33 lymphoma cells were fused with the BW5147 cells.[42]

In the authors' recent studies, the normal T cell partners used for fusion were derived from blast–enriched alloactivated T cell populations. These cells were prepared according to a method established in the laboratory for the production of the lymphokine AEF.[44–46] Thymocytes (1×10^8) are injected i.v. into 650 rad–irradiated syngeneic recipients together with an equal number of irradiated semiallogeneic spleen cells. The alloactivated T cells recovered from the spleens of the recipient mice one week later are placed in a short–term (18 to 24 hr) serum–free culture with irradiated cells of the same F_1 hybrid haplotype used for in vivo activation. The supernatant fluids of these cultures were found to contain, in addition to AEF, other lymphokines such as TCGF,[47] IF,[48] colony stimulating activity,[92] and MAF.[93] Based on these findings, the authors predicted that using such alloactivated T cell populations for hybridization would result in hybridomas that secrete several distinct lymphokines. Furthermore, these hybridomas should allow for the study of the relationship among distinct lymphokine activities.

DBA/2–derived T cell blasts activated against (C3H × DBA/2)F_1 hybrid alloantigens as described above were fused with BW5147 cells at a ratio of 5:1 using 30% PEG.[38] Hybrids were selected in HAT medium and their supernatants were tested for constitutive or mitogen–induced lymphokine activities. Desired hybridomas were cloned and subcloned by limiting dilution techniques and either carried in culture or maintained frozen in liquid nitrogen.

In the following sections the authors' findings will be summarized with respect to the various lymphokine activities secreted by the T cell hybridomas.

III. ALLOGENEIC EFFECT FACTOR (AEF)

A. Biological Effects of AEF

AEF has originally been described as a 45,000 dalton glycoprotein bearing Ia antigenic determinants of the responder haplotype and capable of replacing T helper cells in the in vitro antibody response to particulate or soluble heterologous antigens.[1,44,45,49–51] In later studies it was found that AEF–containing culture supernatants are highly mitogenic for unprimed T cells, can trigger the differentiation of unprimed T cells in the absence of exogenous antigen into CTL that display the Lyt-2$^+$ phenotype, preferentially lyse H–2–identical target cells, and are directed against antigen(s) determined by the K and/or D regions of the murine MHC, and can stimulate the differentiation of unprimed T cells into responding cells of the Lyt–1$^+$ phenotype that can be restimulated in secondary syngeneic mixed lymphocyte reactions (SMLR) that are directed against antigen(s) determined by the *I* region of the *H–2* complex.[46,47,52–54] In addition, AEF–containing culture supernatants were found to promote the long–term growth of murine BM cells with maintenance of stem cell and pre–T cell activity.[55] These latter properties of AEF, namely its ability to trigger differentiation of unprimed T cells into functional effector cells and maintain hematopoietic stem cell activity, distinguish this biologically active mediator from TCGF, since the latter is characterized biologically by its ability to support long–term growth of *primed*, fully mature T lymphocytes previously activated by antigen or otherwise.[56–59] However, since AEF supernatants also contain TCGF in rather high amounts,[47] it is not possible to rule out some contribution by TCGF to the biological effects measured. The authors believe that the elucidation of the relationship among heterogenous biological activities present in a crude lymphokine preparation will be feasible when antibodies specific for various lymphokine activities become available.

B. AEF Secretion by T Cell Hybridomas[38]

1. Biological Activities of Hybridoma Supernatants

After fusion, hybrids were detected in 115 or 288 wells plated and the unstimulated supernatants from these positive wells were screened for B cell–activating capacities. Approximately 1/2 of these supernatants manifested little or no positive biological effects, about 1/3 displayed low to moderate biological activity, and a small number demonstrated rather potent biological effects when tested for their ability to restore the in vitro antibody responses of T cell–depleted B cells following stimulation with SRBC or TNP–SRBC.[38] The hybridoma supernatants tested were obtained in serum–free conditions by washing the cultured hybridoma cells, replating them in serum–free medium, and harvesting the culture supernatants after 24 hr. Culture supernatants from the unfused parental line, BW5147, failed to display any B cell–activating properties in these cultures. Two hybridomas, 27 and 34, that constitutively secreted higher levels of helper activity, were selected for further experimentation. They were found to be true somatic cell hybrids as evidenced by their expression of the relevant Thy–1 and *H–2* alloantigens characteristic of both partner cell types used for fusion.

Because the AEF hybridomas were derived from T cell blasts generated following stimulation by alloantigens, the authors were interested in determining whether the hybridomas themselves displayed any responsiveness to additional stimulation with the original inducing alloantigen. Thus, cells of hybridoma 34 were cultured overnight in the presence of equal numbers of irradiated C3D2F$_1$ target spleen cells and the supernatant recovered from such stimulated hybridoma cultures analyzed for biological activities on both B and T lymphocytes.

As shown in Figure 1, the supernatant from such restimulated hybridoma cells displayed clear B cell–reconstituting effects in in vitro antibody responses to TNP–SRBC (left panel), T cell–activating properties as manifested by its ability to stimulate development of CTL in the absence of exogenous antigen (middle panel), and direct proliferation of unprimed T lymphocytes (right panel). It should be noted that these activities were obtained with a concentration of hybridoma supernatant (1:20) that is well below the activity threshold of supernatants from the same hybridoma not restimulated with alloantigen. Thus, the culture supernatant of the unstimulated hybridoma failed to display B or T cell–activating properties in this experiment when tested at the same 1:20 dilution, but was active at a 1:5 dilution.

2. Inhibition of Biological Activity by Anti–Ia Antibodies

In order to verify that the AEF molecules detected in the T cell hybridoma supernatants were *Ia*–positive, the authors investigated whether the activity of such molecules

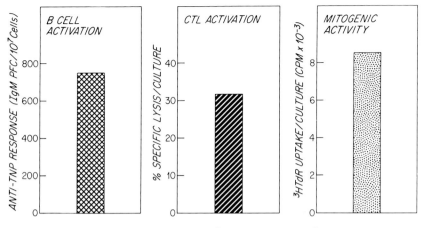

AEF: HYB 34 (1:20 Final Dilution)

FIGURE 1. Biological effects on B and T lymphocytes of AEF hybridoma supernatant obtained after alloantigen restimulation. AEF:Hyb 34 was cultured for 24 hr in the presence of an equal number of fresh, irradiated (1500 rads) C3D2F$_1$ stimulator cells. The supernatant recovered from such stimulation hybridoma cultures was tested at a final dilution of 1:20 for its B cell and T cell–activating properties. B cell–activating properties were measured in terms of capacity to stimulate T cell–depleted DBA/2 spleen cells to respond in vitro to TNP–SRBC. The data are shown in the far left panel as TNP–specific IgM PFC/10^7 cells. Control cultures of the same cells stimulated with TNP–SRBC in the absence of Hyb 34 supernatant yielded no detectable TNA–specific PFC. The T cell–activating properties of AEF: Hyb 34 supernatant at this dilution was measured by stimulation of self–specific CTL (middle panel) and direct mitogenic activity on unprimed T lymphocytes (right panel) using assay systems as described before.[38] The mitogenic activity is expressed as net cpm per culture in experimental cultures after subtraction of background cpm in unstimulated cultures. Background levels for CTL and mitogenic activities, were 6.9% lysis and 5000 cpm, respectively. Supernatants from AEF:Hyb 34 cells not subjected to alloantigen restimulation failed to display significant biological activities at a final dilution of 1:20.

would be sensitive to the effects of anti–*Ia* antibodies. The experiment summarized in Figure 2 demonstrates that this is indeed the case. Anti-Thy-1.2 serum-treated spleen cells of A/J mice were used as responder cells in this experiment, since they are totally disparate at the *I*-region from the DBA/2 strain of origin of the AEF-secreting hybridomas. Moreover, A/J mice are *H-2*-identical to the B10.A mice used for preparation of the anti-*I-A^d* serum employed. This serum was devoid of any reactivity with A/J spleen cells in a C-dependent microcytotoxicity assay (not shown).

As shown in Figure 2, panel A, cultures of such T cell-depleted A/J spleen cells exposed to a conventional AEF preparation developed good primary TNP-specific in vitro responses to TNP-SRBC. Incorporation of anti-*Ia^s* antibodies had no effect on the capacity of this AEF preparation (also derived from DBA/2–activated T cells) in stimulating such B cell responses. In contrast, incorporation of antibodies specific for *I-A^d* determinants substantially inhibited the activity of this AEF preparation on the A/J responder B cells.

As shown in panel B, AEF activity of serum-free supernatant of hybridoma 34 was not significantly affected by the incorporation of normal mouse serum of B10.A origin, whereas incorporation of anti-*I-A^d* antibodies at the same concentration totally abolished the B cell-activating properties of this AEF-secreting hybridoma. Control cultures of untreated (i.e., T cell-containing) A/J spleen cells developed good responses to TNP-SRBC. These responses were not inhibited by the same anti-*I-A^d* antibodies (see Figure 2).

In view of the authors' findings that conventionally-derived AEF bears *Ia* determi-

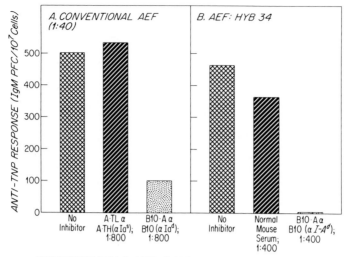

RESPONDER CELLS: ANTI-θ SERUM-TREATED A/J SPLEEN CELLS

FIGURE 2. Inhibition of B cell activating properties of AEF hybridoma super-natant by anti–I-A^d antibodies. Unprimed A/J spleen cells depleted of T lymphocytes by treatment with anti–Thy 1.2 serum + C were cultured (0.5×106 cells per well) for five days in the presence of TNP–SRBC as stimulating antigen and either conventional AEF (final concentration 1:40, panel A) or supernatant from AEF: Hyb 34 (final concentration 1:5, panel B). Cultures contained either no inhibitor serum, normal mouse serum, anti-Ia^s or anti–I-A^d serum at the final concentrations indicated. The data are presented as TNP–specific IgM PFC/10^7 cells assayed in triplicated cultures of each type. Control cultures of T cell–depleted A/J spleen cells cultured in the presence of TNP-SRBC but without any source of AEF yielded no detectable TNP-specific PFC response. Other control cultures of untreated A/J spleen cells produced 516 TNP–specific PFC in response to TNP–SRBC, and this response was not inhibited in the presence of anti– I-A^d serum.

nants[49] and that the biological activity of both the conventional and the hybridoma-derived AEF preparations is inhibited by specific anti-Ia antibodies, it was of importance to determine whether the hybridoma cells express Ia antigens of the normal T cell partner, i.e., Ia^d. Thus, parental and cloned hybridoma cells were incubated with B10.A anti–B10 (anti-I-A^d) or A.TL anti-A.TH (anti-Ia^s) sera, stained with a fluorescent rabbit anti-mouse Ig serum and subjected to analysis on a cell sorter (FACS II). Hybridoma 34 as well as some of its clones were found to express I-A^d determinants in this experiment.[38]

IV. T CELL GROWTH FACTOR (TCGF)

A. Properties of TCGF

TCGF (IL–2) has originally been defined as a T cell-derived lymphokine that allows the long-term culture of activated T cells.[9,10] Studies on the nature of TCGF have been greatly aided by the development of a short-term and sensitive bioassay.[60] This assay takes advantage of the absolute dependence of established activated T cell lines on TCGF for growth. To the extent that TCGF was purified, it has been characterized as a protein with a molecular weight of approximately 30,000 daltons in mice[56-58] and 13 to 15,000 daltons in rats[56-58] and humans.[19,56-58] TCGF exerts a number of biological effects on activated, but not on naive, T cells. These include facilitation of thymocyte responses to T cell mitogens and helper activity for the induction of antibody and CTL responses in vitro. TCGF has also been shown to induce, together with antigen, specific T cell-dependent Ir in spleen cells of athymic nude mice, both in vitro[61–63] and in vivo.[64–66] However, the one property that is clearly unique to TCGF is its ability to maintain the growth of activated T cells.

According to a generally accepted model, stimulation by antigen/lectin activates Mφ to produce a soluble mediator, lymphocyte-activating factor (LAF),[67] termed more recently Interleukin 1 (IL–1),[11] and induces a set of T cells (the so-called T responsive cells) to express specific surface receptors for TCGF molecules. The same antigen/lectin, together with the macrophage-derived LAF, induce another set of T cells (the precursors of T-producer cells) to differentiate into cells that produce TCGF. Once the circuit of TCGF production has been completed, the antigen/lectin is not necessary anymore for T cell proliferation. Binding of TCGF molecules to their respective surface receptors will trigger the T cells into proliferation which will continue as long as TCGF is available.

Many recent studies have focused on TCGF because of its potential application in several areas. First, the biology of TCGF as a hormonal-like mediator regulating the growth of activated T cells is of interest. Secondly, the ability to establish cloned lines of antigen-specific T cells with TCGF makes it possible to use such lines for studying the nature of the T cell receptor for antigen, and immunotherapy (e.g., of tumors). Finally, based on its effects in T cell-deficient nude mice,[61–66] TCGF may have therapeutic potential in immunodeficiencies that involve the T cell compartment. Thus, there is a great need for convenient and homogeneous sources of large quantities of TCGF.

B. TCGF Production by T Cell Hybridomas

1. Cellular Characteristics of TCGF Production

In screening T cell hybridomas (prepared as described above) for TCGF production, the authors have used the TCGF bioassay developed by Gillis et al.[60] Supernatants of unstimulated or mitogen-activated hybridomas were titrated for their ability to support the growth of the TCGF-dependent T cell line CTLL-2[10] in a 24 hr tritiated thymidine (^{3}HTdR) uptake assay. In these titrations a standard TCGF preparation derived from Con A–stimulated rat spleen cells has been included. This standard preparation induced 50% of the maximal ^{3}HTdR uptake by CTLL-2 cells at a dilution of about 1:100 to 1:150 and was arbitrarily assigned a titer of 10 U/ml. This makes the results comparable to those of others[56,57,60] who have assigned a titer of 1 U/ml to a standard preparation that gave 50% of maximal activity at a dilution of approximately 1:10, i.e., it was about 10-fold less active than the standard TCGF preparation used by the authors.

Figure 3 shows the results of TCGF titrations performed on culture supernatants of 5 Con A (10 μg/ml)-stimulated T cell hybridomas. Of these, 2 were negative, another 2 secreted low levels of TCGF, and 1 (#24) secreted relatively high levels of TCGF. The BW5147 tumor line used for fusion failed to secrete detectable amounts of TCGF, either constitutively or following mitogen stimulation. Hybridoma 24 was selected for further analysis and cloned by limiting dilution (0.5 cell per microtiter well). The clones were tested for TCGF production (Figure 4). Of 27 different clones stimulated with Con A, 9 did not produce measurable levels of TCGF. The other clones secreted TCGF at levels ranging from 0.02 to 7.5 U/ml. Ten clones secreted more TCGF than did mouse spleen cells cultured and stimulated under identical conditions (1.2 U/ml).

Clone 24/A10 was subjected to an additional cycle of subcloning in order to verify its true clonal nature. All of 12 subclones selected randomly for screening were found to produce TCGF upon stimulation with Con A (results not shown).

The clones derived from hybridoma 24 were also screened for constitutive TCGF

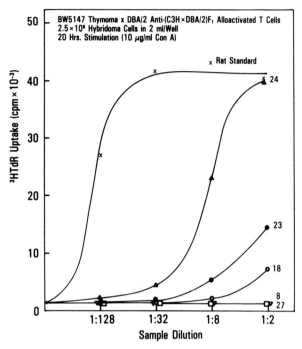

FIGURE 3. TCGF (IL–2) production by T cell hybridoma lines.
Hybridoma cells were cultured in 2 ml cultures at 2.5×10^6 cells
per well in a 24–well (16 mm) tissue culture plate. Supernatants
were harvested after 10 hr of culture with or without 20 μg/ml
Con A. No TCGF activity could be detected in unstimulated hybridoma supernatants.

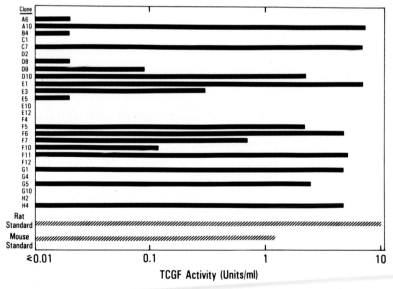

FIGURE 4. TCGF (IL–2) production by clones of T cell hybridoma 24. Hybridoma
cells were cloned at 0.5 cells per well in the presence of 2×10^5 irradiated (2500 rad)
BALB/c thymocytes in flat–bottom microtiter wells (200 μl per well). Growing clones
were transferred to, and expanded in, 16 mm wells. Confluent cultures were split into
two new cultures, one serving as a control and the other one stimulated for 20 hr with
10 μg/ml Con A. Supernatants were then titrated for TCGF activity.

Table 1
CONSTITUTIVE AND CON A-INDUCED TCGF SECRETION BY CLONES OF T CELL HYBRIDOMA 24[a]

Clone	TCGF activity[b] in supernatants of hybridoma clones cultured with:	
	No Con A	10 μg/ml Con A
Gl	6,938 ± 712	50,525 ± 4451
G5	8,311 ± 788	49,385 ± 3146
H4	7,309 ± 830	46,314 ± 7126
A10	4,971 ± 744	50,834 ± 7014
F5	1,568 ± 388	58,802 ± 4833
F12	1,572 ± 193	2,157 ± 2

[a] Hybridoma clones were grown to confluency in 16 mm wells, split between two wells and the cells in one of the wells were stimulated for 20 hr with 10 μg/ml Con A.
[b] 3HTdR uptake by 1×10^4 CTLL-2 cells induced by 50% (v/v) hybridoma supernatant. 3HTdR uptake in the absence of any TCGF source was 1033 ± 94 cpm.

production. Supernatants of 15 out of 27 unstimulated hybridoma clones produced a significant stimulation of growth of the CTLL-2 indicator cells when tested at the highest concentration (50% v/v) and representative results are shown in Table 1. The fact that this activity was produced only by some of the clones suggests that it truly reflects TCGF activity and not some nonspecific growth effect. The authors conclude from these results that some of these T cell hybridoma lines are capable of constitutive TCGF production at very low levels, in agreement with their previously demonstrated ability to secrete AEF without stimulation.[38]

Con A at 10 μg/ml stimulated optimal production of TCGF by hybridoma 24 (Table 1), as compared to 5,20, or 40 μg/ml. Purified PHA (Wellcome) at concentrations of between 2 and 8 μg/ml was a less potent stimulator (not shown). In agreement with findings by others, TCGF production by 24/A10 cells was independent of serum in the culture medium. The ability of these cells to secrete TCGF in the absence of serum should facilitate structural characterization and purification of TCGF molecules.

Clone 24/A10 was also analyzed for its expression of Thy-1 and *H-2* alloantigens by cytofluorographic methods, using the FACS II. As shown in Table 2, this clone expressed Thy 1.2 and *H-2^d* determinants derived from the alloactivated DBA/2 T cells used for fusion, as well as Thy 1.1 and *H-2^k* alloantigens of the BW5147 lymphoma line.

2. Biochemical Analysis

In the authors' studies on the biochemical characterization of the T cell hybridoma-derived TCGF activity procedures similar to those described by others recently have been used. Culture supernatants of 24/A10 cells stimulated for 20 hr with 10 μg/ml Con A in serum-free or FCS (0.5% v/v)–supplemented medium were concentrated by sequential precipitation with 45 and 85% ammonium sulfate. The material precipitated by 85% $(NH_4)_2SO_4$ was depleted of 90 to 95% of the Con A originally present in the culture supernatant (as estimated by residual mitogenic activity on fresh thymocytes or spleen cells) and about 90% of the total protein, while retaining at the same time 85% or more of the TCGF activity. This material was dissolved and extensively dialyzed against PBS (pH 7.0) and further fractionated by DEAE-Sephacel ion exchange and Sephadex G-100 gel filtration chromatographies.

Table 2
FACS II ANALYSIS OF ALLOANTIGEN EXPRESSION BY T CELL HYBRIDOMA CLONE 24/A10[a]

Antibody treatment	Specificity	Fluorescence-positive cells %
None	—	14.1
AKR/Cum anti-AKR/J	Thy 1.1	90.1
F7D5e7 (monoclonal)	Thy 1.2	91.9
C57BL/6 anti-A/J	$H\text{-}2^k$	86.2
B10.BR anti-B10.D2	$H\text{-}2^d$	54.4

[a]Cells were treated with 1:200 dilution of F7D5e7 antibody or 1:20 dilution of the other antibodies, followed by incubation with FITC-conjugated rabbit anti-mouse Ig (1:50). Treatments were performed for 30 min on ice, with 4 washes after each treatment. Cells were analyzed on a FACS II (Becton Dickinson FACS System, Mountain View, Calif.).

Figure 5 depicts the results of a DEAE-Sephacel chromatography of 24/A10-derived TCGF. The material used for this fractionation has previously been subjected to Sephadex G-100 gel chromatography and biologically active fractions were pooled and dialyzed against 0.04 M sodium phosphate buffer pH 8.0. The DEAE-Sephacel column (1.5 × 25 cm) was equilibrated with the same buffer and 30 ml of a TCGF-containing pool were applied to the column. TCGF was eluted with a salt gradient of 0.04 to 0.5 NaCl. Fractions of 4.5 ml were tested for their absorbance at 280 nm, TCGF activity at 1:10 dilution, and conductivity. The results (Figure 5) indicate that TCGF activity was eluted as a relatively broad peak between 30 and 150 mM NaCl (pH 8.0), corresponding to the property of murine TCGF from other cellular sources.

Further fractionation of the DEAE-Sephacel-chromatographed material by Sephadex G-100 gel chromatography indicated (Figure 6) that TCGF activity co-eluted with molecules in the size range of 30 to 45,000 daltons with peak activity at about 35,000 daltons, again in agreement with what has been reported for TCGF derived from other types of murine T cells.

Thus, to the extent that the T cell hybridoma-derived TCGF has been purified, it bears similar properties to TCGF molecules that have been characterized by others. Further purification steps such as PAGE are currently being taken.

V. Mφ ACTIVATING FACTOR (MAF)

A. Properties of MAF

It has become apparent that under certain conditions, the Mφ can express effector cell function toward a variety of intracellular bacterial and microbial pathogens (such as *Listeria monocytogenes,*[68] *Toxoplasma gondii*[69] and *Trypanosoma cruzi*[70]) and neoplastic cells.[71-74] These activities are dependent on a series of reactions that first must alter the functional state of the Mφ to produce an activated mononuclear phagocyte.[68,75-77] Several lines of evidence indicate that this activation process is effected by a T-lymphocyte product denoted Mφ activating factor or MAF. Mφ isolated from *in situ* tumor sites[78] or from mice recovering from bacterial or parasitic infections display the ability to express nonspecific tumoricidal activity in vitro.[73,74] The in vitro interaction of immune T lymphocytes with antigen-pulsed Mφ leads to the elaboration of a soluble factor that can induce cytocidal activity in naive Mφ.[79,80] The generation of this factor is dependent on the same factors that govern T cell Mφ interaction, i.e., a requirement for compatibility between the two cells with respect to Mφ surface markers encoded

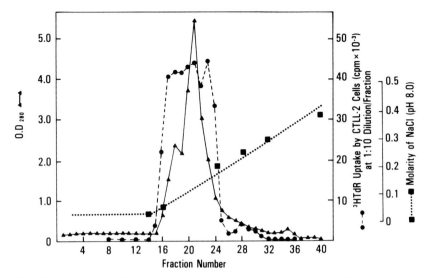

FIGURE 5. DEAE-Sephacel ion–exchange chromatography of T cell hybridoma cell clone 24/A10-derived TCGF (IL–2) activity. Culture supernatants (containing 0.5 percent FCS) of hybridoma cells stimulated for 20 hr with 10 μg/ml Con A were concentrated by $(NH_4)_2SO_4$ precipitation between 45 and 85% (w/v). The dissolved and dialyzed precipitate was fractionated on a 2 × 90 cm Sephadex G–100 column, eluted with phosphate-buffered saline, pH 7.0 and biologically active 5–ml fractions were pooled and concentrated. This material was then chromatographed on a 1.5 × 25 cm DEAE–Sephacel column equilibrated in 0.05 M sodium–phosphate buffer, pH 8.0 with salt gradients from 0.05 to 0.5 M NaCl. 4.5-ml fractions were tested for their O.D.$_{280}$ and biological activity.

by genes in the I region of the MHC and antigen-specificity of the T cell population.[80] MAF activity has also been induced by mitogen stimulation of normal murine spleen cell suspensions. Once formed, MAF action on target Mφ is neither antigen-dependent nor MHC-restricted.[81]

MAF has been reported to alter a number of functional and biochemical properties of Mφ. These alterations include increases in endocytic, biosynthetic, and secretory functions as well as alterations of membrane physiology and composition. However, for the purposes of this discussion, the authors wish to define MAF only as the activity that is responsible for induction of Mφ cytocidal activity toward neoplastic cells.

The current generally held concept is that two signals are required to generate Mφ tumoricidal activity.[82,83] MAF is the first signal that primes the Mφ and makes it susceptible to a "triggering" second signal. Second signals are conveyed by a heterogeneous group of substances and can be of endogeneous as well as exogenous origins. To date, the molecular mechanisms involved in the "priming" and "triggering" steps remain unresolved.

The biochemical identity of MAF is uncertain. Molecular weight values ranging from 28,000 to 300,000 daltons have been reported. On the basis of the largest numbers of reports, however, MAF displays an apparent molecular weight of 45,000 to 55,000 daltons.[84] MAF activity is destroyed upon incubation at or below pH 4.0, above pH 10, and upon heating to 80°C. Conflicting reports exist concerning stability at 56°C. The authors own work indicates that MAF is stable to incubation for 1 hr at 56°C but is destroyed upon incubation at 65°C. The question of whether MAF is identical with other lymphokines is unanswered. While reports exist that indicate that MAF is inseparable from migration inhibition factor (MIF) on the basis of molecular weight and buoyant density,[85] at least one group has reported the separation of the two activities.[86]

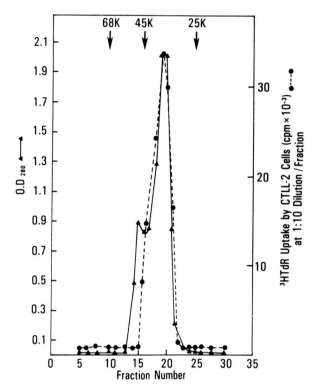

FIGURE 6. Sephadex G–100 gel chromatography of DEAE Sephacel–fractionated TCGF (IL–2) activity derived from T cell hybridoma clone 24/A10. Fractions 16 to 25 recovered from a
DEAE–Sephacel column (See Figure 5) were pooled, concentrated, and rechromatographed on a Sephadex G–100 column.
O.D.$_{280}$ readings and biological activity of 5-ml fractions are
shown.

Partially purified IF preparations have been shown to also induce tumoricidal activity
of Mφ.[87] Because of similarities in molecular weight, pH sensitivity and heat stability,
the possibility arises that MAF and γ-Interferon (γ-IF) are identical. The answers to
these questions must await biochemical purification of MAF. In the past this has proved
difficult since a large amount of MAF-containing starting material was not available.
The identification of T cell hybridoma clones, to be discussed below, that produce
extraordinary levels of MAF should prove to be a solution to this dilemma. The elucidation of the biochemical identity of MAF will then permit the detailed biochemical
analysis of its mechanism of action on Mφ and ultimately lead to an understanding of
the in vivo significance of Mφ effector cell function.

B. MAF Production by T Cell Hybridoma

1. Assays

To screen for the presence of MAF in T cell hybridoma supernatants, the authors
have used a ^{51}Cr-release tumoricidal assay. In this assay 2×10^5 adherent peptone-
elicited peritoneal exudate Mφ are incubated with MAF sources and excess amounts
of heat-killed *Listeria monocytogenes* as a source of second signal. After 4 hr, the
stimuli are washed off and 2×10^4 ^{51}Cr-labeled P815 mastocytoma cells added. After
incubation for 18 hr at 37°C, the specific amount of ^{51}Cr released into the supernatant

Table 3
DEMONSTRATION OF MAF ACTIVITY SECRETED FROM CON A-STIMULATED T CELL HYBRIDOMA 24

Dilution of MAF source	Specific P815 lysis (%)			
	24 + Con A[a]	24[b]	Con A[c]	MAF 8080[d]
1/20	51.4	3.9	0.0	49.8
1/100	43.7	N.D.	N.D.	51.1
1/500	4.2	N.D.	N.D.	29.1
1/2500	0.0	N.D.	N.D.	6.8

[a]Hybridoma 24 incubated for 18 hr with 10 μg/ml Con A.
[b]Supernatant of unstimulated hybridoma 24.
[c]Con A at 10 μg/ml.
[d]Splenic MAF.

is determined. One unit of MAF is defined as the amount of MAF required to effect 50% of maximal ^{51}Cr release.

IF was assayed by the cytopathic effect assay which is based on IF-dependent anti-viral activity. Mouse L-cells (clone 929) were incubated for 24 hr with potential sources of IF. The resulting monolayer of cells were then challenged with purified vesicular stomatitis virus and cultured for an additional 48 hr. Viable monolayers and virus-disrupted monolayers were differentiated by light microscopy. One unit of IF is defined as the reciprocal of the dilution that gave 50% protection of the L-cells from virus.

2. Cellular Characteristics of MAF Production by T Cell Hybridoma

Four parental hybridomas were screened for their ability to release MAF. Only one of the four (hybridoma 24) could be identified as a MAF producer. As seen in Table 3, no MAF activity was detected in the unstimulated cell supernatant. However, upon stimulation with Con A or PHA, MAF activities could be demonstrated and titrated out between dilutions of 1/100 to 1/500. The amount of MAF released was dependent on the Con A concentration used during the stimulation. Maximal release was found between Con A concentrations of 10 to 20 μg/ml. Compared to a standard MAF preparation, the uncloned T cell hybridoma 24 displayed 20 to 30% of lymphokine activity. Stimulated culture supernatants of this hybridoma also contained IF activity.

Upon cloning, 27 clones were obtained. None released MAF or IF constitutively. As seen in Figure 7, 24 clones produced MAF when stimulated with 10 μg/ml Con A. At least seven of the clones produced higher MAF levels than the MAF standard. The MAF content of an additional nine clones had not yet been determined by titration and are indicated by the broken bars labeled N.T., >200. The initial screening indicated that these clones displayed greater than 200 MAF U/ml. Ten clones did not produce IF. One of these clones, G1, produced 55,000 U of MAF per milliliter which is 25 times greater than the MAF standard. No correlation was found between IF levels and MAF levels of the various clones. Of particular importance is the fact that clone G1 failed to secrete IF despite the extraordinarily high quantities of MAF it produced. Taken together these results indicate that MAF and IF can be distinguished on the basis of differential production by clones of the T cell hybridoma.

3. Biochemical Analysis of T Cell Hybridoma MAF

The biochemical analysis of MAF produced by the T cell hybridoma clones 24/G1 has just begun. T cell hybridoma MAF is being produced at the rate of 2 l per week regulatory activities that are not exclusive for the immune system. Moreover, the fact that T cell hybridoma clones produce IF suggests that T cells may secrete molecules that regulate cells outside the reticuloendothelial system. One study[41] suggests that hybridoma variants can be obtained that secrete only TCGF but not CSF. The authors' preliminary studies also suggest that it is possible to select subclones that selectively secrete a given lymphokine. Thus, by analyzing various cloned T cell hybridomas it may be possible to determine whether the genetic machinery for the production of only one, some, or all lymphokines exists in a given T cell. In practical terms, the availability of hybridoma clones selectively secreting one lymphokine will facilitate the purification of such lymphokine free of other lymphokine contaminants.

Additionally, if a cloned T cell hybridoma proves to secrete simultaneously distinct lymphokine activities, it remains to be determined whether the production of different lymphokines is causally related or reflects independent events. For example, it has been shown recently that TCGF-induced development of CTL responses requires IF production.[89] One could, therefore, use the lymphokine-secreting T cell hybridomas to ascertain how various signals modulate the production of biological activities and whether a signal affecting the production of a given lymphokine will simultaneously affect the other ones secreted by the same hybridoma.

Finally, the availability of monoclonal cellular reagents secreting a variety of regulatory molecules provides a convenient tool for molecular genetics studies on such molecules. Thus, the study of these T cell hybridomas will eventually clarify many of the unresolved questions pertaining to the regulation of the reticuloendothelial as well as other systems of the multicellular organism.

ACKNOWLEDGMENTS

We gratefully acknowledge R. Weiner, A. Sferruzza, and P.–M. Paris for their excellent help in performing the experiments described herein and Rebecca Mead for typing this manuscript. This is publication no. 2505 from the Immunology Departments, Research Institute of Scripps Clinic, La Jolla, Calif. This work was supported by USPHS Grants CA-24911, CA-25803, AI-07007 and AI-17354. Altman and Schreiber are recipients of an American Cancer Society, Inc. Junior Faculty Research Award JFRA-17 and an American Heart Association, Inc. Established Investigatorship 77-202, respectively.

REFERENCES

1. **Katz, D. H.,** *Lymphocyte Differentiation, Recognition and Regulation,* Academic Press, New York, 1977.
2. **Altman, A. and Katz, D. H.,** Production and isolation of helper and suppressive factors, *J. Immunol. Methods,* 38, 9, 1980.
3. **Hirai, Y. and Nisonoff, A.,** Selective suppression of the major idiotypic component of an antihapten response by soluble T cell-derived factors with idiotypic or anti-idiotypic receptors, *J. Exp. Med.,* 151, 1213, 1980.
4. **Tada, T., Taniguchi, M., and Okumura, K.,** Regulation of antibody response by antigen-specific T cell factors bearing *I* region determinants, *Prog. Immunol.,* 3, 369, 1977.
5. **Taniguchi, M. and Tokuhisa, T.,** Cellular consequences in the suppression of antibody response by the antigen-specific T-cell factor, *J. Exp. Med.,* 151, 517, 1980.
6. **Mudawwar, F. B., Yunis, E. J., and Geha, R. S.,** Antigen-specific helper factor in man, *J. Exp. Med.,* 148, 1032, 1978.

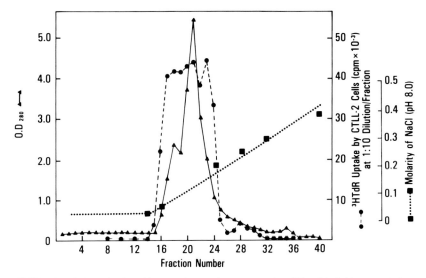

FIGURE 5. DEAE-Sephacel ion–exchange chromatography of T cell hybridoma cell clone 24/A10-derived TCGF (IL–2) activity. Culture supernatants (containing 0.5 percent FCS) of hybridoma cells stimulated for 20 hr with 10 μg/ml Con A were concentrated by $(NH_4)_2SO_4$ precipitation between 45 and 85% (w/v). The dissolved and dialyzed precipitate was fractionated on a 2 × 90 cm Sephadex G–100 column, eluted with phosphate-buffered saline, pH 7.0 and biologically active 5–ml fractions were pooled and concentrated. This material was then chromatographed on a 1.5 × 25 cm DEAE–Sephacel column equilibrated in 0.05 M sodium–phosphate buffer, pH 8.0 with salt gradients from 0.05 to 0.5 M NaCl. 4.5-ml fractions were tested for their O.D.$_{280}$ and biological activity.

by genes in the *I* region of the MHC and antigen-specificity of the T cell population.[80] MAF activity has also been induced by mitogen stimulation of normal murine spleen cell suspensions. Once formed, MAF action on target Mφ is neither antigen-dependent nor MHC-restricted.[81]

MAF has been reported to alter a number of functional and biochemical properties of Mφ. These alterations include increases in endocytic, biosynthetic, and secretory functions as well as alterations of membrane physiology and composition. However, for the purposes of this discussion, the authors wish to define MAF only as the activity that is responsible for induction of Mφ cytocidal activity toward neoplastic cells.

The current generally held concept is that two signals are required to generate Mφ tumoricidal activity.[82,83] MAF is the first signal that primes the Mφ and makes it susceptible to a "triggering" second signal. Second signals are conveyed by a heterogeneous group of substances and can be of endogeneous as well as exogenous origins. To date, the molecular mechanisms involved in the "priming" and "triggering" steps remain unresolved.

The biochemical identity of MAF is uncertain. Molecular weight values ranging from 28,000 to 300,000 daltons have been reported. On the basis of the largest numbers of reports, however, MAF displays an apparent molecular weight of 45,000 to 55,000 daltons.[84] MAF activity is destroyed upon incubation at or below pH 4.0, above pH 10, and upon heating to 80°C. Conflicting reports exist concerning stability at 56°C. The authors own work indicates that MAF is stable to incubation for 1 hr at 56°C but is destroyed upon incubation at 65°C. The question of whether MAF is identical with other lymphokines is unanswered. While reports exist that indicate that MAF is inseparable from migration inhibition factor (MIF) on the basis of molecular weight and buoyant density,[85] at least one group has reported the separation of the two activities.[86]

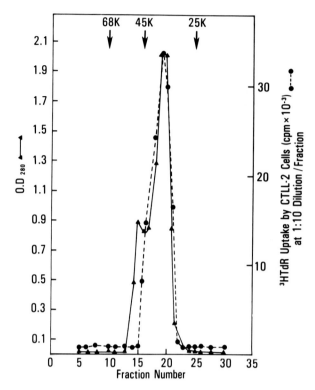

FIGURE 6. Sephadex G–100 gel chromatography of DEAE Sephacel–fractionated TCGF (IL–2) activity derived from T cell hybridoma clone 24/A10. Fractions 16 to 25 recovered from a
DEAE–Sephacel column (See Figure 5) were pooled, concentrated, and rechromatographed on a Sephadex G–100 column.
O.D.$_{280}$ readings and biological activity of 5-ml fractions are
shown.

Partially purified IF preparations have been shown to also induce tumoricidal activity
of Mϕ.[87] Because of similarities in molecular weight, pH sensitivity and heat stability,
the possibility arises that MAF and γ-Interferon (γ-IF) are identical. The answers to
these questions must await biochemical purification of MAF. In the past this has proved
difficult since a large amount of MAF-containing starting material was not available.
The identification of T cell hybridoma clones, to be discussed below, that produce
extraordinary levels of MAF should prove to be a solution to this dilemma. The elucidation of the biochemical identity of MAF will then permit the detailed biochemical
analysis of its mechanism of action on Mϕ and ultimately lead to an understanding of
the in vivo significance of Mϕ effector cell function.

B. MAF Production by T Cell Hybridoma

1. Assays

To screen for the presence of MAF in T cell hybridoma supernatants, the authors
have used a ^{51}Cr-release tumoricidal assay. In this assay 2×10^5 adherent peptone-
elicited peritoneal exudate Mϕ are incubated with MAF sources and excess amounts
of heat-killed *Listeria monocytogenes* as a source of second signal. After 4 hr, the
stimuli are washed off and 2×10^4 ^{51}Cr-labeled P815 mastocytoma cells added. After
incubation for 18 hr at 37°C, the specific amount of ^{51}Cr released into the supernatant

Table 3
DEMONSTRATION OF MAF ACTIVITY SECRETED FROM
CON A-STIMULATED T CELL HYBRIDOMA 24

Dilution of MAF source	Specific P815 lysis (%)			
	24 + Con A[a]	24[b]	Con A[c]	MAF 8080[d]
1/20	51.4	3.9	0.0	49.8
1/100	43.7	N.D.	N.D.	51.1
1/500	4.2	N.D.	N.D.	29.1
1/2500	0.0	N.D.	N.D.	6.8

[a]Hybridoma 24 incubated for 18 hr with 10 μg/ml Con A.
[b]Supernatant of unstimulated hybridoma 24.
[c]Con A at 10 μg/ml.
[d]Splenic MAF.

is determined. One unit of MAF is defined as the amount of MAF required to effect 50% of maximal ^{51}Cr release.

IF was assayed by the cytopathic effect assay which is based on IF-dependent anti-viral activity. Mouse L-cells (clone 929) were incubated for 24 hr with potential sources of IF. The resulting monolayer of cells were then challenged with purified vesicular stomatitis virus and cultured for an additional 48 hr. Viable monolayers and virus-disrupted monolayers were differentiated by light microscopy. One unit of IF is defined as the reciprocal of the dilution that gave 50% protection of the L-cells from virus.

2. Cellular Characteristics of MAF Production by T Cell Hybridoma

Four parental hybridomas were screened for their ability to release MAF. Only one of the four (hybridoma 24) could be identified as a MAF producer. As seen in Table 3, no MAF activity was detected in the unstimulated cell supernatant. However, upon stimulation with Con A or PHA, MAF activities could be demonstrated and titrated out between dilutions of 1/100 to 1/500. The amount of MAF released was dependent on the Con A concentration used during the stimulation. Maximal release was found between Con A concentrations of 10 to 20 μg/ml. Compared to a standard MAF preparation, the uncloned T cell hybridoma 24 displayed 20 to 30% of lymphokine activity. Stimulated culture supernatants of this hybridoma also contained IF activity.

Upon cloning, 27 clones were obtained. None released MAF or IF constitutively. As seen in Figure 7, 24 clones produced MAF when stimulated with 10 μg/ml Con A. At least seven of the clones produced higher MAF levels than the MAF standard. The MAF content of an additional nine clones had not yet been determined by titration and are indicated by the broken bars labeled N.T., >200. The initial screening indicated that these clones displayed greater than 200 MAF U/ml. Ten clones did not produce IF. One of these clones, G1, produced 55,000 U of MAF per milliliter which is 25 times greater than the MAF standard. No correlation was found between IF levels and MAF levels of the various clones. Of particular importance is the fact that clone G1 failed to secrete IF despite the extraordinarily high quantities of MAF it produced. Taken together these results indicate that MAF and IF can be distinguished on the basis of differential production by clones of the T cell hybridoma.

3. Biochemical Analysis of T Cell Hybridoma MAF

The biochemical analysis of MAF produced by the T cell hybridoma clones 24/G1 has just begun. T cell hybridoma MAF is being produced at the rate of 2 l per week

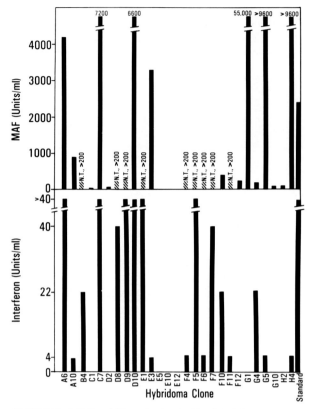

FIGURE 7. MAF and IF production by T cell hybridoma clones.
Levels represent those following stimulation of cultures with 10
µg/ml Con A for 24 hr. Neither MAF nor IF were detectable in
any of the unstimulated culture supernatants. Broken bars represent MAF–containing supernatants identified by screening but not
titrated. These clones contained at least 200 U/ml.

Table 4
COMPARISON OF TEMPERATURE AND pH SENSITIVITIES OF T CELL
HYBRIDOMA MAF AND CONVENTIONAL MAF

Treatment	Original MAF activity (%)	
	T cell hybridoma MAF	Conventional MAF
pH 7.0[a]	100	100
5.0	92	115
4.0	16	18
3.0	16	14
2.0	14	15
4°C[b]	100	100
37°C	100	100
56°C	70	100
65°C	2	2
80°C	0	0

[a]pH treatment by dialysis for 18 hr at 4°C. Samples neutralized by dialysis.
[b]Treatment for 1 hr at the indicated temperatures.

and represents the equivalent in conventional MAF preparations of 4000 mouse equivalents per liter. A comparison of the heat and pH sensitivities of conventional and T cell hybridoma MAF have shown them to be identical. Both are stable to incubation for 1 hr at 56°C but are destroyed upon incubation at 65°C or upon incubation at or below pH 4 for 18 hr at 4°C (Table 4). A comparison of apparent molecular weight on gel permeation columns is currently underway. It is anticipated that this unique reagent will be the source of sufficient amounts of starting material to achieve the purification and identification of MAF.

VI. DISCUSSION AND CONCLUDING REMARKS

Studies described in this communication demonstrate the ability of somatic cell hybrid cell lines, constructed by fusing alloactivated normal T cells with the BW5147 thymoma line, to secrete a number of distinct biological activities, i.e., AEF, TCGF, MAF, and IΓ.

Some of the biologically active mediators, e.g., AEF and TCGF, have been found to be secreted constitutively at low levels and the level of production is increased following stimulation. It is interesting to note that all T cell hybridomas which secrete antigen-specific helper or suppressor factors do so constitutively.[24–36] However, it has not been tested whether production, particularly in the case of the low titer-secreting ones, can be augmented by specific antigen or polyclonal (mitogen) stimulation. In contrast, some,[39–41] but not all[37,38,42] (this chapter as well), of the T cell hybridomas secreting antigen-nonspecific lymphokines are dependent on mitogen stimulation. The reasons for this basic difference are not clear. One possibility to be considered is that the bioassays for antigen-specific factors are much more sensitive than for the antigen–nonspecific ones and thus, antigen-nonspecific lymphokines that may be secreted constitutively can not always be detected by the currently available bioassays. This possibility is supported by findings that indicate that in many cases the biological activity of antigen-specific lymphokines has a much higher titer than that of the antigen-nonspecific ones in conventional preparations. This question may be resolved when direct quantitative assays (e.g., RIAs) of various lymphokines become available.

The studies conducted to date with lymphokine-secreting T cell hybridomas serve to emphasize their usefulness in analyzing some basic unanswered questions regarding the regulation of the immune and hematopoietic systems.

First, such hybridomas enable us to study the relationship between T cells secreting antigen-specific vs. nonspecific lymphokines. Although it is not known whether the same T cell can secrete both types of immunoregulatory activities, there are indications that this may indeed be the case. Thus, in the case of some of the T cell hybridomas secreting nonspecific lymphokines, the normal T cells used for fusion were derived from donors stimulated with specific heterologous[37,40,41] or alloantigens.[37,38] Secondly, cloned antigen-specific T cell hybridomas[88] or TCGF-dependent lines[12] have been found to secrete TCGF and other nonspecific lymphokines[12] upon stimulation with specific antigen in the presence of appropriate antigen-presenting cells. Thus, it is possible that the same T cell, although perhaps at distinct differentiation stages, may secrete both antigen-specific and nonspecific lymphokines.

Secondly, it is not known whether various T cell-derived lymphokines are produced each by a distinct T cell, in "families" of biologically related lymphokines, or all by the same T cell. In addition to various immunoregulatory lymphokines, T cell hybridomas[40,41] or TCGF-dependent lines of cloned T cells[12] have been found to secrete several other molecules that can regulate the differentiation and proliferation of myeloid and erythroid cells. These findings suggest that T cells may exert a broad range of regulatory activities that are not exclusive for the immune system. Moreover, the fact that T cell hybridoma clones produce IF suggests that T cells may secrete molecules that regulate cells outside the reticuloendothelial system. One study[41] suggests that hybridoma variants can be obtained that secrete only TCGF but not CSF. The authors' preliminary studies also suggest that it is possible to select subclones that selectively secrete a given lymphokine. Thus, by analyzing various cloned T cell hybridomas it may be possible to determine whether the genetic machinery for the production of only one, some, or all lymphokines exists in a given T cell. In practical terms, the availability of hybridoma clones selectively secreting one lymphokine will facilitate the purification of such lymphokine free of other lymphokine contaminants.

Additionally, if a cloned T cell hybridoma proves to secrete simultaneously distinct lymphokine activities, it remains to be determined whether the production of different lymphokines is causally related or reflects independent events. For example, it has been shown recently that TCGF-induced development of CTL responses requires IF production.[89] One could, therefore, use the lymphokine-secreting T cell hybridomas to ascertain how various signals modulate the production of biological activities and whether a signal affecting the production of a given lymphokine will simultaneously affect the other ones secreted by the same hybridoma.

Finally, the availability of monoclonal cellular reagents secreting a variety of regulatory molecules provides a convenient tool for molecular genetics studies on such molecules. Thus, the study of these T cell hybridomas will eventually clarify many of the unresolved questions pertaining to the regulation of the reticuloendothelial as well as other systems of the multicellular organism.

ACKNOWLEDGMENTS

We gratefully acknowledge R. Weiner, A. Sferruzza, and P.–M. Paris for their excellent help in performing the experiments described herein and Rebecca Mead for typing this manuscript. This is publication no. 2505 from the Immunology Departments, Research Institute of Scripps Clinic, La Jolla, Calif. This work was supported by USPHS Grants CA-24911, CA-25803, AI-07007 and AI-17354. Altman and Schreiber are recipients of an American Cancer Society, Inc. Junior Faculty Research Award JFRA-17 and an American Heart Association, Inc. Established Investigatorship 77-202, respectively.

REFERENCES

1. **Katz, D. H.**, *Lymphocyte Differentiation, Recognition and Regulation*, Academic Press, New York, 1977.
2. **Altman, A. and Katz, D. H.**, Production and isolation of helper and suppressive factors, *J. Immunol. Methods*, 38, 9, 1980.
3. **Hirai, Y. and Nisonoff, A.**, Selective suppression of the major idiotypic component of an antihapten response by soluble T cell-derived factors with idiotypic or anti-idiotypic receptors, *J. Exp. Med.*, 151, 1213, 1980.
4. **Tada, T., Taniguchi, M., and Okumura, K.**, Regulation of antibody response by antigen-specific T cell factors bearing *I* region determinants, *Prog. Immunol.*, 3, 369, 1977.
5. **Taniguchi, M. and Tokuhisa, T.**, Cellular consequences in the suppression of antibody response by the antigen-specific T-cell factor, *J. Exp. Med.*, 151, 517, 1980.
6. **Mudawwar, F. B., Yunis, E. J., and Geha, R. S.**, Antigen-specific helper factor in man, *J. Exp. Med.*, 140, 1032, 1970.

7. **Kilburn, D. G., Talbot, F. O., Teh, H.-S., and Levy, J. G.,** A specific helper factor which enhances the cytotoxic response to a syngeneic tumor, *Nature (London)*, 277, 474, 1979.
8. **Tada, T. and Okumura, K.,** The role of antigen-specific T cell factors in the immune response, *Adv. Immunol.*, 28, 1, 1979.
9. **Morgan, D. A., Ruscetti, F. W., and Gallo, R.,** Selective *in vitro* growth of T lymphocytes from normal human bone marrows, *Science*, 193, 1007, 1976.
10. **Gillis, S. and Smith, K. A.,** Long term culture of tumour-specific cytotoxic T cells, *Nature (London)*, 268, 154, 1977.
11. **Aarden, L. A. et al.,** Letter to the editor, revised nomenclature for antigen-nonspecific T cell proliferation and helper factors, *J. Immunol.*, 123, 2928, 1979.
12. **Schreier, M. H. and Iscove, N. N.,** Haematopoietic growth factors are released in cultures of *H-2*-restricted helper T cells, accessory cells and specific antigen, *Nature (London)*, 287, 228, 1980.
13. **Farrar, J. J., Fuller-Farrar, J., Simon, P. L., Hilfiker, M. L., Stadler, B. M., and Farrar, W. L.,** Thymoma production of T cell growth factor (Interleukin 2), *J. Immunol.*, 125, 2555, 1980.
14. **Gillis, S., Scheid, M., and Watson, J.,** Biochemical and biologic characterization of lymphocyte regulatory molecules. III. The isolation and phenotypic characterization of Interleukin-2 producing T cell lymphomas, *J. Immunol.*, 125, 2570, 1980.
15. **Shimizu, S., Konaka, Y., and Smith, R. T.,** Mitogen-initiated synthesis and secretion of T cell growth factor(s) by a T-lymphoma cell line, *J. Exp. Med.*, 152, 1436, 1980.
16. **Smith, K. A., Gilbride, K. J., and Favata, M. F.,** Lymphocyte activating factor promotes T-cell growth factor production by cloned murine lymphoma cells, *Nature (London)*, 287, 853, 1980.
17. **MacDonald, A. B., Fraser, C. E. O., and Rubin, A. S.,** Isolation and partial characterization of an antibody enhancing factor from leukaemic owl monkey cell cultures, *Immunology*, 34, 137, 1978.
18. **Gillis, S. and Watson, J.,** Biochemical and biological characterization of lymphocyte regulatory molecules. V. Identification of an interleukin 2-producing human leukemia T cell line, *J. Exp. Med.*, 152, 1709, 1980.
19. **Ruscetti, F. W. and Gallo, R. C.,** Human T-lymphocyte growth factor: regulation of growth and function of T lymphocytes, *Blood*, 57, 379, 1981.
20. **Köhler, G. and Milstein, C.,** Continuous cultures of fused cells secreting antibody of a predefined specificity, *Nature (London)*, 256, 495, 1975.
21. **Hämmerling, G. J.,** T lymphocyte tissue culture lines produced by cell hybridization, *Eur. J. Immunol.*, 7, 743, 1977.
22. **Goldsby, R. A., Osborne, B. A., Simpson, E., and Herzenberg, L. A.,** Hybrid cell lines with T-cell characteristics, *Nature (London)*, 267, 707, 1977.
23. **Köhler, G., Lefkovits, I., Elliott, B., and Coutinho, A.,** Derivation of hybrids between a thymoma line and spleen cells activated in a mixed leukocyte reaction, *Eur. J. Immunol.* 7, 758, 1977.
24. **Kontiainen, S., Simpson, E., Bohrer, E., Beverley, P. C. L., Herzenberg, L. A., Fitzpatrick, W. C., Vogt, P., Torano, A., McKenzie, I. F. C., and Feldmann, M.,** T-cell lines producing antigen-specific suppressor factor, *Nature (London)*, 274, 477, 1978.
25. **Taniguchi, M. and Miller, J. F. A. P.,** Specific suppressive factors produced by hybridomas derived from the fusion of enriched suppressor T cells and a T lymphoma cell line, *J. Exp. Med.*, 148, 373, 1978.
26. **Taussig, M. J. and Holliman, A.,** Structure of an antigen-specific suppressor factor produced by a hybrid T-cell line, *Nature (London)*, 277, 308, 1979.
27. **Taussig, M. J., Corvalan, J. R. F., Binns, R. M., Roser, B., and Holliman, A.,** Immunological activity of a T hybrid line. I. Production of an *H-2*-related suppressor factor with specificity for sheep red blood cells, *Eur. J. Immunol.*, 9, 768, 1979.
28. **Taussig, M. J., Corvalan, J. R. F., Binns, R. M., and Holliman, A.,** Production of an *H-2*-related suppressor factor by a hybrid T-cell line, *Nature (London)*, 277, 305, 1979.
29. **Hewitt, J. and Liew, F. Y.,** Antigen-specific suppressor factors produced by T cell hybridomas for delayed-type hypersensitivity, *Eur. J. Immunol.*, 9, 572, 1979.
30. **Taniguchi, M., Saito, T., and Tada, T.,** Antigen-specific suppressive factor produced by a transplantable I-J bearing T-cell hybridoma, *Nature (London)*, 278, 555, 1979.
31. **Taniguchi, M., Takei, I., and Tada, T.,** Functional and molecular organisation of an antigen-specific suppressor factor from a T cell hybridoma, *Nature (London)*, 283, 227, 1980.
32. **Nelson, K., Cory, J., Hellström, I., and Hellström, K. E.,** T-T hybridoma product specifically suppresses tumor immunity, *Proc. Natl. Acad. Sci. U.S.A.*, 77, 2866, 1980.
33. **Eshhar, Z., Apte, R. N., Löwy, I., Ben-Neriah, Y., Givol, D., and Mozes, E.,** T-cell hybridoma bearing heavy chain variable region determinants producing (T,G)–A—L-specific helper factor, *Nature, (London)*, 286, 170, 1980.

34. **Goodman, J. W., Lewis, G. K., Primi, D., Hornbeck, P., and Ruddle, N. H.,** Antigen-specific molecules from murine T lymphocytes and T cell hybridomas, *Mol. Immunol.,* 17, 933, 1980.
35. **Kapp, J. A., Araneo, B. A., and Clevinger, B. L.,** Suppression of antibody and T cell proliferative responses to L-glutamic acid^{60}-L-alaine^{30}-L-tyrosine^{10} by a specific monoclonal T cell factor, *J. Exp. Med.,* 152, 235, 1980.
36. **Lonai, P., Puri, J., and Hämmerling, G.,** *H-2*-restricted antigen binding by a hybridoma clone that produces antigen-specific helper factor, *Proc. Natl. Acad. Sci. U.S.A.,* 78, 549, 1981.
37. **Neuport-Sautes, C., Rabourdin-Combe, C., and Fridman, W. H.,** T-cell hybrids bear Fcγ receptors and secrete suppressor immunoglobulin binding factor, *Nature (London),* 277, 656, 1979.
38. **Katz, D. H., Bechtold, T. E., and Altman, A.,** Construction of T cell hybridomas secreting allogeneic effect factor (AEF), *J. Exp. Med.,* 152, 956, 1980.
39. **Harwell, L., Skidmore, B., Marrack, P., and Kappler, J.,** Concanavalin A-inducible, interleukin-2-producing T cell hybridoma, *J. Exp. Med.,* 152, 893, 1980.
40. **Schrader, J. W., Arnold, B., and Clark-Lewis, I.,** A Con A-stimulated T-cell hybridoma releases factors affecting haematopoietic colony-forming cells and B-cell antibody responses, *Nature (London),* 283, 197, 1980.
41. **Schrader, J. W. and Clark-Lewis, I.,** T cell hybridoma-derived regulatory factors. I. Production of T cell growth factor following stimulation by concanavalin A, *J. Immunol.,* 126, 1101, 1981.
42. **Stull, D. and Gillis, S.,** Constitutive production of Interleukin 2 activity by a T cell hybridoma, *J. Immunol.,* 126, 1680, 1981.
43. **Watanabe, T., Kimoto, M., Maruyama, S., Kishimoto, T., and Yamamura, Y.,** Regulation of antibody response in different immunoglobulin classes. V. Establishment of T hybrid cell line secreting IgE class-specific suppressor factor, *J. Immunol.,* 121, 2113, 1978.
44. **Armerding, D. and Katz, D. H.,** Activation of T and B lymphocytes *in vitro.* II. Biological and biochemical properties of an allogeneic effect factor (AEF) active in triggering specific B lymphocytes, *J. Exp. Med.,* 140, 19, 1974.
45. **Eshhar, Z., Armerding, D., Waks, T., and Katz, D. H.,** Activation of T and B lymphocytes *in vitro.* V. Cellular locus, metabolism and genetics of induction and production of the allogeneic effect factor, *J. Immunol.,* 119, 1457, 1977.
46. **Altman, A., Cardenas, J. M., Bechtold, T. E., and Katz, D. H.,** The biological effects of allogeneic effect factor on T lymphocytes. I. The mitogenic activity and the autonomous induction of cytotoxic T lymphocytes by AEF, *J. Immunol.,* 124, 105, 1980.
47. **Altman, A. and Katz, D. H.,** Stimulation of autoreactive T lymphocytes by allogeneic effect factor (AEF): relevance to normal pathways of lymphocyte differentiation, *Immunol. Rev.,* 51, 3, 1980.
48. **Altman, A., Cardenas, J. M., Welsh, R. M., Jr., and Katz, D. H.,** The biological effects of allogeneic effect factor on T lymphocytes. III. Interferon does not contribute to the biological activities displayed by AEF on both T and B lymphocytes, *Ann. Immunol.,* 131C, 335, 1980.
49. **Armerding, D., Sachs, D. H., and Katz, D. H.,** Activation of T and B lymphocytes *in vitro.* III. Presence of *Ia* determinants on allogeneic effect factor (AEF), *J. Exp. Med.,* 140, 1717, 1974.
50. **Armerding, D., Kubo, R. T., Grey, H. M., and Katz, D. H.,** Activation of T and B lymphocytes *in vitro:* presence of β$_2$-microglobulin determinants on allogeneic effect factor, *Proc. Natl. Acad. Sci. U.S.A.,* 72, 4577, 1975.
51. **Armerding, D., Eshhar, Z., and Katz, D. H.,** Activation of T and B lymphocytes *in vitro.* VI. Biochemical and physiochemical characterization of the allogeneic effect factor, *J. Immunol.,* 119, 1468, 1977.
52. **Altman, A., Bechtold, T. E., Cardenas, J. M., and Katz, D. H.,** The biological effects of allogeneic effect factor on T lymphocytes: *in vitro* induction of cytotoxic T lymphocytes manifesting preferential lytic activity against *H-2*-identical tumor cells, *Proc. Natl. Acad. Sci. U.S.A.,* 76, 3477, 1979.
53. **Altman, A., Cardenas, J. M., Bechtold, T. E., and Katz, D. H.,** The biological effects of allogeneic effect factor on T lymphocytes. II. The specificity of AEF induced cytotoxic T lymphocytes, *J. Immunol.,* 124, 114, 1980.
54. **Altman, A. and Katz, D. H.,** Existence of T cells manifesting self-reactivity indistinguishable from alloreactivity, *J. Immunol.,* 125, 1536, 1980.
55. **Altman, A., Gilmartin, T. D., and Katz, D. H.,** Bone marrow stem cell differentiation *in vitro:* promotion of long term growth by a soluble lymphocyte-derived mediator, *Science,* 211, 65, 1980.
56. **Watson, J. and Mochizuki, D.,** Interleukin 2: a class of T cell growth factors, *Immunol. Rev.,* 51, 257, 1980.
57. **Smith, K. A.,** T cell growth factor, *Immunol. Rev.,* 51, 337, 1980.
58. **Watson, J., Mochizuki, D., and Gillis, S.,** T-cell growth factors: Interleukin 2, *Immunology Today,* 1, 113, 1980.

59. **Altman, A.,** T-cell growth factor (Interleukin 2), *Immunology Today,* 2, 1, 1981.
60. **Gillis, S., Ferm, M. M., Ou, W., and Smith, K. A.,** T cell growth factor: parameters of production and a quantitative microassay for activity, *J. Immunol.,* 120, 2027, 1978.
61. **Gillis, S., Union, N. A., Baker, P. E., and Smith, K. A.,** The *in vitro* generation and sustained culture of nude mouse cytolytic T-lymphocytes, *J. Exp. Med.,* 149, 1460, 1979.
62. **Hunig, T. and Bevan, M. J.,** Specificity of cytotoxic T cells from athymic mice, *J. Exp. Med.,* 152, 688, 1980.
63. **Gillis, S. and Watson, J.,** Interleukin-2 induction of hapten-specific cytolytic T cells in nude mice, *J. Immunol.,* 126, 1245, 1981.
64. **Wagner, H., Hardt, C., Heeg, K., Rollinghoff, M., and Pfizenmaier, K.,** T cell derived helper factor (Interleukin 2) allows the *in vivo* induction of cytotoxic T cells in thymus deficient nu/nu mice, *Nature (London),* 284, 278, 1980.
65. **Stotter, H., Rude, E., and Wagner, H.,** T cell factor (Interleukin 2) allows *in vivo* induction of T helper cells against heterologous erythrocytes in athymic (nu/nu) mice, *Eur. J. Immunol.,* 10, 719, 1980.
66. **Reimann, J. and Diamantstein, T.,** Interleukin-2 allows *in vivo* induction of anti-erythrocyte autoantibody production in nude mice associated with the injection of rat erythrocytes, *Clin. Exp. Immunol.,* 43, 641, 1981.
67. **Gery, I., Gershon, R. K., and Waksman, B. H.,** Potentiation of the lymphocyte response to mitogens. I. The responding cell. *J. Exp. Med.,* 136, 218, 1972.
68. **Mackaness, G. B.,** Cellular immunity, in *Mononuclear Phagocytes,* van Furth, R. Ed., Oxford University Press, New York, 1970, 641.
69. **Murray, H. W. and Cohn, Z. A.,** Macrophage oxygen-dependent antimicrobial activity. III. Enhanced oxidative metabolism as an expression of macrophage activation, *J. Exp. Med.,* 152, 1596, 1980.
70. **Nogueira, N. and Cohn, Z. A.,** *Trypanosoma cruzi:* An *in vitro* induction of macrophage microbicidal activity, *J. Exp. Med.,* 148, 288, 1978.
71. **Granger, G. A. and Weiser, R. S.,** Homograft target cells: specific destruction *in vitro* by contact interaction with immune macrophages, *Science,* 145, 1427, 1964.
72. **Evans, R., and Alexander, P.,** Cooperation of immune lymphoid cells with macrophages in tumor immunity, *Nature (London),* 228, 620, 1970.
73. **Hibbs, J. B., Lambert, L. H., and Remington, J. S.,** Resistance to murine tumors conferred by chronic infection with intracellular protozoa *Toxoplasma gondii* and *Binsonita jellisoni, J. Infect. Dis.,* 124, 587, 1971.
74. **Cleveland, R. P., Meltzer, M. S., and Zbar, B.,** Tumor cytotoxicity *in vitro* by macrophages from mice infected with *Mycobacterum bovis* strain BCG, *J. Natl. Cancer Inst.,* 52, 1887, 1974.
75. **North, R. J.,** The concept of the activated macrophage, *J. Immunol.,* 121, 806, 1978.
76. **Karnovsky, M. L. and Lazdino, J. K.,** Biochemical criteria for activated macrophages, *J. Immunol.,* 121, 809, 1978.
77. **Cohn, Z. A.,** The activity of mononuclear phagocytes: fact, fancy and future, *J. Immunol.,* 121, 813, 1978.
78. **Russell, S. W., Gillespie, G. Y., and Pace, J. L.,** Evidence for mononuclear phagocytes in solid neoplasms and appraisal of their nonspecific cytotoxic capabilities, in *Contemporary Topics in Immunobiology,* Vol. 10, Witz, I. P. and Hanna, M. G., Eds., Plenum Press, New York, 1980, 143.
79. **Ruco, L. P. and Meltzer, M. S.,** Macrophage activation for tumor cytotoxicity. Induction of tumoricidal macrophages by supernatants of PPD-stimulated bacillus Calmette-Guerin-immune spleen cell culture, *J. Immunol.,* 119, 889, 1977.
80. **Farr, A. G., Wechter, W. J., Kiely, J.-M., and Unanue, E. R.,** Induction of cytocidal macrophages following *in vitro* interactions between Listeria-immune T cells and macrophages: role of *H-2, J. Immunol.,* 122, 2405, 1979.
81. **Fidler, I. J.,** Activation *in vitro* of mouse macrophages by syngeneic, allogeneic or xenogeneic lymphocyte supernatants, *J. Natl. Cancer Inst.,* 55, 1159, 1975.
82. **Weinberg, J. B., Chapman, H. A. and Hibbs, J. B.,** Characterization of the effect of endotoxin on macrophage tumor cell killing, *J. Immunol.,* 121, 72, 1978.
83. **Ruco, L. P. and Meltzer, M. S.,** Macrophage activation for tumor cytotoxicity: development of macrophage cytotoxic activity requires completion of a sequence of short-lived intermediary reactions, *J. Immunol.,* 121, 2035, 1978.
84. **Leonard, E. J., Ruco, L. P., and Meltzer, M. S.,** Characterization of macrophage activation factor, a lymphokine that causes macrophages to become cytotoxic for tumor cells, *Cell. Immunol.,* 41, 347, 1978.

85. **Nathan, C. F., Remold, H. G., and David, J. R.,** Characterization of a lymphocyte factor which alters macrophage functions, *J. Exp. Med.,* 137, 275, 1973.

86. **Kniep, E. M., Kickhofen, B., and Fischer, H.,** Macrophage cytotoxicity factor purification and separation from MIF, in *Biochemical Characterization of Lymphokines,* de Weck, A. L., Kristensen, F., and Landy, M., Eds., Academic Press, New York, 1980, 149.

87. **Schultz, R. M.,** Macrophage activation by interferons, in *Lymphokine Reports,* Vol. 1, Pick, E., Ed., Landy, M., Advisory Ed., Academic Press, New York, 1980, 63.

88. **Kappler, J., Skidmore, B., White, J., and Marrack, P.,** Antigen-inducible *H-2*-restricted, interleukin-2-producing T cell hybridomas. Lack of independent antigen and *H-2* recognition, *J. Exp. Med.,* 153, 1198, 1981.

89. **Farrar, W. L., Johnson, H. M., and Farrar, J. J.,** Regulation of the production of immune interferon and cytotoxic T lymphocytes by Interleukin 2, *J. Immunol.,* 126, 1120, 1981.

90. **Altman, A. and Haas, M.,** Manuscript in preparation.

91. **Altman, A., Sferruzza, A., Weiner, R. G., and Katz, D. H.,** Constitutive and mitogen-induced production of T cell growth factor by stable T cell hybridoma lines, *J. Immunol.,* 128, 1365, 1982.

92. **Altman, A., Gilmartin, T. D., and Katz, D. H.,** Unpublished observations.

93. **Schreiber, R. D., Altman, A., and Katz, D. H.,** Identification of a T cell hybridoma which produces extraordinary quantities of macrophage activating factor, *J. Exp. Med.,* in press.

Chapter 7

FUNCTIONAL T CELL HYBRIDOMAS PRODUCING ANTIGEN-SPECIFIC IMMUNOREGULATORY FACTORS

Zelig Eshhar

TABLE OF CONTENTS

I. Introduction 134

II. Generation of T Cell Hybridomas 135
   A. Choice of Lymphoma Line 135
   B. Enhancement of the Frequency of Functional Hybridomas by
      Enrichment of Activated T Lymphocytes 135
   C. Selection Strategy for Antigen–Specific Functional Hybridomas ...137

III. Monoclonal T Cell–Derived Soluble Factors That Mediate Specific
   T Helper Cell Function 138
   A. (T,G)-A--L-Specific Helper Factor Replacing T Cells in
      Antibody Response 138
   B. Establishment of R-9, (T,G)–A--L–Specific Hybrid Line
      Expressing Surface V_H Determinants 139
      1. Fine Antigenic Specificity of R-9–Derived ThF. 140
      2. Possession by the (T,G)–A--L–Specific R-9 Factor
         of V Region–Like and MHC–Encoded Determinants 141
   C. Production of CGG–Specific ThF by T Cell Hybridoma 143
   D. Production of Factors Augmenting T Cell–Dependent Help in
      Antibody Responses by T Cell Hybridoma 143

IV. Suppressor T Cell Factors—Generation and Characterization of Hybrid
   Lines Producing Antigen–Specific Suppressor Factor(s) 144
   A. TsF Specific to Protein Antigens and SRBC 144
   B. TsF Specific to Synthetic Polypeptide Antigens 147
      1. GAT– and GT–Specific TsF 147
      2. (T,G)–A--L–Specific Suppressor T Cell Hybridoma 147
   C. TsF Specific to Defined Haptenic Groups 148
      1. ABA–Specific T Cell Hybridomas 149
      2. NP–Specific T Cell Hybridomas 149

V. Molecular Organization of Monoclonal T Cell Factors and Its
   Relationship to the T Cell Receptor 150
   A. Id and V_H Determinants on T Cell Factors 150
   B. Comparison Between the T Cell Factor and Antibody–Binding Site 151
   C. Association of MHC Gene Products in the T Cell Factors 152
   D. Molecular Organization of T Cell Factors 152
   E. Structural Scheme for Antigen-Specific *Ia*–Bearing T Cell Factors 155
   F. Comparison of T Cell Factors and Receptors 157

VI.   Mechanism(s) of T Cell Factor Activity 158
       A.   Genetic Restriction of Factor Activity 158
       B.   Site(s) of Factor Interaction 159
             1.   Helper Factors 160
             2.   Suppressor Factors 160

VII.   Concluding Remarks 162

Acknowledgment 164

References 164

I. INTRODUCTION

Helper and suppressor cells that regulate the function of effector cells play a central role either by cell–to–cell interaction or by soluble macromolecular factor(s) in the control mechanism of immunological responses. Over the past few years it has been shown that such immunoregulatory helper and suppressor cells belong to different subsets of T lymphocytes, are equipped with receptors for antigens and are capable of recognizing autologous MHC–encoded molecules.

As a consequence of antigenic stimulation in vitro, activated T cells release factor(s) that can specifically replace the T cells' regulatory function in the process of antibody production. Currently there is much evidence indicating that factors that function in an antigen–specific manner bind antigen with specificity comparable to that of antibodies. However, they do not contain Ig–constant structures, but possess determinants that are similar to heavy chain variable region *(V_H)* gene products. Factors manifesting different regulatory activities exhibit distinct *I* subregion encoded determinants such as helper factors bearing *I–A* and suppressor factors *I–J*. Recent comprehensive reviews[1–5] summarize the information concerning antigen–specific factors that has been accumulated during the last 10 years since the report about the first antigen-specific factor.[6]

Although the mode of action of the soluble immunoregulatory mediators and their physiological role is not well–understood, the factors usually considered as the soluble analogues of the T cell receptor can serve as an invaluable functional source for studies and characterization of the antigen recognition unit of T cells. The chemical approach aimed at purifying and analyzing the T cell factors has been hampered, however, by the minute amounts of active material recovered from the heterogenous cell population serving to produce the factors. To overcome this and other limitations and to immortalize functional T cells, various approaches have been attempted recently, such as somatic cell hybridization,[7–15] viral transformation,[16] and establishment of continuous lines dependent on constant antigenic stimulation or supply of TCGF.[17–19]

In this chapter the author shall review the recent attempts to establish T cell hybridomas producing antigen–specific helper or suppressor factors. The information gathered from several model systems will be compared and discussed with particular regard to the nature of the T cell receptor. Upon stimulation with antigen, activated T cells also release nonspecific immunoregulatory mediators in addition to the antigen–specific factors. These factors are the subject of another chapter in this volume (Altman, Schreiber, and Katz), therefore this account shall be restricted to antigen–specific factors only.

II. GENERATION OF T CELL HYBRIDOMAS

The first report describing the successful establishment of functional T hybridomas was by Parkman and Merler,[20] who fused mouse thymocytes and fibroblasts. They found that some of the hybrid cell lines were capable of acting as helper T cells in the restoration of irradiated and BM–reconstituted mice in the production of PFC. However, no continuation of this study was reported and it was only after the successful generation of B cell hybridomas producing mAbs by Köhler and Milstein[21] that many attempts were made to establish functional T cell hybridomas. The initial experiments[7,8] did not yield active hybridomas because there was most likely inadequate fusion with the partner tumor cell line and insufficient enrichment of the functional T cell partners that were not in the right activation stage to allow fusion. However, more recent attempts to establish functional hybridomas appeared fruitful,[9–15,22,23] mainly due to the improved fusion technology employing various T lymphoma lines and the use of PEG as fusing agent, the use of enriched populations of T lymphocytes, and the employment of sensitive, fast, and reliable assay systems that permitted selection of active hybrid clones.

A. Choice of Lymphoma Line

The initial failure to establish functional T cell hybridomas raised the possibility of inherited repression imposed on the activated lymphocyte by the tumor cell fusion partner. It now appears that few tumor cell lines can yield active hybridomas. Table 1 lists the lymphoma lines that served as the tumor partner in successful fusion experiments. The most common is the AKR/J–derived thymoma line BW5147, that was derived by Hyman at the Salk Institute. This cell line served in fusions yielding functional hybridomas that manifested specific suppression,[9–13] helper,[14,15] and cytotoxic[22,23] activities. The functional diversity of hybrid clones derived from the BW5147 line implies that BW cells can be used to immortalize different activities. Nonetheless, additional tumor lines that would improve the yield and activity of the resulting hybridomas or result in preferential fusion of certain functional T cells subsets would be advantageous.

B. Enhancement of the Frequency of Functional Hybridomas by Enrichment of Activated T Lymphocytes

Since there are few active T cells in a population of immune lymphocytes, it is crucial to enrich the activated cells prior to fusion. Because of their avid antigen–binding receptors, specific T–suppressor subpopulations can be purified on antigen–coated columns, petri dishes,[10,11,26,27] and on RBC (by rosetting).[26,27] As surface antigens are expressed preferentially by certain subsets of functional T lymphocytes, they can be differentiated by antibody stains. Thus, Taniguchi and collaborators[10,12] stained *I–J*–bearing suppressor cells and hybridomas with fluorescent anti–*I–J* antibodies and selected positively stained cells with FACS.

Furthermore, the differentiation stage of the T lymphocytes affects their tendency to undergo fusion and dictates the activity of the resultant hybridomas. The selected activation of certain subsets of regulatory or effector T cells is dependent on the mode of antigen presentation and use of adjuvants. Thus, T cells activated prior to fusion with large doses of soluble antigens, hapten–modified syngeneic cells, or autologous Ig, yielded suppressor hybridomas,[9–13] whereas T cells activated in the presence of adjuvant and stimulated in vitro by antigen–bearing adherent cells, yielded helper hybridomas.[14] A scheme of the procedure used for the establishment of (T,G)–A--L–specific helper T cell hybridomas is shown in Figure 1. T cells were first activated to antigen ((T,G)–A--L) in irradiated recipient mice. After a week, the activated cells harvested

Table 1
TUMOR CELL LINES USED FOR FUSION WITH T CELLS

Cell line	Characteristics	Surface antigens	Ref.
BW5147	AKR/J thymoma; HGPRT[−(a)]	Thy1.1; H-2^k; Ly1$^-$, 2$^-$, 3$^-$, 6$^+$	R. Hyman, Salk Institute
EL-4	C57BL/6 T lymphoma; TK[−(b)]	Thy1.2; H-2^b; Ly2$^+$	24
L5178	DBA/2 leukemia; HGPRT[−(a)]	Thy1.2; H-2^d,	25
AKR-A	AKR/J thymoma; HGPRT[−(b)]	Thy1.1; H-2^k	23 (Herberman, NIH)

[a]Hypoxanthine: guanine phosphorylosyl transferase deficient line (grows in the presence of 8-azoguanine, dies in the presence of aminopterin).
[b]Thymidine kinase deficient line (grows in the presence of bromodeoxyuracil, dies in aminopterin).

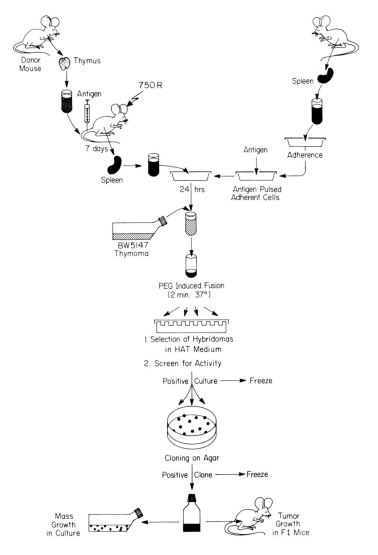

FIGURE 1. Scheme for the activation of antigen–specific T cells and establishment of hybrid clones.

from the spleens of the mice were rechallenged on antigen–bearing splenic adherent cells, a procedure that has been found to potentiate activated cells.[28] After overnight incubation, the enriched and activated T cells were fused in a 1:1 ratio with BW cells, with PEG as the fusing agent.[14]

C. Selection Strategy for Antigen–Specific Functional Hybridomas

The screening procedure to select for the few active hybridomas among the many hybrid cultures usually obtained following fusion must be fast and simple enough to allow screening of many samples, and must be unequivocal. In principle, the methods mentioned above that serve to enrich activated T cells can also be employed for selecting the antigen–reactive hybrid cells. Thus, suppressor hybrids bearing *I–J* determinants were sorted out by the cell sorter[10,12] and antigen–binding hybrid cells were identified and separated from the rest of the cells by their ability to bind to antigen–coated plates,[26,27] or by the rosetting technique.[26,27]

While suppressor T cells bind nominal antigen with high avidity, helper T cells do not. However, helper T cells do bind antigens that were previously "processed" by Mφ.[29,30] Such processed antigens consist of fragments of the antigen complexed with "self" *I*–subregion gene products. Lonai et al.[15] have recently used radiolabeled processed antigen (*Ia*–associated antigen complex) to identify and enumerate specific chicken gamma globulins (CGC)–binding helper hybridomas.

Hybrid cells or their culture supernate can be used for functional assays, although the assay of cell–free supernates is easier and more convenient. The most common assay for helper cell function or factor activity is the in vitro antibody production assay,[31] a microculture modification of the Mishell–Dutton system. In this assay system, the ability of the factor to replace carrier–primed helper cells and provide help to hapten-primed spleen cells is measured after 4 to 5 days of incubation in culture. Likewise, the suppressor factor activity is determined by the ability of hybridoma supernates to specifically inhibit antibody production of primed spleen cells in vitro.[31] The most common assay employs a factor directed at a specific protein carrier that suppresses the antibody response elicited by the hapten–protein conjugate.[9,10,12] The preferential suppression of some antibody classes by certain antigen–specific factors[32,36] can be attributed to specific suppression of class–specific helper T cells, as reported for the allotype suppression phenomenon.[37] Another system where both suppressor cells and factors inhibited the activity of effector T cells is in delayed type hypersensitivity (DTH) response.[38-41] Hewitt and Liew[13] generated T cell hybridomas producing factors that suppress DTH responses to SRBC. They could differentiate between factors that specifically suppressed the induction phase and factors that suppressed the elicitation phase of DTH. Another T cell response that is impeded by hybridoma–derived T cell factor is the antigen–specific lymphoproliferative response. Recently, Kapp et al.[42] have generated GAT–specific suppressor hybridomas that produced factors that inhibited both antibody responses and proliferation of GAT–primed cells. Finally, stimulated T cell hybridomas can be detected because they secrete nonspecific lymphokines, which affects Mφ function–like MIF and MAF to become cytotoxic.[43]

III. MONOCLONAL T CELL–DERIVED SOLUBLE FACTORS THAT MEDIATE SPECIFIC T HELPER CELL FUNCTION

Antigen–specific helper factors (ThF) have been studied in fewer systems and are less common than the suppressor factors (TsF), mainly due to the fact that it is more difficult to enrich specifically and monitor the helper cells and their responses. The avidity of antigen binding to helper cells is very low and occurs only in the presence of "self"–*Ia* antigens.[29,30] In addition, when activated T cells are challenged with antigen, they may mask specific ThF activity by releasing nonspecific T cell replacing factor(s) (TRF)[44] together with a specific helper factor.

Two types of antigen–specific T cell factors that finally augment the B cell response have been described. One is the ThF that can replace the function of the antigen–specific helper T cell.[5,45-47] The second class is the T cell augmenting factor (TaF) that augments the antibody response only in the presence of helper T cells.[48]

A. (T,G)–A--L–Specific Helper Factor Replacing T Cells in Antibody Response

Taussig and Munro[45,49,50] and Mozes and co–workers[5,46,51,52] carried out most of the studies on "conventional" ThF. They mainly studied the antibody response to the branched polypeptide (T,G)–A--L in animals, while the group of Howie, Feldmann, and coworkers[4,47,53] mainly studied the responses to (T,G)–A--L in vitro. The Ir to (T,G)–A--L,[54] the most studied branched–synthetic polypeptide antigen, is genetically

Table 2
PROPERTIES OF (T,G)-A--L-SPECIFIC ThF PREPARED IN IN VIVO OR IN VITRO SYSTEMS

1. Released into the culture supernate of in vivo and in vitro activated T cells upon restimulation with (T,G)-A--L.
2. Bind specifically to (T,G)-A--L affinity columns and the activity can be recovered in the eluates.
3. Help BM cells in adoptive transfer and unprimed or hapten primed B cells in vitro in antibody responses.
4. React with target B cells (and probably Mφ) that exhibit appropriate acceptor site.
5. Ir genes control the production and/or acceptance by B cells of the ThF signal.
6. T cells of low responder H-2^k mice produce active factor that interacts with B cells across H-2 barrier.
7. Carry I-A-subregion–coded determinants.
8. Do not express Ig constant region determinants, but variable region framework (V_H) and Id–like determinants.
9. Glycoprotein with molecular weights of 50,000 to 70,000 that may be composed of two chains.

controlled by Ir genes located within the I-A subregion of the MHC.[55,56] The "conventional" (T,G)-A--L–specific ThF studied by Taussig and Mozes, was derived from T cells that had been activated to (T,G)-A--L in irradiated recipient mice and then removed and cultured in the presence of antigen. The helper activity of the cell–free supernates was analyzed by their ability to help BM cells to exercise anti–(T,G)-A--L response in adoptive transfer experiments.

The (T,G)-A--L–specific ThF, studied by Howie and Feldman,[47,53] was prepared from spleen cells that were primed in vitro for four days with a low dose of (T,G)-A--L (1 μg/ml), harvested and then cultured with fresh antigen. They analyzed the helper function of the cell–free supernates by co–culturing the factor with unprimed spleen or B cells plus (T,G)-A--L or TNP–(T,G)-A--L and monitoring the development of specific IgM PFC. It is notable that the overall effect and properties of the (T,G)-A--L–specific ThF prepared in different ways, were similar. The properties of the "conventional" (T,G)-A--L–specific ThF are summarized in Table 2. The following common properties can be outlined: both factors are secreted from activated T cells, they bind to and assist unprimed B cells to produce mostly IgM antibodies, and they express I-A subregion encoded Ia determinant,[52,53] and Ig variable region–encoded determinants.[57] Finally, the in vivo and in vitro (T,G)-A--L–specific ThF exhibited similar antigenic specificities as determined by their ability to bind or react with related polypeptide antigens.[46,47]

All the studies described above dealt with (T,G)-A--L–specific helper factor(s) derived from a heterogeneous population of activated cells. For a better understanding of the fine specificity, molecular organization, and mechanism of function of T cell factor and receptors, homogeneous T cell lines are necessary. To achieve this, a (T,G)-A--L–specific hybrid line has recently been established and denoted R–9, which produced helper factor.[14,31] Here are described the properties of this hybridoma and its products, and compare it to other nonclonal and monoclonal ThF.

B. Establishment of R-9, A (T,G)–A--L–Specific Hybrid Line Expressing Surface V_H Determinants

The scheme describing the procedure employed for the in vivo activation of (T,G)–A--L–specific T cells, the short in vitro stimulation on (T,G)–A--L–bearing splenic adherent cells and the fusion with BW5147 thymoma cells is described in Figure 1 and discussed in section II.B. The activation procedure used was very efficient, has been shown to potentiate specific helper cells activity,[28] and may be the prime cause for the high frequency of potent hybridomas obtained in this fusion. Out of 21 independent hybrid lines established, one line (R–9) released factor that specifically enhanced the antibody response to (T,G)–A--L. Another line (R–17) augmented the response in a nonantigen specific manner, while a third line (R–11) produced factor that specifically suppressed the anti–(T,G)–A--L–specific response. Experiments with two hybrid lines, R–9–helper hybrid line and R–11 suppressor line, will be described in more detail below. Both lines are true hybrids since they contain an uneuploid number of chromosomes (around 65), express surface antigen (*H–2;* Thy 1.) of both parental cells, and grow as tumors in (C3H.SWxAKR/J)F$_1$ mice. The hybridoma cells grew in vitro with a generation time of about 10 hr and were not dependent for their growth and activity on any known external stimuli such as antigen or TCGF. R–9 and R–11 hybridomas retained their specific activity after continuous growth for six months. However, in order to avoid variation and select for stable clones, after a certain period in culture (usually two to three months), new cultures were initiated from frozen batches, re-cloned, and selected for positive clones.

The hybrid cells did not exhibit Ig determinants when tested with fluorescent antibodies against the Ig constant region. However, rabbit antibodies against the variable region of the V_H of myeloma protein M.315,[58] stained the majority of the R–9 and R–11 hybrid cells, while anti–V_L antibodies[14,36,60] did not. These reagents, developed by Ben–Neriah and Givol against the V_H and V_L fragments of myeloma proteins, reacted specifically with heavy or light chains of a number of myeloma proteins. Thus they are specific to the invariant portion (framework) of the Ig variable regions.[58,59] Another reagent tested for reactivity against the hybridoma surfaces was the Id antibodies directed against (T,G)–A--L–specific idiotypes that have been reacted with 30 to 40% of anti–(T,G)–A--L antibodies.[61] Such anti–Id antibodies were also efficient in the absorption of the active moiety of "conventional" ThF,[57] caused proliferation of (T,G)–A--L–activated T lymphocytes,[62] and replaced antigen in triggering activated T cells in DTH response.[63] Both R–9 and R–11 cell lines stained positively with the anti–Id antibodies. More recently a series of anti–(T,G)–A--L mAbs have been prepared, two of which expressed the major (T,G)–A--L Id.[64] Antiserum that had been raised in mice against one anti–(T,G)–A--L mAb and was proven to contain anti–(T,G)–A--L Id, stained R–9 and R–11 cells specifically. Thus, it is suggested that the functional R–9 and R–11 hybridomas do not express determinants encoded by the Ig constant region and light chains on their surfaces, but bear antigenic molecules identical or crossreactive with the variable region framework *(V_H)* or Id determinants. It should be noted that many attempts to demonstrate the presence of V_H gene products on heterogeneous activated cells by binding experiments were unsuccessful,[152] nor was this author able to stain cytolytic T–hybridomas[22] by the anti–V_H antibodies. Thus, the expression of V_H antigens on the functional R–9 and R–11 hybridomas reflects their monoclonality and specific activation stage.

1. Fine Antigenic Specificity of R–9–Derived ThF

R–9 hybridoma secreted (T,G)–A--L–specific ThF into the culture supernate without the necessity of external stimulus. Relatively high activity of factor was also detected in the ascites fluid of R–9–bearing mice. The (T,G)–A--L–specific T cell replacing activity of the factor was demonstrated on (T,G)–A--L or hapten-primed B cells, either in vivo in adoptive transfer experiments or in antibody production assay in vitro.[14,36,66] The activity of the factor was specific to (T,G)–A--L, since it did not support antibody responses to other unrelated carriers. To test the fine antigenic specificity, the factor's reactivity toward different polypeptide antigens was determined. A "conventional" ThF preparation produced by heterogeneous (T,G)–A--L–activated cells reacted with various (T,G)–A--L–related polypeptides[46] to the same degree as anti–(T,G)–A--L antibodies.[67] Both factor and antibodies reacted with (T,G)–A--L, (Phe,G)–A--L, (H,G)–A--L, and G–A--L, however antibodies, but not factor, could bind (T,G)–Pro--L. One interpretation of these data is that the factor, like antibodies, is a mixture of heterogeneous molecules, each endowed with a binding site specific for a certain epitope. However, since in later experiments it was found that most of the factor activity could be removed by absorption on different affinity columns, this explanation is not likely. An alternative possibility is that the factor's binding site recognizes one determinant common to all the polypeptide antigens with which it reacted, such as the G–A--L polypeptide. This was verified with R–9–hybrid–derived factor whose antigen–binding site is probably a product of one gene. Absorption experiments[66] on affinity columns made of the different polypeptide antigens clearly demonstrated that the active moiety in R–9 supernate binds to and can be recovered from columns of (T,G)–A--L, (Phe,G)–A--L and G–A--L, and binds to a lesser extent to immunoabsorbents of (H,G)–A--L and (T,G)–Pro--L. This observation (see also Table 4) supports the concept of a single cross–reactive determinant that is recognized by all the factor molecules. It is pertinent to indicate that the fine specificity of monoclonal anti-(T,G)–A--L antibodies expressing the major (T,G)–A--L Id.[64] was similar to that observed for the monoclonal (T,G)–A--L–specific ThF.

2. Possession by the (T,G)-A--L-Specific R-9 Factor of V Region–Like and MHC–Encoded Determinants

The (T,G)-A--L–specific, R-9-factor possesses V region–like and MHC–encoded determinants. Since the antigen–binding specificity of the T cell–derived helper factors and the antibodies are similar, it has been suggested that T cells utilize the same V region genes, coding for the antigen–binding site of antibodies and for their antiantigen receptor or factor. Support for this concept comes from a large body of evidence that antigen–specific T cells and their factors contain determinants shared with the antibody idiotype or with the framework of the Ig V_H (discussed in section V.A). The anti-V_H reagent that binds to R-9 and R-11 cells inhibited antigen binding to T cells[68] and interfered with helper T cell activity.[69] Therefore it was of interest to analyze whether the R-9 hybridoma–derived soluble ThF also contain determinants crossreacting with the Ig-variable region gene products. To test this assumption, R-9 factor that was purified from a (T,G)-A--L column was passed over immunoabsorbents made of anti-V_H and anti-(T,G)-A--L Id.[31,66] Almost all the activity could be recovered in eluates from the affinity columns and no factor activity was detected in the effluent from the columns (Figure 2). Because the (T,G)–A--L helper activity was not absorbed on columns of anti-V_L (κ or λ) or antiwhole Ig,[66] it was suggested that V_H-like products are shared by the (T,G)–A--L–specific monoclonal helper factor. Expression of MHC gene products in the R-9 helper factor was studied by affinity chromatography with immunoabsorbents using "conventional" and monoclonal anti–H-2^b columns.[66] Antibodies against the whole H-2^b region, anti-I-A^b + I-B^b, and anti-I-A^b + I-B^b + I-C^b removed the helper factor activity, while anti-K^b, anti-H-2^k and anti-I-A^k failed to bind and remove the active moiety. Hence, the R-9 ThF expressed I-A antigenic determinants in addition to V_H gene product and antigen–binding site. It is noteworthy that the anti-Ia^b mAbs provided by Dr. G. Hämmerling, failed to absorb the factor's activity. It is possible that these mAbs are directed against Ia specificities, which are not expressed on the monoclonal R-9 ThF. However, it is tempting to speculate that the Ia determinant possessed by the T cell factor belongs to a T cell–specific class of Ia molecules, detected by polyclonal anti-I^b antisera and not by the monoclonal reagents. The existence of such T cell–specific Ia molecules on specific T cells and their factors has been demonstrated previously by Taniguchi, Tada, and their groups.[70–72] Since the R-9 is a hybrid between

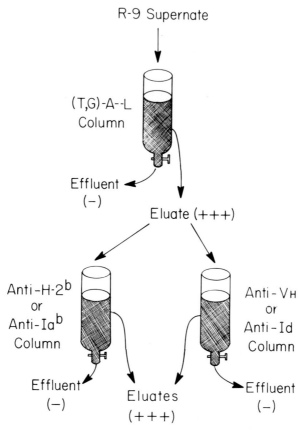

FIGURE 2. Expression of both *I-A^b* and *V_H* determinants on the same active complex by (T,G)-A--L-specific helper factor.

AKR/J(*H-2^k*) thymoma and activated T cells of C3H.SW (*H-2^b*), it is interesting to note that only anti-*H-2^b* (and not anti-*H-2^k*) absorbents could remove the factor activity. Assuming that the R-9 hybrid cell is capable of synthesizing both *Ia^b* and *Ia^k*, these observations indicate that the helper factor of this clone possesses only *Ia^b* in its active moiety. Lonai et al.[15] found that the ThF derived from CGG-specific hybridoma contains both *Ia^b* and *Ia^k* antigenic determinants. This also implies that free recombination and segregation of the *V_H* part with the two Ia molecules can occur.

Since Ig heavy chain and MHC genes are located in different chromosomes (12 and 17 in the mouse), it is difficult to envisage the V gene product and *Ia* antigen on the same polypeptide chain. A model of each determinant expressed on separate molecules that are complexed to form the active and specific factor, seems more plausible. To check whether free molecules can be detected, inactive effluents, obtained after affinity chromatography of R-9 supernate on either anti-*H-2^b* or anti-*Id* columns, were mixed together and tested for factor activity (see Figure 3). The recombined effluents yielded active factor.[65,66] The simplest explanation for this experimental observation is that the *V_H* and *Ia*–bearing molecules are not covalently bound (at least in part of the monoclonal ThF). Therefore after immunoabsorption, free chains might exist in the effluents and recombine to yield active factor complex after mixing the effluents. The data of Taniguchi et al.,[73,74] who performed similar experiments with hybridoma-derived suppressor cell factor, fits the model of recombination of antiantigen and antiself parts into

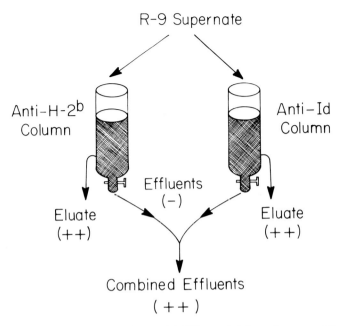

FIGURE 3. Expression of V_H and MHC–encoded determinants on different polypeptide chains.

functional factor. More detailed analysis of the molecular composition of helper and suppressor factors will be presented in section V.

C. Production of CGG-Specific ThF by T Cell Hybridoma

Recently, Lonai, Puri, and Hämmerling[15] have generated CGG-specific hybridomas by the fusion of BW5147 cells with either C57BL/6 or B10.BR NP-CGG–immunized spleen cells. Out of 500 fusion lines, 11 were selected on the basis of binding of radioiodinated Ia–associated antigen complex (IAC). The IAC was obtained by incubation of syngeneic splenic macrophages with radiolabeled antigen. For antigen binding, the hybrid cells require a monokine similar to IL-1.[29,30] The binding affinity of the IAC to the T hybrid cells is higher than that of the antigen alone and could be inhibited by anti-V_H, anti-H-2 or monoclonal anti-I-A. Anti-V_L and antinonrelevant H-2 did not inhibit the antigen binding to cells. Six hybrid lines were found to secrete CGG-specific helper factor. The factor, like the hybrid cells, contains both V_H determinants and Ia antigens. Both hybrid cells and factor functioned in a self H-2 genetically restricted manner, i.e., the hybridoma–bound antigen processed by macrophages possessing the homologous Ia antigens, and the factor affected or was absorbed only by B cells containing the same Ia antigens. One of the hybrid lines originated from C57BL/6xBW fusion–produced factor that could be removed by anti-Ia^k and anti-Ia^b, suggesting that although not functional, the BW I–A subregion product can be assembled into active factor together with V_H molecule.[75] The significance of this observation and its relevance to the molecular model of the factor will be discussed in the following sections.

D. Production of Factors Augmenting T Cell–Dependent Help in Antibody Responses by T Cell Hybridoma

Tokuhisa et al.[48] have described another type of ThF extracted from antigen–primed T cells that enhances in vitro hapten carrier antibody response only in the presence of T cells having the same specificity. This TaF did not enhance humoral responses in the absence of T cells. In the presence of T cells, it augmented the in vitro antibody response only when it was added 24 to 48 hr after the culture was started. Another difference from the (T,G)-A--L–specific ThF described before is that the TaF acted in an *H-2* restricted manner; i.e., it affected T cells of only *I-A* subregion compatible strains. Otherwise, the physicochemical and serological properties are similar to those described for the ThF. Of specific interest is the observation made by Tokuhisa et al.[48] that the TaF possesses *Ia* antigens that are not common to B cells, but are exclusively expressed on activated T cells. A unique locus has been proposed that controls the polymorphic T cell Ia antigen on the factors.

Tada et al.[71,72] have recently generated hybridomas between BW5147 cells and T cells that bind to KLH–coated plates. Hybrid cells expressing *Ia^k* antigens were selected by the FACS. The activity of factor extracted from one clone (FL10) was antigen–specific and functioned in an *I-A* restricted manner. There is evidence that both hybridomas and the factor derived from them possess *Ia* antigen that is encoded by the *I-A* subregion, but its specificities are serologically distinct from those of B cell *Ia* antigens.[71,72] Based on this observation it was suggested that ThF and TaF carry *Ia* antigen unique to the T cell that is associated with the antigen-specific augmenting molecule.

IV. SUPPRESSOR T CELL FACTORS—GENERATION AND CHARACTERIZATION OF HYBRID LINES PRODUCING ANTIGEN–SPECIFIC SUPPRESSOR FACTOR(S)

TsF have been described in numerous experimental systems. Most of the studies dealt with either the suppression of antibody responses to protein and polypeptide antigens, or with suppression of DTH response to proteins, red cells, or contact sensitivity reaction to haptens (for reviews see references 1 to 4). TsF have been described in many more systems than ThF, mainly due to the relative ease with which TsF can be induced, enriched, and detected. The most common methods to induce tolerance and suppressor cells involve high doses of soluble protein (aggregate-free) antigens in the absence of adjuvant,[32,76,77] or in the presence of incomplete adjuvants,[78] and the use of reactive haptenic groups,[79] hapten modified syngeneic cells,[80,81] or autologous Ig[82] (for reviews, see references 83, 84). The high affinity of suppressor cell receptors to antigens allows their enrichment from cell-free extracts of primed or tolerant animals by absorption and elution from immobilized antigen columns.

Unlike ThF, TsF is usually extracted from suppressor cells, although it can be found also in the culture supernate of TsF. Some differences in activity and structure reported for various TsF preparations can be related to the mode of TsF derivation (received by Taussig[3]). It is beyond the scope of this chapter to review all the information regarding "conventional" TsF, and it has been amply reviewed elsewhere.[1-4] Table 3 summarizes most of the functional and structural features of the TsF. In most respects TsF is similar to ThF (compare Tables 2 and 3). However, they differ at least in their Ia antigens; i.e., while TsF usually expresses Ia antigens encoded in the *I-J* subregion, the ThF *Ia* antigen is encoded in the *I-A* subregion. More detailed characterization of monoclonal TsF produced by suppressor cell hybridomas is described and discussed in the following sections.

A. TsF Specific to Protein Antigens and SRBC

The first functional T cell hybridomas reported were those that produced TsF specific to human gamma globulin (HGG) (Taniguchi and Miller[10]) and KLH (Kontiainen et al.,[9] Taniguchi, Saito, and Tada[12]). At the same time, Taussig and collaborators[11] established a hybrid T cell line that produced an SRBC–specific factor, capable of sup-

Table 3
PROPERTIES OF ANTIGEN-SPECIFIC SUPPRESSOR FACTORS

1. Extracted from or secreted by antigen–primed suppressor T cells.
2. Bind specifically to the antigen served for their production.
3. Suppress antibody production, DTH, and cytotoxic T cell responses in antigen–specific manner.
4. Most of the factors act on T cells to induce second type of suppressor cells. Some directly suppress B cells or effector T cells.
5. Lack constant region determinants but may express variable region framework and Id–like determinants.
6. Carry determinants coded by *I-J* and some *I-C* subregion genes.
7. Most of the suppressor factors interact in *H-2* or Id–restricted manner.
8. 50,000 to 70,000 mol wt, composed in many cases from two polypeptide chains: one carries V_H and antigen–binding site, the other is MHC gene product.

pressing IgM and IgG antibody responses. Hewitt and Liew[13] described the establishment and properties of a factor derived from T hybrid cells that suppresses the specific DTH response to SRBC. The suppressor cells induced by Taniguchi et al.[10,12] were obtained from mice injected with relatively high amounts of deaggregated soluble HGG or KLH. They removed the B cells by adhering the tolerized splenocytes onto anti–Ig coated plates. They enriched for suppressor T cells by binding them to antigen–coated plates and then eluting them at low temperatures. This enriched population (0.5% of the unfractionated population and about 100–fold more active) was fused with EL-4[10] or BW5147[12] lymphomas. Following selection in HAT medium, hybridomas were sorted for *I-J^b*–bearing cells by the FACS. After in vitro screening for suppressive activity of either culture supernates or cell-free extracts, three groups of *I-J*–bearing hybrid lines could be classified according to their TsF activity:

1. KLH–specific suppressor hybridomas
2. Antigen-nonspecific suppressor and non–*H-2* restricted lines
3. Nonfunctional hybridomas

The hybridomas generated by Taniguchi and Miller by fusion with EL-4 cells appeared to be unstable.[10]

More recently, in a series of elegant studies, the groups of Taniguchi and Tada characterized the properties of suppressor hybrid cells and the functional TsF produced by them.[12,70–74,85–87] Both hybrid cells and factor bound KLH specifically. The binding of radioactive and fluorescent KLH was dependent on the cell cycle.[85] Thus, after synchronization in culture, about 70% of suppressor hybrid cells in the M phase bound KLH but not NP–MGG, whereas less than 30% of the cells bound antigen in the S phase. Interestingly, the expression of *I-J* products on the cells and amount of suppressive activity extracted from the cells was also cell cycle-dependent, maximal during the M phase and minimal at the S phase of the synchronized hybrid cells.[85] The C57BL/6 KLH–specific TsF bound specifically to immunoadsorbents composed of KLH, anti-*I-J^b*, and anti-V_H, but not to other antigens, anti-*I-J^k*, anti-Ig, or anti-V_L.[70,72–74,85] In recent experiments, the factor was found to be composed of two separate polypeptide chains, covalently associated by disulfide bonds in the secreted TsF, and present in a nonassociated form in extracts from the suppressor hybrid lines.[73,74,85] These conclusions were derived from the results of absorption experiments with cell–free extracts, purified on affinity columns composed of KLH and of anti–*I-J^b*. The effluents from these columns were pooled and assayed for their suppressive activity. All the activity could be removed by both columns. However, mixing the effluents from KLH and *I-J^b* columns resulted in active and specific TsF. The same results were obtained from secreted Tsf (culture supernate or ascites fluid) only if the TsF was reduced with 5 m*M* dithiothreitol (DTT) before absorption on columns.[74] To eliminate the possibility of an additive effect of residual intact TsF in the effluents, double absorption experiments were performed that clearly indicated that there are three components in the hybridoma extract: the antigen–binding chain, the *I-J* product, and the associated form of the two polypeptide chains. The possible mode of association of the two chains and its molecular nature will be discussed in section V.D.

The functionally different types of hybridomas obtained enabled Taniguchi et al.,[70,72,85] to observe and specify heterogeneity in the *I-J* gene product as expressed on the suppressor cells, and in the TsF derived from them. Such heterogeneity was first detected using anti–*I-J^b* alloantiserum (B10.A(5R) anti–B10.A(3R)) preabsorbed on specific or nonspecific hybridomas, and testing the residual cytotoxic activity on the different hybrid cells. The conventional alloanti–*I-J^b* antibodies detected on the hybridoma cells at least two different antigenic determinants. Absorption by a specific hybridoma resulted in decrease of reactivity against the homologous and other antigen–specific hybridomas without affecting the cytotoxic activity towards nonspecific hybridomas. Conversely, antiserum absorbed by the nonspecific hybridoma still bound and lysed the specific hybridoma. Additional confirmation for the existence of different *I-J* determinants expressed on the subsets of T cell suppressor hybridomas was obtained with two different anti–*I-J^b* mAbs prepared by Taniguchi et al.[85] Hence, the activity of one anti–*I-J^b* mAb (D7) could be eliminated only by absorption by the antigen–specific hybridomas, while the activity of another anti–*I-J^b* mAb (C5) could be removed by absorption by the nonspecific hybridomas. These results suggest that the *I-J* subregion accomodates a few subloci, in accord with previous observations by Tada et al.,[88] who demonstrated different *I-J* products on Lyl^+ subclass of T helper cells (Th_2) adherent to nylon and on Ly2^+, 3^+ T-suppressor (Ts_2) cells.

In a similar system, Kontiainen, Feldmann, and collaborators[9,89] established a few stable suppressor cell hybridomas by the fusion of BW5147 and in vitro induced suppressor cells specific to KLH. The supernates of these hybridomas specifically suppressed DNP-PFC responses to DNP-KLH when cultured, in vitro. The active factor could be bound specifically to KLH and anti-*I-J* immunoabsorbent. However, it differed from the TsF reported by the groups of Taniguchi and Tada mentioned above in its non-MHC restricted function and its direct effect of Ly1^+2^- T helper cells and not on the secondary T suppressor cells (Ts_2).

Another member of the family of MHC nonrestricted TsF is the SRBC–specific factor produced by hybridomas that were established by Taussig et al.[11,90-93] The culture supernate of one T hybridoma suppresses primary and secondary antibody responses to SRBC. The factor binds specifically to SRBC and to immunoabsorbents made against antigens coded in the *I–E/C* subregion. Accordingly, the SRBC TsF can be absorbed onto B cells carrying acceptor molecules coded in the *I–E/C* subregion. As reported for the KLH–specific TsF, this factor is also composed of two separate polypeptide chains, however the active unit is of higher molecular weight than that reported for the other factors (see Table 5).

Another SRBC TsF released from T hybrid lines is the DTH–suppressor factor generated by Hewitt and Liew.[13] A few hybridomas were obtained by the fusion of SRBC–primed splenocytes and BW5147 cells that release TsF into their culture supernates or ascitic fluid. This TsF is suppressed in non H 2 restricted manner, during either the induction phase or the expression of DTH. Interestingly, the TsF *Ia* determinants have been claimed to be of carbohydrate nature.[94]

B. TsF Specific to Synthetic Polypeptide Antigens

The hybridoma-derived monoclonal suppressor factors to protein antigens described in the previous section recognize undefined determinants on the antigenic molecules, so that the characterization of their fine specificity is limited. From this point of view, antigens that are composed of simple and chemically defined molecules, such as synthetic polypeptide antigens or haptenic groups are an advantage. Of special interest are the antigens that elicit responses characterized by antibodies expressing common or cross-reactive idiotype.

1. GAT- and GT-Specific TsF

One of the most extensively studied model systems is the specific suppression induced by the random co–polymers GAT and GT. It was demonstrated by Benacerraf's group (Kapp et al.,[77,95] Debre et al.,[96,97] Waltenbaugh et al.[98]) that nonresponder strains of mice primed with GAT or GT develop suppressor–T cell responses. GAT–specific suppressor factor could be extracted from the suppressor cells and analyzed for its ability to suppress the response to GAT-MBSA either in vivo or in vitro. A few of the properties of the GAT–specific TsF are similar to those described above for KLH: it bears *I-J* encoded determinant, binds antigen, and lacks constant Ig determinants. Notably, GAT–specific TsF expresses the cross-reactive idiotype CGAT that is common to all strains of mice producing anti–GAT antibodies.[99] However, unlike the KLH factor described by Tada and Taniguchi, the GAT– and GT–specific factors function efficiently across *H-2* barriers. Moreover, studies to elucidate the mechanism and targets for GAT–TsF activity revealed a new class of suppressor T cells (Ts$_2$) that are induced by the TsF$_1$ (Waltenbaugh[98,100]). This induction of Ts$_2$ occurred across *I-J* barriers, the cells expressed anti-Id activity, and produced suppressor factor designated TsF$_2$.[101]

More recently, Kapp, Araneo, and Clevinger[42,102] have established T cell hybridoma between BW5147 cells and nonresponder DBA/1 spleen cells, primed with GAT, and induced for suppressor cells with cortisone acetate. The hybrid cells produced a factor that suppressed GAT–specific PFC and proliferative responses. The monoclonal TsF was very active (culture supernates still suppressed at $1:10^4$ dilution) and resembled in all aspects the conventional GAT-TsF extracted from primed T cells.

2. (T,G)-A--L–Specific Suppressor T Cell Hybridoma

In a similar system, the author was recently able to generate a hybridoma that secreted (T,G)-A--L-specific suppressor factor.[60,65,103] This hybridoma (denoted R-11) was established in the same fusion experiment as that described in section III.B, for the preparation of the (T,G)-A--L–specific helper hybridoma. R-11 hybrid cells, derived from high responder mice (C3H.SW, *H-2^b*) activated T cells that were triggered in vitro,[14] expressed V_H determinants, as was verified using both rabbit anti-V_H antibodies and anti–(T,G)-A--L idiotypes.[60,65,103] The factor(s) secreted by these cells also carried the same V_H determinant in addition to *H-2^b* encoded antigens. The presence of *I-J^b* determinants on both cells and soluble factor is yet to be established. The activity of R-11 factor was monitored either in vivo in adoptive transfer, or by its ability to suppress anti–(T,G)-A--L antibody responses in vitro. The fine specificity of the TsF was analyzed using affinity columns constructed of different synthetic polypeptides. The suppressive activity of R-11 supernate could be completely removed by columns of (T,G)-A--L and (T,G)-Pro--L, and to a lesser extent by (H,G)-A--L and G-A--L, while (Phe,G)-A--L failed to absorb the TsF activity (see Table 4). These results are similar, but not identical, to those obtained with R-9 factor (see section III.B-2) that bound (T,G)-Pro--L to a lesser degree. In the light of their identity in expression of Id and

Table 4
**FINE SPECIFICITY OF (T,G)-A--L-SPECIFIC ANTIBODIES
AND T CELL FACTORS** [a]

	T cell factor			Antibodies	
Antigen	Activated T-cells	R-9 helper hybridoma	R-11 suppressor hybridoma	Conventional	Monoclonal Id–positive
(T,G)-A--L	+	+	+	+	+
(Phe,G)-A--L	+	+	−	+	+
(H,G)-A--L	N.D.	±	±	+	+
G-A--L	+	+	±	+	+
(T,G)-Pro--L	−	±	+	+	−
(T-T-G-G)-A--L	N.D.	N.D.	N.D.	+	+
(T-G-T-G)-A--L	N.D.	N.D.	N.D.	±	+

[a] (T,G)-A--L-specific helper and suppressor activity was assayed in effluents and eluates obtained from affinity columns constructed with the different synthetic antigens.

similarity in the binding of synthetic polypeptides, it can be concluded that the antigen-binding sites of R-9 helper hybrid and R-11 are closely related.

C. TsF Specific to Defined Haptenic Groups

T cells can be activated specifically to small haptenic groups such as DNP, NP, ABA, and PC. In most of the hapten–reactive systems, the response exhibited by certain strains of mice is characterized by cross–reactive idiotypes, which are very helpful for genetic and molecular studies of the T cell factors and receptors. The main response elicited by the chemically reactive haptens is skin contact sensitivity, a DTH–like response where both effector and regulatory cells are of the T cell lineage. Suppressor cells specific to the haptenic groups are usually induced by either i.v. administration of the chemically reactive haptenic groups,[38,79] or after coupling them to isologous carrier proteins[82] or cells.[39,70,80,81,40,41] Asherson and Zembala[38,79] were the first to demonstrate specific TsF activity in contact sensitivity by harvesting soluble factor from cultured lymph node cells obtained from mice given picrylsulfonic acid i.v.[79] This suppressor factor was subsequently proven to be a glycoprotein of about 50,000 daltons that bound the antigen and contained *H-2*-coded determinants.[38] Green et al.[81] later demonstrated that the TNP-TsF possesses *I-J*–coded determinants. A similar approach was attempted by Moorhead and collaborators utilizing dinitrophenyl sulfonic acid to induce suppressor cells and TsF that specifically inhibited the development and transfer of contact sensitivity to dinitrofluorobenzene.[39,80,104] Interestingly, the activity of this factor was *H-2* restricted to the *H-2K* or *H-2D* subregions of MHC,[104] and the DNP-TsF was found to possess *I-C* subregion coded determinants. So far, no functional hybridoma was reported in these systems. The cloning approach should be encouraged in haptenic systems of this kind, since there is cumulative experience of sophisticated techniques and reagents that have been used to study the active site of DNP–specific antibodies. This experience can be utilized for immunochemical studies of monoclonal DNP or TNP–specific T cell factors.

Another extensively studied model system is the specific suppression of DTH response to the hapten azobenzenarsonate (ABA). ABA–specific TsF can be extracted from suppressor cells induced by i.v. administration of ABA coupled syngeneic cells.[40,105,106,116] Both suppressor cells and TsF possess the cross-reactive idiotype (CRI)[105,107,116] of the anti–ABA antibodies of the A/J mice, as characterized by Nisonoff and co-workers.[108] Expression of the CRI defined on the factor, like the antibody idiotype, was coded by the Ig heavy chain allotype–linked genes. The ABA system has been used to investigate the mode of action of ABA–specific suppressor cells and TsF.[106] Briefly, as in the GAT system,[98,100] antigen–induced and specific suppressor cells secreted TsF_1, which induced a second set of suppressor T cells (Ts_2)–bearing antiidiotypic receptor in untreated mice (reviewed in reference 2).

1. ABA-Specific T Cell Hybridomas

Few groups have produced ABA–specific T hybridomas. Ruddle and collaborators[26,27] have established T cell hybridomas, that bound preferentially ABA coupled to sheep and mouse erythrocytes. These rosettes can be inhibited by ABA albumin and not by albumin alone. Three hybrid lines stained for the ABA CRI in an immunofluorescence assay. Cultured supernates of these lines could suppress specifically primary anti–ABA antibody response. Another ABA–specific T hybridoma was generated by Pacifico and Capra[109,110] by the fusion of BW5147 with spleen cells of mice, treated by the administration of ABA lymphocytes. Hybrid lines secreting component(s) that inhibited the binding to ABA of CRI–positive monoclonal anti–ABA antibodies were selected for further characterization of ABA–binding T cell product. For this purpose biosynthetically labeled hybrid supernate was passed through various affinity columns and the eluates were subjected to chemical analyses. It was found that the hybridomas secrete or shed 62,000–dalton, antigen–specific product, that bind to rabbit antisera against the CRI. In addition, the ABA–specific molecules contain I–region–encoded determinants. Since both anti–CRI and anti–I precipitated only one type of molecule, it was suggested that the two determinants are expressed on the same molecule. Analysis by high pressure liquid chromatography (HPLC) of tryptic peptides from material obtained from two ABA–binding hybridomas revealed that the majority of the peptides was shared by both T cell products. However, few peptides were clearly distinguishable, indicating that in addition to their remarkable structural similarity, unique differences also exist between the two monoclonal T cell products. So far no functional activity was reported for these ABA–binding molecules, and additional information is required before excluding the existence of a second chain that might be radiolabeled to a lesser degree, and therefore is not revealed in the detection procedure employed. The one chain–vs.–two chain model and its implications will be discussed in section V.D.

2. NP-Specific T Cell Hybridomas

An additional haptenic system that is widely used as an experimental model for studying the mechanism of the immunosuppressive circuit is the response to 3-nitro-4-hydroxyphenacetyl (NP) in mice of the Igl^b allotype. The primary antibody response to NP is characterized by the heteroclitic fine specificity,[111] defined clonotype,[112] and idiotypic marker comprising the predominant antibody population of C57BL/6 mice.[113] NP–specific molecules carrying idiotypic determinants were isolated and characterized from T cells adhering to antigen–coated nylon nets,[114,115] however, those molecules did not display any activity. Therefore, Weinberger et al.[41] elicited NP–specific suppressor cells essentially as described for the ABA system, using NP–modified syngeneic spleen cells. The restriction elements of the interactions of these suppressor cells with effector cells studied in NP–specific, DTH responses were controlled by both IgH–V and I–A genes.

Kontiainen et al.[89] have generated NP–specific suppressor hybridomas, secreting potent TsF that could be absorbed on NP columns. Interestingly, the factor derived from BWxC57BL/10 (H-2^k × H-2^b) hybridoma, possessed determinants coded by the I-J^k subregion that originated from the nonfunctional BW–parental tumor cells. This finding supports the hypothesis that the V-gene and I-gene products are expressed on separate polypeptide chains.

More recently, Tada and coworkers[72,117] established another NP–specific suppressor hybridoma in a procedure similar to that described before for the KLH system. One of the hybridomas obtained expressed on its surface NP^b Id and $I\text{-}J^k$ determinants. The binding of the anti-Id to these hybrid cells was inhibited by lower concentration of NIP (4-hydroxy-5-iodo-3-nitro-phenyl) than NP, thus demonstrating the heteroclicity properties, also shared by certain T cells and B cells in primary anti–NP responses.[111] Using TsF extracted from the NP and Id–specific hybridoma, Tada demonstrated that anti-Id T cells are required for Id suppression.[117] Thus, after removal of anti-Id T cells by plating of primed helper cells on NP^b–Id coated dishes, NP–specific TsF no longer suppressed the Id expression as was detected by co–culturing the suppressor factor with NP–primed B cells and the depleted T cells. These results substantiate the conclusion put forward by Sy et al.[106,116] in the ABA system and Weinberger et al.[41] in the NP system, that anti-Id-specific suppressor T cells (Ts_2) can be activated by Id–bearing TsF_1.

V. MOLECULAR ORGANIZATION OF MONOCLONAL T CELL FACTORS AND ITS RELATIONSHIP TO THE T CELL RECEPTOR

Following the successful precedent with antibodies, it was hoped that chemical characterization of the T cell receptor would be accomplished after the establishment of functional homogeneous T cell lines or hybridomas. It is clear today however, almost four years after the generation of the first functional hybridomas, that this task is still an arduous one. A dim light can be seen at the end of the tunnel, however. The monoclonal functional T cells factors have proven highly instrumental in analysis of the nature of cellular interactions governing the immunoregulatory circuits. Furthermore, the immunochemical information obtained so far from studies with hybridoma-derived T cell factors confirmed and substantiated the data originating from factors extracted from heterogeneous T cell populations. At present, sufficient homogeneous material is being accumulated that will soon allow precise chemical analysis. It is generally accepted today that the following elements constitute the functional antigen-specific T cell factors:

1. Antigen-binding site
2. *V*-region gene product
3. *I*-subregion gene product

In the next sections the nature of each element and their interrelationship in composing the active factor will be discussed.

A. Id and V_H Determinants on T Cell Factors

The presence of Id markers on functional T cell factors was verified in most of the systems where Id responses could be demonstrated. When the Id expression was linked to Igh allotypic genes, the factor also exhibited the same linkage. Thus, (T,G)-A-- L–specific factors produced by activated cells,[57] continuous lines,[103] and helper or suppressor hybridomas,[66] could be specifically absorbed on antibodies to C3H.SW-derived anti-(T,G)-A--L Id. Similar results were obtained in the ABA system.[105,109] Another set of antibodies, the rabbit antibodies directed against the variable region of the Ig heavy chain[58] V_H, have proved to be very useful reagents for the detection of *V*-region gene products on both ThF[15,66,103] and TsF.[85] Until now, the presence of V_H gene determinants on the T cell factors was inferred by serological studies. This information suggests that the factors might be coded by V_H genes. However, since the factors and antibodies bind the same antigen, the possibility exists that the anti-Id antibodies recognize similar or cross–reactive structures in the factor that are not necessarily coded by the same V_H genes dictating the antibody structure. The well–known anti-anti-insulin antibodies that cross–react with the insulin receptor on cells[118] exemplify this kind of situation.

In contrast to the presence of V-gene like products, no constant region determinants, nor known V_L or constant region markers could be detected on functional factors and activated T cells. The possibility that the V_H-positive factors bear constant region with some effector functions analogous to Ig is still unknown and awaits more precise analysis of the T cell factor.

B. Comparison Between the T Cell Factor and Antibody-Binding Site

The shared or cross–reactive idiotypic and V_H determinants and the similar antigen–binding specificity of T cell factors and antibodies suggest homology between the factor and antibody–binding sites. Careful analysis of the fine specificity of factors and antibodies reacting with the same antigens has revealed some differences in the antigen–binding capacity and the repertoire of those two components. Differences in antigen–binding capacity, reflected in differences in avidity and degree of cross–reactivity between factors and antibodies sharing the same Id, may be due to the fact that the factors lack the Ig light chain that contributes to both Id determinants and binding specificity of antibodies. It is tempting to suggest that the *I* subregion–encoded molecule might, among other functions, participate in the tertiary structure of the factors' binding site. However, there is no solid information to validate this hypothesis. The ideal system to compare the binding site of T cell factor and antibody should use monoclonal factors and antibodies sharing the same Id. An attempt to compare the fine antigenic specificity of (T,G)-A--L–specific antibodies to that of helper factors (derived from R-9 hybridoma or activated cell line) and suppressor factor (R-11) is outlined in Table 4. The degree and pattern of binding to various synthetic polypeptide antigens (all of which reacted with anti–(T,G)-A--L antibodies) is not identical in all the factors. While all the factors reacted with (T,G)-A--L, G-A--L, and to some degree with (H,G)-A--L (judged by the ability of the active moiety to specifically bind to, and be recovered from, affinity columns), only R-9 and R-11 reacted with (T,G)-Pro--L. R-11 TsF did not bind to (Phe,G)-A--L, while all the helper factors did. The anti-(T,G)-A--L antibodies produced in C3H.SW mice reacted with all the synthetic antigens listed in the table, and partially also with (T-G-T-G)-A--L, reflecting the heterogeneity of the response. Recently, a series of mAbs specific to (T,G)-A--L and its ordered determinant (T-T-G-G)-A--L have been prepared.[64] Four different groups of antibodies could be identified, distinct in their binding of various (T,G)-A--L related polypeptides. Interestingly, only two antibodies expressed the major anti–(T,G)-A--L Id, as determined by the ability of guinea-pig anti-Id antisera to inhibit the binding of ^{125}I-(T,G)-A--L to the mAbs. These antibodies reacted with (T,G)-A--L, (H,G)-A--L, (Phe,G)-A--L, G-A--L, (T-T-G-G)-A--L, and (T-G-T-G)-A--L, but not with (T,G)-Pro--L or (T-T-G-G)-Pro--L, demonstrating G-A--L specificity. To summarize, the Id-positive monoclonal anti–(T,G)-A--L antibodies, and the monoclonal ThF and TsF exhibit different specificity towards some of the antigens tested. There is a closer relationship between ThF and antibodies than between the TsF and ThF. It should be noted that similar observations were made in the GAT–specific TsF, which is only partially bound to GT, whereas anti–GAT antibody is completely cross–reactive.[119] How can such differences in specificity be reconciled with the sharing of Id? One explanation is that the factors and antibodies share the same binding site, coded by the same V_H gene, but due to lack of light chain there are varying degrees of flexibility of the factors' binding site that can therefore accommodate some cross–reactive antigens in a different manner than the antibody. Another possibility is that each component has its own distinct antigen–combining site, but nevertheless expresses similar structure as detected by cross–reaction with the Id antibodies. The third possibility is that the anti-Id antibodies are a heterogeneous mixture and might recognize different specificities on the factors and the antibodies. Hopefully, anti-Id mAbs will soon be available that might help to resolve this issue. A more conclusive solution would be from sequence comparison between purified factors and antibodies or their cloned genes.

C. Association of MHC Gene Products in the T Cell Factors

All the antigen–specific immunoregulatory factors described in this chapter bear determinants coded for by genes in the *I* region of the MHC. It appears that factors exhibiting certain biological activity are products of a defined subregion within the *I* region, i.e., helper and augmenting T cell factors possess *I-A* subregion gene products, while suppressor factors express *I-J* or *I-C* subregion-coded determinants. Moreover, as discussed in the previous sections and described by Tada, Taniguchi, and coworkers,[1,71,72] the *Ia* antigens expressed on ThF and TaF appear to be distinct for T cells. Furthermore, studies with either absorbed conventional anti–*I* antisera or mAbs[85] revealed that antigen–specific hybridomas and their factors express different *Ia* antigens from those expressed by nonspecific hybridomas. These and other results demonstrate the serological heterogeneity of *Ia* antigens on different subsets of functional T cells. Both *I-A* and *I-J* subregion encoded molecules detected on helper and suppressor–antigen–specific T cells, their hybridomas, and functional factors are different molecules from those detected on B cells and Mϕ. All together, these studies indicate functional significance for the *Ia* molecules in the active factors. The observation of Kontiainen et al.,[89] who detected association of *Ia* molecules of BW genotype with functional suppressor factor derived from hybrid clone, clearly implies that the *Ia* molecules do not determine the specificity of the factor. These results do not exclude the possibility that the *Ia* molecule helps to maintain the conformation of the factors' combining site in an active form. The fact that *Ia* molecules serve as the main restriction elements in the systems where MHC restriction of factor activity was observed, suggests that *Ia* molecules serve as interacting molecules whose sole function is either to recognize or to be recognized by the acceptor or target cell.

D. Molecular Organization of T Cell Factors

A minimum model of T cell factor has to accomodate the antigen–combining site, V_H determinants, and *Ia* antigens on one molecule. There is sound information from several independent studies that these three elements co–purify and behave as a linked entity after immunoabsorption. Both helper and suppressor factors eluted from antigen columns can subsequently be readsorbed and eluted form anti–*H-2* or anti–V_H immunoabsorbents.[66,103] The genes coding for V_H determinants and *Ia* antigens are located on different chromosomes (12 and 17 in the mouse). Thus, to assume that these gene products are co–expressed on a single polypeptide chain will require an unprecedented mechanism of interchromosomal rearrangment. However, if one considers the carbohydrate moiety of *Ia* antigens as the polymorphic element, a model can be suggested of a glycoprotein molecule whose peptide backbone is dictated by V_H genes and carbohydrate sidechains constructed by specific glycosyltransferases that are controlled by the *I*-region. In fact, both Liew[94] and Howie et al.,[53] have recently described the removal of factor activity by rabbit antibodies to "carbohydrate" *Ia*[120] antigen.

A survey of the structural characteristics of "conventional" antigen-specific T cell factors has been reported elsewhere.[1-3] Table 5 summarizes additional information concerning monoclonal factors that is currently available. In general, two main types of factors or antigen–binding molecules have been described using extracts or culture supernates derived from heterogeneous or cloned populations of T cells. One type of antigen-specific material, composed of a single chain with molecular weight of about 70,000 was usually reported to lack *Ia* determinants.[114,115,121,124] Representative of this group is the monoclonal SRBC–specific suppressor factor derived from TCGF–dependent cloned lymphocytes.[125,126] This highly purified glycoprotein binds specifically to SRBC and completely suppresses the in vitro production of anti–SRBC PFC, due to inactivation of Ly-1 helper cells. The 70,000 dalton protein undergoes degradation into 45,000 and 24,000 mol wt peptides,[126] the large peptide mediates nonspecific suppression, and the small peptide retains antigen–binding activity but is not reactive. An exception from the single polypeptide group is the 62,000 dalton molecule derived from the ABA–specific hybridoma, recently described by Pacifico and Capra.[109,110] It was claimed that the same peptide that binds ABA specifically also exhibits the arsonate cross–reactive Id and *Ia* antigens. Although so far no function could be assigned to this T cell product, Pacifico and Capra consider four possibilities to explain the unprecedented expression of I and V gene products on a single polypeptide molecule:

1. The *V* region loci have been duplicated and they, or structures related to them, are encoded on chromosome 17;
2. The *I*–region loci have been duplicated and exist on chromosome 6 and/or 12 as well as on chromosome 17;
3. Protein or RNA ligase exists that splices either nucleic acids or protein from different chromosomes;
4. The *I*–loci do not contain the structural genes for the polypeptide chains in question, but rather encode modifying enzymes that actually dictate the serological specificities.

This latter possibility is supported by the suggestion that the serologically detectable *Ia* antigens on factors may be of carbohydrate nature.[53,120]

The second type of antigen–specific T cell molecule is composed of two chains: one that binds antigen and a second that bears *Ia* determinants. In this type of molecule, the two gene products are expressed on separate polypeptide chains that are covalently or noncovalently associated. Most of the experimental data in favor of the two–chain model is derived from studies that analyzed the molecular organization of T cell factors. Taniguchi and associates studied KLH–specific TsF, obtained from either cell–free extracts or culture supernates of suppressor hybrid cells.[12,70,73,74,85-87] As described in section IV.A–1, both KLH and anti–I-J affinity columns removed the TsF activity. Mixing the effluents of the two columns reconstituted most of the activity. Reconstitution of secreted TsF was not obtained unless reduction preceeded the absorption.[74] These results indicate that the extractable TsF is composed of two noncovalently bound chains,[73] and that in the secreted form the V_H-bearing chain and the *I-J*–encoded chain are bound through disulfide bond(s).[74] More recently, Taniguchi et al.[85] have repeated this experiment with ^{35}S–methionine labeled TsF, obtained from KLH–specific hybridoma. Three significant major bands of 45,000, 25,000, and 16,000 dalton were apparent after gel electrophoresis of material eluted from either KLH or anti-*I-J*[b] columns. Upon repeated absorption of the acid eluate from the first columns on a second set of immunoabsorbents only the 45,000 dalton band was obtained in the eluate from the second KLH column, and therefore appears to be the antigen–binding polypeptide chain. The

Table 5
MOLECULAR CHARACTERISTICS OF MONOCLONAL HELPER AND SUPPRESSOR FACTOR

Factor type	Antigenic specificity	MHC restriction	Mol wt	Chain composition	I-region determinants	V-region determinants	Ref.
14							
ThF	(T,G)-A--L	N.T.[a]	55—70,000	V-chain + I-chain	I-A	V_H; Id	14, 65, 66
ThF	CGG	Yes (I-A)	N.T.	Probably 2 chains	I-A	V_H	15, 75
TaF	KLH	Yes (I-A)	60—70,000	N.T.	I-A	N.T.	71
TsF	KLH	Yes (I-J)	70,000	V-chain (45,000) + I-chain (25,000)	I-J	V_H	12, 70, 73, 74, 85
TsF (in vitro)	KLH	No	80,000 (?)	Probably 2 chains	I-J	V_H	9, 89
TsF (in vitro)	NP	No	N.T.	Probably 2 chains	I-J	V_H	89
TsF	(T,G)-A--L	N.T.	50—70,000	Probably 2 chains	I-J	V_H; Id	60, 65
TsF	SRBC	No	200,000	V-chain (85,000) + I-chain (25,000)	I-E/C	V_H negative	11, 90, 91, 92
TsF(DTH)	SRBC	No	<50,000	N.T.	I-J	N.T.	13, 94
TsF(TCGF)	SRBC	N.T.	70,000	Breaks into 24,000 and (45,000)	No	N.T.	125, 126
TsF	GAT	No	24,000	One chain	I-J	Id	42, 102
TsF	ABA	N.T.	92,000 (?)	N.T.	N.T.	Id	26, 121
T_F	ABA	Activity unknown	62,000	One chain	I-J	Id	109, 110

[a]N.T.: not tested at the time the manuscript was submitted for publication.

component of 25,000 dalton was retained on the second anti–*I-J^b* column and most likely corresponds to the *I-J* product. The third peak of 16,000 daltons appeared to be nonspecific material that could also be obtained from BW5147 cell extract. Since in nondissociating conditions, both monoclonal and "conventional" TsF activity was chromatographed in a fraction between 45,000 to 70,000 mol wt, it was suggested by Taniguchi et al.[85] that the antigen–binding and *I-J*–encoded polypeptide chains make up one single unit of the active form of TsF, having a molecular weight of around 68,000. Another two–chain TsF of higher molecular weight is the SRBC–specific monoclonal TsF obtained by Taussig et al.,[91,92] which has a mol wt of about 200,000 as determined by gel filtration. This molecule dissociates into two nondisulfide–linked polypeptide chains of about 85,000 and 25,000 daltons, respectively. Before dissociation, both chains could be bound to SRBC or anti–*H-2* antibodies. However, NP–40 extracts of [^{3}H]-leucine labeled cells analyzed in the same way showed only the 85,000 chain that was not precipitable by anti–*H-2* but bound specifically to SRBC.

Molecular analysis of monoclonal ThF and TaF revealed essentially the same properties described above for the suppressor factors. The (T,G)-A--L–specific helper factor derived from R-9 hybridoma[14,66,103] is a glycoprotein composed of two chains noncovalently associated. The results of experiments, reconstituting effluents obtained from anti–*H-2* and anti-Id immunoabsorbents described in more detail in section III. B–3 are depicted in Figure 3. The conclusion reached from such experiments is that the factor molecule that usually occurs in associated form is composed of two chains, and therefore most of the activity is absorbed by both anti–V_H and anti–*H-2* immunoabsorbents. However, a certain proportion of free independent polypeptide chains do also exist. Such chains would not bind to the irrelevant column. Thus, noncovalently associated, free Ia chains are found in the effluent of anti-Id, and free V-chains are present in the effluent of anti–*H-2* column. Upon mixing the effluents, some of the free chains associate and make up active factor. So far this observation could not be confirmed by structural analysis of the components obtained after the immunoabsorption because of the tendency of some membrane proteins present in the supernates to adhere nonspecifically to the affinity columns. This fact also hampered the affinity purification and biochemical characterization of the (T,G)-A--L–specific ThF obtained from (T,G)-A--L columns. Analysis by gel filtration and absorption on a lentil–lectin column indicated that the factor is a glycoprotein of 50,000 to 70,000 mol wt.

Genetic support for the two separate chains model discussed above for both TsF and ThF is also provided by the studies of Kontiainen et al.[89] As a result of the fusion of BW5147 cells with C57BL/10–activated cells, one hybrid cell line was obtained that yielded factor–bearing *I-J^k* determinants originating from the BW5147 cells. Such factor is therefore composed of entities derived from both parental cells. A similar observations was made by Lonai et al.[75] who showed that one of the CGG–specific helper hybridomas produced a factor that contained both *Ia^b* and *Ia^k* specificities. The factors' V_H moiety derived from the *H-2^b* parental cells, and yet can recombine freely with *Ia^k*, indicating again that the factor is made up of at least two polypeptide chains.

E. Structural Scheme for Antigen-Specific, *Ia*-Bearing T Cell Factors

In the light of all the information described and discussed in the previous sections, a minimal structural scheme of antigen-specific T cell factors can be proposed. As depicted in Figure 4, the functional factor is composed of two polypeptide chains: the structure of one chain (V) is most likely coded by the variable region gene that determines the antigen-binding specificity of the molecule. The second chain (I) is coded by specialized loci in the *I* region of the MHC, located on chromosome 17 in mice. The variable region gene product expresses framework determinants defined by anti–V_H

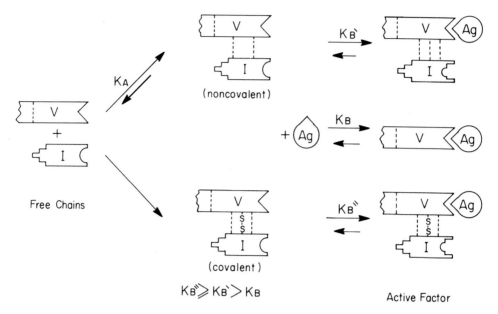

$$K_B'' \gg K_B' > K_B$$

V = Variable Region Product (V_H and Idiotype)

I = MHC I Region Product I-A: Helper Factor

I-J or I-C: Suppressor Factor

FIGURE 4. Model for I–chain and V–chain association in functional T cell factor(s).

antibodies. In certain systems, major or cross–reactive Id markers are also detected on
the factor molecule. Some of them are closely linked to the heavy chain allotypes,
implying that the factors' chain is most likely coded by genes located on chromosome
12 in mice. The factors' two polypeptide chains are synthesized independently and
became associated in the cytoplasm in covalent or nonocovalent complex that comprises the active unit. The noncovalently associated complex (like that shown in Figure
4), exists in equilibrium with the free chains. The antigen–binding site can be similar
(but not identical) to the antibody site. The differences seen in the fine specificity of
antigen binding between factors and antibodies can be attributed to the lack of light
chain that participates in constructing the antibody–binding site, and in many cases
constructs the idiotypic determinants. Possible compensation for the lack of light chain
in the factor can be achieved by association between two adjacent *V* chains, or by
proper attachment of the *I* chain to the factors' *V* chain. Although the mode of such
association is not yet known, it is suggested in the scheme that the associated forms
of the factors have higher avidity to the antigen. It is also possible that interaction with
the antigen stabilizes the active conformation of the binding site, although the *V* chain
of TsF per se can bind antigen, as was shown by Taniguchi et al.[85] and Taussig et al.[92]
To date, it is not yet known if the V_H chain also contains constant region, which by
analogy to the Ig Fc is responsible for the effector properties of different isotypes.
Another possibility is that the *I*–coded chain is responsible for the effector properties
of the factor, thus the *I-A* region is coding for the helper activity and the *I-J* for the
suppressive one. Experiments are presently in progress aimed at determining whether
the I chain of the suppressor factor from R-11 hybridoma will confer specific suppressive activity on the separated V chain, derived from the helper R-9 hybridoma, or vice
versa. The *Ia* antigens expressed on functional T cells and factors differ not only from

the "conventional" B cell *Ia* antigens, but also among various T cell subsets and even between specific and nonspecific hybridoma.[85,87] Although the role and mode of action of *Ia* antigens is not clear as yet, it has been suggested by Tada, Taniguchi, and associates[72] that the *I* region product selects the target cell type to be activated, by virtue of its endowed-restriction specificity. If the heterogeneity of T cell and factor *Ia* antigens is associated with the antigen–binding site, this can be recognized by the acceptor cell to be activated. It is also possible that the binding of antigen to the factor induces conformational changes in the *Ia* molecule, as depicted in Figure 4. This tertiary structure is recognized by other T cells capable of identifying *Ia*–antigen complexes. The molecular mechanism of these interactions, whether they are of "self–self" or "self–anti–self" kind of interaction, and whether the α or the β chains of the *Ia* antigens are exclusively expressed and involved in this intercellular recognition, have to await further analysis of purified components derived from both inducer and acceptor cells. The monoclonal factors described herein and acceptor hybrid cells similar to those described by Taniguchi et al.[85,87] are significant steps towards this aim.

F. Comparison of T Cell Factors and Receptors

Are the antigen–specific factors a soluble version of the T cell receptors? The information available to date is insufficient and does not provide a conclusive answer. Although monoclonal factors and active T cell clones are available, the amounts of active material are so small that the properties of the antigen–reactive molecules could be compared until now only by functional assays.

In some respects the factors' properties are similar to those of the cell-bound receptor. The fine specificity of antigen binding and reactivity toward cross–reacting antigens and the V chain products (framework and Id determinants) appear to be similar in both soluble factors and cell–bound receptors. Additional indirect support for the similarity between the soluble factor and the antigen receptor on T cells comes from the correlation observed by Taniguchi et al.,[85] between the degree of cellular expression of *I-J* and the antigen–binding site of synchronized cultures of suppressor cell hybridoma as well as the level of activity of extracted TsF. Finally, the same restriction elements have been described in some experimental systems for both cloned T cell populations and their monoclonal factors. In these systems the MHC or allotype–restricted or nonrestricted factor activity may correlate to different subsets of the regulatory T cells producing the factor(s).

In spite of the similarities discussed above, few differences are observed between the soluble factors and cell–bound receptors. First, there is the well–known fact that helper T cells do not bind or respond to antigen unless it is presented together with *Ia* antigens. On the other hand, soluble helper factors do bind to immobilized antigens.[14,15] In view of the low functional affinity suggested for the antigen–binding site(s) of the cellular receptor, it is possible that the soluble factor binds to the high density of antigen accessible on the affinity columns with increased avidity. Alternatively, it is possible that soluble Ia antigens present in crude factor preparations or which copurify with the active moiety of the factor, will compensate for the "*Ia*-antigen complex" that binds in higher affinity to helper T cells.[29,30] It is of interest therefore, to verify whether separate helper factor V chains (obtained in the effluent of anti–*H-2* absorbed factor, Figure 3), is still capable of binding to antigen columns. A second phenomenon that is not readily observed with antigen-reactive T cells is that the soluble factor can be absorbed by acceptor cells in the absence of antigen.[75,85,93] It is possible that by dissociating the receptor from its membraneous milieu, such properties of "like–like" interaction became more apparent. In this regard, a group of antigen–binding molecules[114,121–124] derived from T cell but that are devoid of any functional activity has to be mentioned. These molecules display molecular weights in the range described for the soluble functional factors, however, most of them are composed of only one polypeptide chain and lack the *Ia* antigens. The relationship between these molecules and the functional soluble factor(s) or the T cell receptor is also obscure.

Taken together, it appears as if there is enough solid information today in favor of the hypothesis that the soluble factors are products of the same genes coding for the antigen recognition moiety of T cells. How these molecules exert their immunoregulatory function is still an open question and more detailed information obtained from sequence comparison of isolated factor and receptors is needed before any final conclusion can be made.

VI. MECHANISM(S) OF T CELL FACTOR ACTIVITY

A. Genetic Restriction of Factor Activity

One of the most characteristic functional features of T cells is the genetic restriction of their interaction. At least two elements were found to be involved in the genetic restriction: MHC and V_H gene products. The concept of the MHC restriction stems from the general rule that T cells recognize antigen in association with "self"–MHC antigens. This phenomenon is well–established and it is now generally accepted that Ir gene products are "self"–MHC antigens or Ia antigens (for recent discussion see references 127, 128). Less explored is the phenomenon of Ig or idiotype recognition by certain populations of T cells. Id–specific helper[129-133] or suppressor[41,106,107] cells have been described. Some of them, specific for particular Id, are generated by exposure to antigen in the context of that Id and are not generated in the absence of that Id.[131,134,135] While most of the cellular interactions are genetically restricted, only some of the T cell factors react with syngeneic or *I* region compatible target cells. In many experimental systems the ability of TsF and ThF to exert their regulatory function was not genetically restricted. Among the restricted ThF are the RGG helper factor described by Shiozawa et al.,[136] the KLH augmenting factor,[48] the CGG helper factor,[15,71] and the soluble human factor described by Geha.[137] Among the genetically restricted suppressor factors are the KLH specific TsF of Tada and Taniguchi's groups (reviewed in reference 1), the FDNB TsF in contact sensitivity described by Moorhead,[104] and the OVA–specific human TsF.[138]

The second category is of non–MHC restricted factors, such as the in vitro–produced helper and suppressor factors to KLH, GAT, or (T,G)-A--L, reported by Feldmann's group,[41,47,139] the GAT–specific suppressor factor[95-98,102] and the ABA[105-107] TsF described by Benacerraf's group, and the (T,G)-A--L helper factor[50,51] that cooperated with B cells across an *H-2* barrier. It has however to be emphasized, that part of the non–*H-2* restricted factors are acting in fact in V_H compatible manner. In the GAT system, the TsF bearing the anti–GAT cross–reactive Id, present in all mouse strains,[140] is therefore reacting in all these strains in a V_H–restricted manner. Similarly, the non–MHC–restricted ABA–specific TsF suppressed only DTH responses in V_H matched recipient mice that express the ABA cross–reactive Id.[106,107] Similar results have been also obtained in the NP haptenic system.[41]

Because self–MHC restriction is a mandatory characteristic of primed T cells, the question arises as to why certain T cell replacing factors do function in a non–MHC restricted manner. As already stated above, such behavior may indicate that the factor is not the same molecule as the T cell receptor, therefore it functions according to a different and independent mechanism. If so, it is envisaged that the physiological effect of the MHC nonrestricted factors is negligible, since the overall behavior of T cells is restricted. Another explanation is that the apparent MHC nonrestricted factors actually originate from restricted cellular components, but due to their dissociation from the cellular matrix, the soluble factor can also recognize or be recognized by allogenic target cells. This can be due to exposure of cryptic determinants that are common or cross–reactive with the acceptor cell. Finally, the author would like to suggest another explanation, based on the model of the antigen–specific factor depicted in Figure 4. If the two chains composing the factor molecule are not covalently bound and may exist under a certain equilibrium constant also in nonassociated form, it is possible that the antigen–specific V chain will associate with other (not autologous) I chain and form an active factor unit with the new I–region restriction element. Experimentally, such an I–chain could be derived from the target cell population, and if in excess on factors' I–chain, a mixed molecule could be assembled consisting of the antigen–specific V chain of the factor donor and the I–chain of the acceptor cells. The validity of this hypothesis can be examined experimentally. It predicts that in the MHC–restricted factors, there is covalent or tight association between the I– and V–chains. As has been shown by Taniguchi et al.,[74,85] such complexes can be dissociated under reducing conditions and the isolated chains can be obtained from anti–*Ia* and antigen or anti-Id affinity columns. Mixing of such isolated chains derived from allogeneic donors and analysis the *H-2* restriction of the mixed chain factor by its ability to interact with different primed acceptor cells, are feasible experiments with the monoclonal factors available today. In fact, as was shown by Lonai et al.[75] and Kontiainen et al.,[89] mixed assembled monoclonal factor molecules with new restriction elements are obtained from somatic T-cell hybrids.

B. Site(s) of Factor Interaction

The simplest explanation to account for the activity of the antigen–specific T cell factor(s) is by their interaction with the antigen and then focusing the complex composed of *Ia*–bearing factor and antigen onto reactive acceptor sites of the target cell. Nothing is yet known about the molecular events accompanying such interactions and its outcome can be either an inductive (turn-on) or a suppressive (turn-off) signal. The immunoregulatory T cell factor binds to acceptor cells also in the absence of antigen. However, the role of antigen might be in directing the factor onto cells of corresponding specificity and possibly increasing the affinity of binding. The recognition and selection of the cell type to be activated can be accomplished by interaction between the I–region products of both factor and target cell. It is likely that the interaction between T cell factor(s) and target cells mimics the recognition by T cells of antigen presented by Mφ. The elements that participate in these similar recognition events are the antigen, or even Id, associated with the target cell *Ia* antigen. Since the interaction of the T cell factor(s) and acceptor cell was found to be strain–restricted, various mechanisms have been proposed to account for the mode of action between the two MHC products, whether by like–like type of interaction or by complementarity interaction. In view of the polymorphism of *Ia* antigens suggested by Tada,[72] the two interacting molecules are controlled by closely linked multiple I–region loci. Since *I-A* encoded helper factor reacts with cells carrying *I-A* coded acceptors and *I-J* positive suppressor factors further induce other *I-J* T cells to become suppressor (see below) it was suggested[3] that the products of the *I* region themselves have defined biologic acitivity as those of the Fc portion of Ig molecules. Alternatively, the factor molecules can just serve as antigen carriers that are focused onto the appropriate acceptor cell by virtue of their restriction elements. The interaction itself then induces the target cell to function according to what it is programed for.

1. Helper Factors

Helper T cell factors in antibody responses replace T cells and act on B cells in the presence of Mφ.[4,141-143] To identify the target cell that bears the acceptor molecule(s) and directly interacts with the factor, absorption studies were performed utilizing various cell populations. Both B cells[144] and Mφ[142] have been indicated as capable of absorbing the helper activity of conventional and monoclonal[75] ThF. Based on absorption studies and the dependency of factor activity on Mφ,[6] Feldmann suggested that the Mφ serve as integrating cells that are essential as intermediary concentrating devices for ThF. A major question in this context is how ThF, when bound with antigen to accessory cells, is immunogenic for B cells. So far, it was found that direct cellular interaction is required for this process, and that it can be inhibited by anti–*Ia* antisera.[6]

There are also T helper factors that can recruit other T cells. The T cell augmenting factor described by Tokuhisa et al.[48] acts on primed T cells and can be absorbed by T cells. In view of the pathway suggested for the helper T cell induction and function[109] suggested by Feldmann et al.,[145] it is possible that TaF is a product of an amplifier Ly1$^+$ T cell that acts on another Ly1$^+$ effector helper cell. After being triggered by TaF and antigen, the activated effector cell releases ThF that acts on Mφ and B cells. The interaction of TaF with the target T cell is antigen–specific and *I–A*–restricted[48] while the second antigen–specific factor in the helper cell circuit is not MHC–restricted,[47,50] although *H-2* restriction has been observed for the CGG–specific monoclonal ThF.[15,75] The MHC restriction was mapped in the *I–A* subregion. Tada and collaborators[71,72] have observed unique *Ia* antigens on the KLH–specific TaF and the hybridoma producing it. This I-A gene product was shown to be distinct from the *Ia* antigens on B cells or Mφ. The genetic relationship between the helper factor and its acceptor molecule has been studied by Taussig and colleagues in the genetically controlled system of antibody response to (T,G)-A--L.[144] As was reported in a series of studies that also analyzed human ThF,[116] the control over the production of (T,G)-A--L–specific ThF and its acceptor expression were found to be genetically independent. A four–gene model describing the factor–acceptor relationships has been suggested.[3,144] Two of the genes coding for T cell factor and its appropriate acceptor are closely related MHC genes. The products of the two background genes were suggested as either contributing to the structure or controlling the production of the factor and acceptor.[3]

In accordance with Jerne's network theory,[147] which proposed the significance of Id–anti–Id interactions in the physiologic regulation of Ir and the occurrence of T cells with anti-Id specificity,[132] the existence of helper factors lacking antigen–binding site with anti-Id specificity has been indicated.[148] Such factors were identified in the supernate of SRBC– or HRBC–activated cells stimulated in vitro by Con A. The anti-Id specificity of the factors was demonstrated by the ability of red cells coated with antibodies to absorb the factors' activity. Since the B cell receptor for antigen consists of Id, similar mechanism of B cell triggering by antigen–specific and anti-Id–specific factors could be envisaged.

2. Suppressor Factors

Antigen–specific suppressor factors regulate the Ir in a few stages. In antibody responses they can directly block B cells, inhibit helper T cells, or induce the activation of a second population of suppressor cells. Likewise, in cellular responses as DTH and cell–mediated lymphotoxicity (CML), TsF can act on T cells involved in the induction or in the effector phase of the response. Indeed, factors exerting antigen–specific suppression in each of the aforementioned phases have been described and thoroughly discussed.[1-4] The monoclonal TsF described in this chapter is preferable to the heterogeneous TsF derived from supernates or extracts of suppressor cells, since it allows analysis of the mechanism underlying the activity of each individual factor. In most of the systems the activity described for "conventional" factor can be now manifested by cloned lines.

In antibody responses, some monoclonal factors have been reported that interact with B cells, although most of the TsF described acts in carrier–specific manner. In this way, it does not directly block antigen–recognition by B cells. Among the factors affecting B cells is the hybridoma-derived SRBC-specific TsF described by Taussig et al.[90-93] that is being absorbed by unprimed B cells and suggested as acting on B cells, although the participation of Mφ was not convincingly excluded. Another monoclonal factor that suppresses B cells in a class–specific manner is the IgE–specific TsF described by Watanabe et al.[35] that can be absorbed on primed B cells.

More common is the effect of TsF on primed helper T cells in antibody responses. The KLH– and GAT–specific factor prepared from in vitro–activated suppressor cells[4,36,139] acted on nylon wool nonadherent $Ly1^+2^-$ T cells and could be completely absorbed by target T cells.[139] The hybridoma cells established from the in vitro–primed suppressor cells secreted TsF that functioned in a fashion similar to the parental cells' TsF.[9,89] Direct activity on $Ly1^+$ unprimed cells was also manifested by the cloned TsF prepared from TCGF–dependent line by Fresno et al.[125,126] A similar target for the suppressive effect also involved in T–T cell interaction, is shown by the monoclonal TsF active in the elicitation phase of DTH to SRBC.[13] Likewise, the "conventional" hapten–specific TsF studied by Zembala and Asherson[38] and Moorhead[39] directly suppressed primed effector T cells mediating contact sensitivity.[80,104,149] However an alternative mechanism can also be considered in which the TsF can act by passively sensitizing ("arming") Mφ that in turn release nonantigen–specific factor when triggered by the specific antigen (the bystander effect).[79,149,150]

The third mechanism of TsF action, and probably the most studied one, is by induction of further suppressor T cell populations. The KLH–specific TsF studied by Tada, Taniguchi, and their groups[1,12,32,33,70-74,85-88,117] resembles the factors acting in the GAT, GT, ABA, and NP models studied by Benacerraf and his collaborators.[2,40-42,77,81,95-102,105-107,119,128] Although denoted by different numbers, the two groups have described similar complex pathways, consisting of a sequence of activating interactions between the cell types as discussed in detail in references 1 to 4. According to Tada and Taniguchi, TsF derived from $Ly2^+,3^+$ suppressor T cells acts on syngeneic or *H-2*–compatible $Ly1^+2^+,3^+$ acceptor cells. These latter cells are involved as intermediaries in the induction of nylon wool adherent, *I-J*–positive Ts$_2$ cells[151] ($Ly1^-,2^+,3^+$) to mature into suppressor Ts$_2$. Upon encounter with the antigen, the Ts$_2$ cells suppress antibody responses across *H-2* barriers by antigen–nonspecific factors (TsF$_2$).[85]

In the scheme put forward by Benacerraf's laboratory, activated–*I-J* and Id–positive T cells produce TsF$_1$ that is not MHC–restricted, but is functionally restricted by V_H genes. TsF$_1$ induces pre–Ts$_2$ ($Ly1^+2^+,3^+$) to mature Ts$_2$ cells, which are the anti-Id-specific cells that produce TsF$_2$.[106,107] By appropriate cell transfer experiments, it was found that TsF$_2$ acts in an *I-J* or *I-C*-restricted manner and in an antigen- or Id–specific manner on a third set of suppressor T cells (Ts$_3$).[107] Ts$_3$, when triggered with antigen, secretes nonantigen-specific factor TsF$_3$.[2,128,107]

The main difference between the two schemes described above is that induction of Ts$_2$ in the KLH system was strictly MHC–restricted, while no restriction was found in this phase for the other TsF. Such distinction might reflect variations in the mode of factor preparation and the assay system used to detect the factors' activity. It was also suggested[152] that the prevalence of common or cross–reacting Id in the GAT, ABA, and NP responses might replace the *I-J*–restriction reported in the KLH response. Thus, in certain cases, *I-J* products would serve as cell-interaction elements, while Ig-V_H gene compatibility would be a prerequisite in other systems.

The *I-J*–positive hybridomas established by Taniguchi et al.[86] served as an ideal tool to study the factor–acceptor interaction at the molecular level.[85–87] The KLH–specific $V_H{}^+$, *I-J*$^+$, TsF produced by one hybridoma (34S-18) could be absorbed by another T cell hybridoma (34S-281) that expresses only *I-J*^{b}. Coincubation of TsF with the acceptor hybridoma induced the formation of KLH–specific factor that suppressed antibody responses in *H-2*–restricted manner. This TsF$_2$ expressed *I-J*^{b}, but could not be absorbed on KLH affinity columns. Since it acted in KLH–specific manner, Taniguchi et al.[85] suggested that this factor most likely possesses the Id receptor for the antigen–binding structure of TsF.

The studies with the KLH–specific monoclonal TsF did not allow analysis of the involvement of anti-Id suppressor cells and factors, as suggested and studied by Nisonoff and Green[107] and Sy et al.[106] Tada's group recently established NP–specific hybridoma that produces TsF, and carries the Np^b Id. When cultured together with NP–KLH–primed T cells and NP B cells, the factor suppressed formation of the NP Id.[117] However, when the NP–KLH T cells anti-Id–bearing cells were removed (by absorption onto an Id–coated plate), from the NP–KLH T cells no suppression of the Id expression could be demonstrated. This observation supports the aforementioned studies in the GAT and ABA systems about the activation of anti-Id T cells by Id–bearing TsF. Thus, suppressor T cells (Ts$_2$) and factors (TsF$_2$) bearing anti-Id receptors, can interact with Id–bearing T or B cells in the absence of antigen and without the involvement of Ig, and therefore take part in the Id network.[147]

It seems that there is no single mechanism by which the immunoregulatory T cell factors exert their function. The multiplicity of action sites observed for different factors is not due to heterogeneity in the factor preparation, since monoclonal factors displayed a similar pattern of reactivity to that observed for the ''conventional'' factor preparation. Alternatively, it is likely that the different cellular interaction sites reflect the complexity of the T cell circuit. Thus, it is possible that specific factors derived from different cell populations in the circuit will function accordingly and affect various target cells.

Although the molecular basis of factor–acceptor cell interaction is still obscure, the monoclonal approach has provided us with both homogeneous factor preparation and cloned acceptor cells that enabled definition of the restriction elements controlling this interaction. The monoclonal reagents should be a valuable asset for further analysis of the molecular mechanism underlying the antigen recognition, activation, and regulation of T cells.

VII. CONCLUDING REMARKS

The major advantage of functional T cell hybridomas is that they are the ideal source for mass production, purification, and molecular characterization of immunoregulatory T cell factors. The monoclonal factors described in this review reflect the progress that has already been achieved. Large amounts of crude material that contain homogeneous factors are readily available from hybridoma supernates or ascites fluid. The factors' active components can be isolated by conventional methods but affinity chromatography is a more effective method particularly for TsF. This is because TsF expresses higher affinity to antigen than ThF. Although purification to homogeneity of T cell factor in amounts sufficient for detailed physicochemical analysis–like sequence and subunit organization and affinity determination has not yet been reported, the author believes that within the next year basic information will be available. Nevertheless, the constitutive production of factor by hybrid clones enables the analysis of biosynthetically radiolabeled factor molecules in conditions that ascertain the integrity of the molecule that otherwise appears to be easily degraded. However, one cannot yet construct a structural model for the antigen–specific factors. Basically, two types of molecules are apparent: one that accomodates the antigen–binding site, V_H determinants, and the *I*–region product on a single peptide chain, and the second that associates two polypeptide chains. The first bears the V–gene product and the second the I–gene products. A plausible alternative to the two–chain model for the two separate gene products, is the one-chain model where *Ia* determinants are carbohydrates bound to the polypeptide V_H chain (coded by a *V* region-like gene). Resolution between these models will require sequence information. Currently, most of the information related to the presence of variable region determinants on the T cell factors comes indirectly from serologic determinations (e.g., from Id or antiframework [V_H] antibody reactions). Although suggestive, serologic cross–reactivity does not necessarily imply that T cells are utilizing the same B cell pool of V genes to construct their antigen–recognition unit. Final approval for V–gene identity between T cell products and antibodies still awaits direct evidence that should emerge from the sequence analysis of monoclonal V_H and Id–positive factors on both protein and genomic level. To this end, monoclonal T cell factors and antibodies that display similar antigenic specificity and shared idiotypicity, such as in the (T,G)-A--L system or the ABA and NP systems, are greatly advantageous. The issue of *I*–region polymorphism demonstrated by Tada and Taniguchi, using serologic analysis of T cells and their products should also be resolved by sequence comparison of B and T cell Ia antigens or by using DNA recombination techniques when an I–gene cDNA probe will be available. The preparation of mAbs that will preferentially react with T cell *Ia* antigens also should be helpful in analyzing the molecular organization of soluble factors and cell–bound receptors.

Although considerable information is known with regard to the sites of factor interaction within the different stages of the immunological circuits, nothing is known about the molecular events participating and controlling the factor/acceptor interactions. It is assumed that *I*–region products are the recognition elements and that either Id–antigen or Id-anti-Id interactions are necessary for triggering the response. Monoclonal factors and cloned acceptor cells are an ideal system to study the mechanism of action of these factors.

As to the mechanism underlying the different regulatory effects of helper vs. suppressor factors, we can only speculate. The major difference between these factors is that they express and interact with cells carrying different *I*-region products: *I-A* for helper and *I-J* or *I-C* for suppressor factors. Perhaps each factor recognizes (or is recognized by) its appropriate acceptor T cell via the *I*–region restriction elements. Such interaction when accompanied by antigen-Id, or Id–antiidiotype interaction, transmits a specific signal that induces the target cell to differentiate further than for which it was programed. Still, the possibility remains that factors mediating different effects are endowed with different effector molecules (analogous to Fc portion of different Ig classes). The availablility of monoclonal ThF and TsF demonstrating similar antigenic specificities and the same *V* region (akin to those in the (T,G)-A--L system) should enable an analytical comparison of the different components composing the factors.

Many questions remain unanswered: what is the relationship between the soluble T cell factors and the antigen–specific, membrane–bound T cell receptor? what is the physiological role of the factors in vivo? and finally, are factors involved in such disorders as immunodeficiency or autoimmune disease? Since it was demonstrated that both ThF and TsF can be obtained from activated human T cells in vitro, perhaps one can induce antigen–specific factors that will suppress effector cells in autoimmune diseases, allergies, or allograft rejection. Specific helper factors can replace defective or deficient T cells and can facilitate or increase immunity when necessary. The results in model systems have been encouraging, especially for TsF, which when injected into animals in minute amounts rendered them nonresponsive. It has been more difficult to suppress an ongoing response, but it is hoped that with the help of hybridoma–derived monoclonal factors, the right conditions will be established to allow clinical application.

ACKNOWLEDGMENT

I thank Dr. Gerald Hillman for helpful comments and Ms. Esther Gross for excellent secretarial assistance. I am an incumbent of the Recanati Career Development Chair in Cancer Research.

REFERENCES

1. **Tada, T. and Okumura, K.,** The role of antigen-specific T cell factors in the immune response, *Adv. Immunol.,* 28, 1, 1979.
2. **Germain, R. N. and Benacerraf, B.,** Helper and suppressor T cell factors, in *Springer Seminars in Immunopathology,* Vol. 3, Eichmann, K., Ed., Springer-Verlag, Basel, 1980, 93.
3. **Taussig, M.,** Antigen-specific T-cell factors, *Immunology,* 41, 759, 1981.
4. **Feldmann, M. and Kontiainen, S.,** The role of antigen-specific T-cell factors in the immune response, in *Lymphokines,* Vol. 2, Academic Press, New York, 1981, 87.
5. **Mozes, E.,** The nature of antigen-specific T cell factors involved in the genetic regulation of immune responses, in *The Role of Products of the Histocompatibility Gene Complex in Immune Responses,* Katz, D. H. and Benacerraf, B., Eds., Academic Press, New York, 485, 1976.
6. **Feldmann, M. and Basten, A.,** Cell interactions in the immune response *in vitro.* III. Specific cooperation across a cell impermeable membrane, *J. Exp. Med.,* 136, 49, 1972.
7. **Hämmerling, G. J.,** T lymphocyte tissue culture lines produced by cell hybridization, *Eur. J. Immunol.,* 7, 743, 1977.
8. **Goldsby, R., Osborne, B. A., Simpson, E., and Herzenberg, L. A.,** Hybrid cell lines with T-cell characteristics, *Nature (London),* 267, 707, 1977.
9. **Kontiainen, S., Simpson, E., Boherer, E., Beverley, P. C. L., Herzenberg, L. A., Fitzpatrick, W. C., Vogt, P., Torano, A., McKenzie, I. F. C., and Feldmann, M.,** *Nature (London),* 274, 477, 1978.
10. **Taniguchi, M. and Miller, J. F. A. P.,** Specific suppressor factor produced by hybridomas derived from the fusion of enriched suppressor T cells and a lymphoma cell line, *J. Exp. Med.,* 148, 373, 1978.
11. **Taussig, M., Corvalán, J. R. F., Binns, R. M., and Holliman, A.,** Production of an H-2 related suppressor factor by a hybrid T cell line, *Nature (London),* 277, 305, 1979.
12. **Taniguchi, M., Saito, T., and Tada, T.,** Antigen-specific suppressor factor produced by a transplantable I-J bearing T cell hybridoma, *Nature (London),* 278, 555, 1979.
13. **Hewitt, J. and Liew, F. Y.,** Antigen-specific suppressor factors produced by T cell hybridomas for delayed type hypersensitivity, *Eur. J. Immunol.,* 9, 572, 1979.
14. **Eshhar, Z., Apte, R. N., Löwy, I., Ben-Neriah, Y., Givol, D., and Mozes, E.,** T cell hybridoma bearing heavy chain variable region determinants producing (T,G)-A--L specific factor, *Nature (London),* 286, 270, 1980.
15. **Lonai, P., Puri, J., and Hämmerling, G. J.,** H-2 restricted antigen binding by a hybridoma clone that produces antigen-specific helper factor, *Proc. Natl. Acad. Sci. U.S.A.,* 78, 549, 1981.
16. **Finn, O. J., Boniver, J., and Kaplan, H. S.,** Induction, establishment in vitro and characterization of functional antigen-specific, carrier-primed murine T-cell lymphomas, *Proc. Natl. Acad. Sci. U.S.A.,* 76, 4033, 1979.

17. **Julius, M. H. and Augustin, A. A.,** Helper activity of T cells stimulated in long-term culture, *Eur. J. Immunol.,* 9, 671, 1979.
18. **Möller, G.,** Ed., T cell stimulating growth factors, *Immunol. Rev.,* 51, 1980.
19. **Möller, G.,** Ed., T cell clones, *Immunol. Rev.,* 54, 1981.
20. **Parkman, R. and Merler, E.,** Thymus dependent functions of mouse thymocyte-fibroblast hybrid cells, *Nature (London),* 245, 14, 1973.
21. **Köhler, G. and Milstein, C.,** Continuous cultures of fused cells secreting antibody of predefined specificity, *Nature (London),* 256, 495, 1975.
22. **Kaufmann, Y., Berke, G., and Eshhar, Z.,** Cytotoxic T lymphocyte hybridomas which mediate specific tumor cell lysis *in vitro, Proc. Natl. Acad. Sci. U.S.A.,* 78, 2502, 1981.
23. **Nabholz, M., Cianfriglia, M., Acuto, O., Conzelmann, A., Haas, W., Böehmer, H. V., Mc-Donald, H. R., Pohlit, H., and Johnson, J. P.,** Cytolytically active murine T-cell hybrids, *Nature (London),* 287, 437, 1980.
24. **Gorer, P. A. and Kaliss, N.,** The effect of isoantibodies *in vivo* on three different transplantable neoplasms in mice, *Cancer Res.,* 19, 824, 1959.
25. **Fisher, G. A.,** Studies of the culture of leukemic cells *in vitro, Ann. N.Y. Acad. Sci.,* 76, 673, 1958.
26. **Whitaker, R. B. and Ruddle, N. H.,** Antigen-specific T-cell hybrids. I. Ovalbumin binding T-cell hybrid, *Cell. Immunol.,* 55, 56, 1980.
27. **Ruddle, N. H., Beezley, B., and Eardley, D.,** Regulation of self recognition by T cell hybrids, *Cell. Immunol.,* 55, 42, 1980.
28. **Apte, R. N., Dayan, M., and Mozes, E.,** Modulation of the helper activity of educated T cells to synthetic polypeptide poly(Tyr,Glu)-poly(DLAla)-Poly(Lys) by adherent cell bound antigen, *Cell. Immunol.,* 61, 104, 1981.
29. **Puri, J. and Lonai, P.,** Mechanism of antigen binding by T cells. H-2(I-A)-restricted binding of antigen plus Ia by helper cells, *Eur. J. Immunol.,* 10, 273, 1980.
30. **Puri, J., Shinitzky, M., and Lonai, P.,** Concomitant increase in antigen binding and in T cell membrane lipid viscosity induced by the lymphocyte activating factor, LAF, *J. Immunol.,* 124, 1937, 1980.
31. **Apte, R. N., Eshhar, Z., Löwy, I., and Mozes, E.,** Growth and function of antigen-specific immortalized helper T cell lines, in *Experimental Hematology Today, 1980,* Baum, S. J., Ledney, G. D., and Khan, A., Eds., Springer-Verlag, Basel, 1, 1981.
32. **Tada, T., Okumura, K., and Taniguchi, M.,** Regulation of hemocytotropic antibody formation in the rat. VIII. An antigen specific T cell factor that regulates anti-hapten homocytotropic antibody response, *J. Immunol.,* 111, 952, 1973.
33. **Takemori, T. and Tada, T.,** Properties of antigen-specific suppressive T cell factor in the regulation of antibody response of the mouse. 1. *In vivo* activity and immunochemical characterization, *J. Exp. Med.,* 142, 1241, 1975.
34. **Suemura, M., Kishimoto, T., Hirai, Y., and Yamamura, Y.,** Regulation of antibody response in different immunoglobulin classes. III. *In vitro* demonstration of IgE class-specific suppressor functions of DNP-Mycobacterium primed T cells and the soluble factor released from these cells, *J. Immunol.,* 119, 149, 1977.
35. **Watanabe, T., Kimoto, M., Maruyama, S., Kishimoto, T., and Yamamura, Y.,** Regulation of antibody response in different immunoglobulin class. V. Establishment of T hybrid cell line secreting IgE class-specific suppressor factor, *J. Immunol.,* 121, 213, 1978.
36. **Kontiainen, S. and Feldmann, M.,** Suppressor cell induction *in vitro.* III. Antigen-specific suppression by supernatants of suppressor cells, *Eur. J. Immunol.,* 7, 310, 1977.
37. **Herzenberg, L. A., Okumura, K., Cantor, H., Sato, V. L., Shen, F-W., Boyse, E. A., and Herzenber, L. A.,** T cell regulation of antibody response: demonstration of allotype-specific helper T cells and their specific removal by suppressor T cells, *J. Exp. Med.,* 144, 330, 1976.
38. **Asherson, G. L., Zembala, M., and Noworolski, J.,** The purification of specific anti-picryl T suppressor factor which depresses the passive transfer of contact sensitivity: affinity chromatography on antigen and concanavalin A Sepharose and specific elution with hapten and α-methylmannoside, *Immunology,* 35, 1051, 1978.
39. **Moorhead, J. W.,** Soluble factors in tolerance and contact sensitivity to DFNB in mice. II. Genetic requirements for suppression of contact sensitivity by soluble suppressor factor, *J. Immunol.,* 119, 1773, 1977.
40. **Green, M. I., Bach, B. A., and Benacerraf, B.,** Mechanisms of regulation of cell-mediated immunity. III. The characterization of azobenzenearsonate-specific suppressor T cell derived factors, *J. Exp. Med.,* 149, 1069, 1979.
41. **Weinberger, J. Z., Benacerraf, B., and Dorf, M. E.,** Hapten-specific T cell responses to 4-hydroxy-3-nitrophenyl acetyl. III. Interaction of effector suppressor T cells is restricted by H-2 and Igh-V genes, *J. Exp. Med.,* 151, 1413, 1980.

42. **Kapp, J. A., Araneo, B. A., and Clevinger, B. L.,** Suppression of antibody and T cell proliferative responses to L-glutamic^{60}-L-alanine^{30}-L-tyrosine^{10} by a specific monoclonal T cell factor, *J. Exp. Med.,* 152, 235, 1980.

43. **Jones, C. M., Braatz, J. A., and Herberman, R. B.,** Production of both macrophage activating and inhibiting activities by a murine T-lymphocyte hybridoma, *Nature (London),* 291, 502, 1981.

44. **Schrier, M. H. and Tees, R.,** Clonal induction of helper T cells: conversion of specific signals into nonspecific signals, *Int. Arch. Allergy Appl., Immunol.,* 61, 227, 1980.

45. **Taussig, M. J.,** T cell factor which can replace T cells *in vivo, Nature (London),* 248, 234, 1974.

46. **Isac, R. and Mozes, E.,** Antigen-specific T cell factors: a fine analysis of specificity, *J. Immunol.,* 118, 584, 1977.

47. **Howie, S. and Feldmann, M.,** *In vitro* studies on H-2 linked unresponsiveness to synthetic polypeptides. III. Production of an antigen-specific T helper cell factor to (T,G)-A--L., *Eur. J. Immunol.,* 7, 417, 1977.

48. **Tokuhisa, T., Taniguchi, M., Okumura, K., and Tada, T.,** An antigen-specific I-region gene product that augments the antibody response, *J. Immunol.,* 120, 414, 1978.

49. **Munro, A. J., Taussig, M. J., Campbell, R., Williams, H., and Lawson, Y.,** Antigen-specific T cell factor in cell co-operation. Physical properties and mappings in the left hand (K) half of H-2, *J. Exp. Med.,* 140, 1579, 1974.

50. **Taussig, M. J., Munro, A. J., Campbell, R., David, C. S., and Staines, N. A.,** Antigen-specific T cell factor in cell co-operation. Mapping within the I region of the H-2 complex and ability to co-operate across allogeneic barriers, *J. Exp. Med.,* 142, 697, 1975.

51. **Mozes, E.,** Some properties and functions of antigen-specific T cell factors, in *Ir Genes and Ia Antigens,* McDevitt, H. O., Ed., Academic Press, New York, 475, 1978.

52. **Isac, R., Dorf, M. E., and Mozes, E.,** The T cell factor specific for poly(Tyr,Glu)-poly-Pro-poly-Lys is an I-region gene product, *Immunogenetics,* 5, 467, 1977.

53. **Howie, S., Parish, C. R., David, C. S., McKenzie, I. F. C., Maurer, P. H., and Feldmann, M.,** Serological analysis of antigen-specific helper factors specific for poly-L-(Tyr,Glu)-poly-DL-Ala-poly-L-Lys (T,G)-A--L and LGlu^{60}-LAla^{30}-LTyr^{10} (GAT), *Eur. J. Immunol.,* 9, 501, 1979.

54. **Sela, M., Fuchs, S., and Arnon, R.,** Studies on the chemical basis of the antigenicity of proteins. V. Synthesis, characterization and immunogenicity of some multichain and linear polypeptides containing tyrosine, *Biochem. J.,* 85, 223, 1962.

55. **Mozes, E. and Shearer, G. M.,** Genetic control of immune responses, *Curr. Top. Microbiol. Immunol.,* 59, 167, 1972.

56. **McDevitt, H. O. and Chinitz, A.,** Genetic control of the antibody response: relationship between immune response and histocompatibility (H-2) type, *Science,* 163, 1207, 1969.

57. **Mozes, E. and Haimovich, J.,** Antigen-specific T cell helper factor cross reacts idiotypically with antibodies of the same specificity, *Nature (London),* 278, 56, 1979.

58. **Ben-Neriah, Y., Wuilmart, C., Lonai, P., and Givol, D.,** Preparation and characterization of anti-framework antibodies to the heavy chain variable region (V$_H$) of mouse immunoglobulins, *Eur. J. Immunol.,* 8, 797, 1978.

59. **Ben-Neriah, Y., Lonai, P., Gavish, M., and Givol, D.,** Preparation and characterization of antibodies to the λ chain variable region (V$_λ$) of mouse immunoglobulins, *Eur. J. Immunol.,* 8, 792, 1978.

60. **Eshhar, Z., Apte, R., Löwy, I., and Mozes, E.,** T cell hybridomas producing (T,G)-A—L specific helper and suppressor factors, in, *Monoclonal Antibodies and T cell Hybridomas,* Hämmerling, G., Hämmerling, U., and Kearney, J. F., Eds., Elsevier/North–Holland, Amsterdam, 1981, 469.

61. **Schwartz, M., Lifshitz, R., Givol, D., Mozes, E., and Haimovich, J.,** Cross reactive idiotypic determinants on murine anti-(T,G)-A—L antibodies, *J. Immunol.,* 121, 421, 1978.

62. **Lifshitz, R., Parhami, B., and Mozes, E.,** Enhancing effect of murine anti-idiotypic serum on the proliferative response specific for poly(Tyr,Glu)-poly(DLAla)-poly(Lys), *Eur. J. Immunol.,* 11, 27, 1981.

63. **Strassmann, G., Lifshitz, R., and Mozes, E.,** Elicitation of delayed type hypersensitivity responses to (T,G)-A--L by anti-idiotypic antibodies, *J. Exp. Med.,* 152, 1448, 1980.

64. **Parhami, B., Eshhar, Z., and Mozes, E.,** Production and characterization of monoclonal antibodies specific to (T,G)-A--L and its ordered analogue (T-T-G-G)-A--L, *Isr. J. Med. Sci.,* in press.

65. **Eshhar, Z., Apte, R. N., Löwy, I., and Mozes, E.,** (T,G)-A--L specific immunoregulatory factors produced by T-hybridomas, in *Mechanisms of Lymphocytes Activation,* Resh, K. and Kirchner, H., Eds., Elsevier/North Holland, Amsterdam, 1981, 557.

66. **Apte, R. N., Eshhar, Z., Löwy, I., Zinger, H., and Mozes, E.,** Characterization of a poly(Tyr,Glu)-poly(DLAla)—poly(Lys) specific helper factor derived from a T cell hybridoma, *Eur. J. Immunol.,* 11, 931, 1981.

67. **Mozes, E., McDevitt, H. O., Jaton, J.-C., and Sela, M.,** The nature of the antigenic determinant in the genetic control of the antibody response, *J. Exp. Med.,* 130, 493, 1969.

68. **Lonai, P., Ben-Neriah, Y., Steinman, L., and Givol, D.,** Selective participation of immunoglobulin V region and major histocompatibility complex products in antigen binding by T cells, *Eur. J. Immunol.,* 8, 827, 1978.

69. **Eichmann, K., Ben-Neriah, Y., Hetzelberger, D., Polke, C., Givol, D., and Lonai, P.,** Correlated expression of V_H framework and V_H idiotypic determinants on T helper cells and on functionally undefined T cells binding group A streptococcal carbohydrate, *Eur. J. Immunol.,* 10, 105, 1980.

70. **Taniguchi, M., Takei, I., Saito, T., Hiramatsu, K., and Tada, T.,** Functional organization of I-J subregion gene products on T cell hybridomas, in *Biochemical Characterization of Lymphokines,* deWeck, A. L., Kristansen, F., and Landy, M., Eds., Academic Press, New York, 577, 1980.

71. **Hiramatsu, K., Miyatani, S., Kim, M., Yamada, S., Okamura, K., and Tada, T.,** Unique T cell Ia antigen expressed on a hybrid cell line producing antigen specific augmenting T cell factor, *J. Immunol.,* 127, 1118, 1981.

72. **Tada, T., Taniguchi, M., Okumura, K., Hayakawa, K., Hiramatsu, K., and Suzuki, G.,** Ia antigens on T cell factors produced by hybridomas, in *Proc. 7th Conv. Immunology, Immunobiology of Major Histocompatibility Complex, No. 9,* Zaleski, M. B., Ed., S. Karger, Basel, 1980, 1.

73. **Taniguchi, M. and Takei, I.,** Functional and molecular organization of an antigen-specific suppressor factor from a T cell hybridoma, *Nature (London),* 283, 227, 1980.

74. **Taniguchi, M., Saito, T., Takei, I., and Tokuhisa, T.,** Presence of interchain S-S bonds between the gene products that compose the secreted form of an antigen-specific suppressor factor, *J. Exp. Med.,* 153, 1672, 1981.

75. **Lonai, P., Puri, J., and Hämmerling, G. J.,** T hybridoma cells which produce genetically restricted helper factors and bind the carrier in association with Ia, in *Lymphokine Reports,* Feldmann, M. and Schrier, M., Eds., Academic Press, New York, in press.

76. **Jones, T. B. and Kaplan, A. M.,** Immunologic tolerance to HGG in mice. I. Suppression of the HGG response in normal mice with spleen cells or spleen cell lysate from tolerant mice, *J. Immunol.,* 118, 1880, 1977.

77. **Kapp, J. A., Pierce, C. W., De La Croix, F., and Benacerraf, B.,** Immunopressive factor(s) extracted from lymphoid cells of nonresponder mice primed with L-glutamic acid[60]-L-alanine[30]-L-tyrosine[10] (GAT). I. Activity and antigen specificity, *J. Immunol.,* 116, 305, 1976.

78. **Swierkosz, J. E. and Swanborg, R. H.,** Suppressor cell control of unresponsiveness to experimental allergic encephalomyelitis, *J. Immunol.,* 115, 631, 1975.

79. **Zembala, M. and Asherson, G. L.,** T cell suppression of contact sensitivity in the mouse. II. The role of soluble suppressor factor and its interaction with macrophages, *Eur. J. Immunol.,* 4, 799, 1974.

80. **Moorhead, J. W.,** Soluble factors in tolerance and contact sensitivity to 2,4-dinitrofluorobenzene in mice. I. Suppression of contact sensitivity by soluble suppressor factor released *in vitro* by lymph node cells, *J. Immunol.,* 119, 315, 1977.

81. **Green, M. I., Pierres, A., Dorf, M. E., and Benacerraf, B.,** The I-J subregion codes for determinants on suppressor factor(s) which limit the contact sensitivity response to picryl chloride, *J. Exp. Med.,* 146, 293, 1977.

82. **Borel, Y.,** Hapten bound to self IgG induce immunologic tolerance, while when coupled to syngeneic spleen cells they induce immune suppression, *Immunol. Rev.,* 50, 71, 1981.

83. **Gershon, R. K.,** T cell control of antibody production, *Contemp. Top. Immunobiol.,* 3, 1, 1974.

84. **Möller, G.,** Ed., Suppressor T lymphocytes, *Transp. Rev.,* 26, 1975.

85. **Taniguchi, M., Saito, T., Takei, I., Kanno, M., Tokuhisa, T., and Tomioka, H.,** Suppressor T cell hybridomas and their soluble products, in *Lymphokine Reports,* Vol. 5, Feldmann, M. and Schrier, M. Eds., Academic Press, New York, in press.

86. **Taniguchi, M., Saito, T., Takei, I., and Tada, T.,** The establishment of T cell hybridomas with specific suppressive function, in *T and B Lymphocytes: Recognition and Function,* Bach. F., Bonavida, B., and Vitetta, E., Eds., Academic Press, New York, 667, 1979.

87. **Taniguchi, M., Takei, I., Saito, T., and Tokuhisa, T.,** Activation of an acceptor T cell hybridoma by a V_H^+ I-J$^+$ monoclonal suppressor factor, in *Immunoglobulin Idiotypes and Their Expression,* Janeway, C., Sercraz, E., and Wigzell, H., Eds., Academic Press, New York, in press.

88. **Tada, T., Nonaka, M., Okumura, K., Taniguchi, M., and Tokuhisa, T.,** in *Cell Biology and Immunology of Leukocyte Function,* Quastel, M., Ed., Academic Press, New York, 353, 1979.

89. **Kontiainen, S., Cecka, J. M., Culbert, E., Simpson, E., and Feldmann, M.,** T cell hybrids producing antigen-specific factors, in *Protides of the Biological Fluids,* Vol. 28, Peeters, H., Ed., Pergamon Press, Oxford, 451, 1980.

90. **Taussig, M. J., Corvalan, J. R. F., Binns, R. M., Roser, B., and Holliman, A.,** Immunological activity of a hybrid line. I. Production of an H-2 related suppressor factor with specificity for sheep red blood cells, *Eur. J. Immunol.,* 9, 768, 1979.

91. **Taussig, M. J. and Holliman, A.,** Structure of an antigen-specific suppressor factors produced by a hybrid T cell line, *Nature (London),* 277, 308, 1979.

92. **Taussig, M. J., Corvalan, J. R. F., and Holliman, A.,** Characterization of an antigen-specific factor from hybrid T cell line, *Ann. N.Y. Acad. Sci.,* 332, 316, 1979.

93. **Taussig, M. J.,** Antigen specific suppressor factor from a T hybrid line and its B cell acceptor, in *Protides of the Biological Fluids,* Vol. 28, Peeters, H., Ed., Pergamon, Oxford, 529, 1980.

94. **Liew, F. Y., Sia, D. Y., Parish, C. R., and McKenzie, I. F. C.,** Major histocompatibility gene complex (MHC) coded determinants on antigen-specific suppressor factor for delayed type hypersensitivity and surface phenotypes of cells producing the factor, *Eur. J. Immunol.,* 10, 305, 1980.

95. **Kapp, J. A., Pierce, C. W., Schlossman, S., and Benacerraf, B.,** Genetic control of immune responses *in vitro.* V. Stimulation of suppressor T cells in nonresponder mice by the terpolymer L-glutamic acid^{60}-L-alanine^{30}-L-tyrosine^{10} (GAT), *J. Exp. Med.,* 140, 648, 1974.

96. **Debré, P., Kapp, J. A., Dorf, M. E., and Benacerraf, B.,** Genetic control of immune suppression. I. Experimental conditions for the stimulation of suppressor cells by the copolymer L-glutamic acid^{50}-L-tyrosine^{50} (GT) in nonresponder BALB/c mice, *J. Exp. Med.,* 142, 1436, 1975.

97. **Debré, P., Waltenbaugh, C., Dorf, M. E., and Benacerraf, B.,** Genetic control of specific immune suppression. III. Mapping of H-2 complex complementing genes controlling immune suppression by the random copolymer, L-glutamic acid^{50}-L-tyrosine (GT), *J. Exp. Med.,* 144, 272, 1976.

98. **Waltenbaugh, C., Thézé, J., Kapp, J. A., and Benacerraf, B.,** Immunosuppressive factor(s) specific for L-glutamic acid^{50}, L-tyrosine^{50} (GT). III. Generation of suppressor T cells by suppressive extract derived from GT-primed lymphoid cells, *J. Exp. Med.,* 146, 970, 1977.

99. **Germain, R. N., Ju, S.-T., Kipps, T. J., Benacerraf, B., and Dorf, M. E.,** Shared idiotypic determinants on antibodies and T-cell-derived suppressor factor specific for the random terpolymer L-glutamic acid^{60}-L-alanine^{30}-L-tyrosine^{10}, *J. Exp. Med.,* 149, 613, 1979.

100. **Waltenbaugh, C. and Benacerraf, B.,** Specific suppressor extract stimulates the production of suppressor T cells, in *Proc. 3rd Ir Gene Workshop,* McDevitt, M. O., Ed., Academic Press, New York, 1978, 549.

101. **Germain, R. N., Thézé, J., Kapp, J. A., and Benacerraf, B.,** Antigen-specific T-cell-mediated suppression. I. Induction of L-glutamic acid^{60}-L-alanine^{30}-L-tyrosine^{10} specific suppressor T cell *in vitro* requires both antigen-specific T-cells suppressor factor and antigen, *J. Exp. Med.,* 147, 123, 1978.

102. **Webb, D. R., Krupen, K., Araneo, B., Kapp, J., Nowowiejski, I., Healy, C., Wieder, K., and Stein, S.,** Chemical characterization of antigen specific suppressor lymphokines, in *Potential Utilization of Lymphokines in Cancer Therapeutics,* Raven Press, New York, in press.

103. **Mozes, E., Eshhar, Z., and Apte, R. N.,** Soluble products of functional T cell continuous lines and hybridomas specific to the synthetic polypeptide (T,G)-A--L, in *Lymphokine Reports,* Vol. 5, Feldmann, M. and Schrier, M., Eds., Academic Press, New York, in press.

104. **Moorhead, J. W.,** Soluble factors in tolerance and contact sensitivity to 2,4-dinitrofluorobenzene in mice. III. Histocompatibility antigens associates with the hapten dinitrophenol serve as target molecules on 2,4-dinitroflurobenzene immune T cells for soluble suppressor factor, *J. Exp. Med.,* 150, 1432, 1979.

105. **Bach, B. A., Greene, M. I., Benacerraf, B., and Nisonoff, A.,** Mechanism of regulation of cell mediated immunity. IV. Azobenzenearsonate specific suppressor factor(s) bear cross reactive idiotypic determinants the expression of which is linked to the heavy chain allotype linkage group of genes, *J. Exp. Med.,* 149, 1084, 1979.

106. **Sy, M.-S., Dietz, M. H., Germain, R. N., Benacerraf, B., and Green, M. I.,** Antigen and receptor driven regulatory mechanisms. IV. Idiotype bearing suppressor T cells factor (TsF) induces second order suppressor cells (Ts2) which express anti-idiotypic receptors, *J. Exp. Med.,* 151, 1183, 1980.

107. **Nisonoff, A. and Green, M. I.,** Regulation through idiotypic determinants of the immune response to the P-azophenylarsonate hapten in strain A mice, in *Progress in Immunology,* Vol. 4, Fougereau, M. and Dausset, J., Eds., Academic Press, New York, 1980, 57.

108. **Nisonoff, A., Ju, S.-T., and Owen, F. L.,** Studies of structure and immunosuppression of a cross reactive idiotypes in strain A mice, *Immunol. Rev.,* 34, 89, 1977.

109. **Pacifico, A. and Capra, J. D.,** T cell hybrids with arsonate specificity. I. Initial characterization of antigen-specific T cell products that bear a cross-reactive idiotype determinants encoded by the murine major histocompatibility complex, *J. Exp. Med.,* 152, 1289, 1980.

110. **Estess, P., McCumber, L., Siegelman, M., Waldschmidt, T., Pacifico, A., and Capra, J. D.,** in *Progress in Immunology,* Vol. 4, Fougereau, M. and Dausset, J., Eds., Academic Press, New York, 1980, 3.

111. **Imanishi-Kari, T. and Mäkëla, O.,** Inheritance on antibody specificity. I. Anti-(4-hydroxy-3-nitro-phenyl) acetyl of the mouse primary response, *J. Exp. Med.,* 140, 1498, 1974.

112. **Karjalainen, K. and Mäkëla, O.,** A mendalian idiotype is demonstrable in the heteroclitic anti-NP antibodies of the mouse, *Eur. J. Immunol.,* 8, 105, 1978.

113. **Jack, R. S., Imanishi-Kari, T., and Rajewsky, K.,** Idiotypic analysis of the response of C57BL/6 mice to (4-hydroxy-3-nitrophenyl) acetyl groups, *Eur. J. Immunol.,* 7, 559, 1977.

114. **Krawinkel, U., Cramer, M., Imanishi-Kari, T., Jack, R. S., Rajewsky, K., and Mäkëla, O.,** Isolated hapten-binding receptors of sensitized lymphocytes. I. Receptors from nylon wool-enriched mouse T lymphocytes lack serological markers immunoglobulin constant domains but express heavy chain variable portions, *Eur. J. Immunol.,* 7, 566, 1977.

115. **Krawinkel, U., Cramer, P., Melchers, I., Imanishi-Kari, T., and Rajewsky, K.,** Isolation of hapten-binding receptors of sensitized lymphocytes. III. Evidence for idiotypic restriction of T cell receptors, *J. Exp. Med.,* 147, 1341, 1978.

116. **Sy, M.-S., Dietz, M., Nisonoff, A., Germain, R. N., Benacerraf, B., and Greene, M. I.,** Antigen and receptor-drived regulatory mechanisms. V. The failure of idiotype-coupled spleen cells to induce unresponsiveness in animals lacking the appropriate V_H genes is caused by the lack of idiotype-matched targets, *J. Exp. Med.,* 152, 1226, 1981.

117. **Tada, T., Okumura, K., Hayakawa, K., Suzuki, G., Abe, R., and Kumagai, Y.,** Immunological circuitry governed by MHC and V_H gene products, in *Immunoglobulin Idiotypes and Their Expression,* Janeway, C., Sercraz, E., and Wigzell, H., Eds., Academic Press, New York, in press.

118. **Sege, K. and Peterson, P. A.,** Use of anti-idiotypic antibodies as cell surface receptor probes, *Proc. Natl. Acad. Sci. U.S.A.,* 75, 2443, 1981.

119. **Thézé, J., Kapp, J. A., and Benacerraf, B.,** Immunosuppressive factor(s) extracted from lymphoid cells of non responder mice primed with L-glutamic acid^{60}-L-alanine^{30}-L-tyrosine^{10} (GAT). III. Immunochemical properties of the GAT-specific suppressive factor, *J. Exp. Med.,* 145, 839, 1977.

120. **Parish, C. R., Jackson, D. C., and McKenzie, I. F. C.,** Low molecular weight Ia antigens in normal mouse serum. III. Isolation and partial chemical characterization, *Immunogenetics,* 3, 455, 1976.

121. **Goodmann, J. W., Lewis, G. K., Primi, D., Hornbeck, P., and Ruddle, N. H.,** Antigen-specific molecules from murine T lymphocytes on T cell hybridomas, *Mol. Immunol.,* 17, 933, 1080.

122. **Binz, H. and Wigzell, H.,** Shared idiotypic determinants on B and T lymphocytes reacting against the same antigenic determinants. V. Biochemical and serological characteristics of naturally occurring soluble antigen-binding T-lymphocyte-derived molecules, *Scand. J. Immunol.,* 5, 559, 1976.

123. **O'Connor, S., Eardly, D., Shen, F.-W., Gershon, R. K., and Cone, R. E.,** Isolation and partial characterization of antigen binding molecules produced by in-vitro educated T cells, *Mol. Immunol.,* 17, 913, 1980.

124. **Rubin, B., Suzan, M., Kahn-Perles, B., Boyer, C., Schiff, C., and Bourgois, A.,** Isolation, and biochemical characterization of idiotype bearing T cell receptors which express private allotype and/or isotypes: a review, *Bull. Inst. Pasteur, Paris,* 78, 305, 1980.

125. **Fresno, M., Nabel, G., McVay-Boudreau, L., Furthmayer, H., and Cantor, H.,** Antigen-specific T lymphocyte clones. I. Characterization of a T lymphocyte clone expressing antigen-specific activity, *J. Exp. Med.,* 143, 1246, 1981.

126. **Fresno, M., McVay-Boudreau, L., Nabel, G., and Cantor, H.,** Antigen-specific T lymphocyte clones. II. Purification and biochemical characterization of an antigen-specific suppressive protein synthesized by cloned T cells, *J. Exp. Med.,* 143, 1260, 1981.

127. **Janeway, C. A. and Jason, J. M.,** How T lymphocytes recognize antigen, in *Critical Reviews in Immunology,* Vol. 1, Atassi, M. Z., Ed., CRC Press, Boca Raton, Fla., 133, 1980.

128. **Benacerraf, B.,** Genetic control of the specificity of T lymphocytes and their regulatory products, in *Progress in Immunology,* Vol. 4, Fougereau, M. and Dausset, J., Academic Press, New York, 1980, 419.

129. **Hämmerling, G. J., Black, S. J., Berek, C., Eichmann, K., and Rajewsky, K.,** Idiotypic analysis of lymphocytes *in vitro.* II. Genetic control of T-helper cell responsiveness to anti-idiotypic antibody, *J. Exp. Med.,* 143, 861, 1976.

130. **Eichmann, K., Falk, I., and Rajewsky, K.,** Recognition of idiotypes in lymphocyte interactions. II. Antigen-independent cooperation between T and B lymphocytes that possess similar and complementary idiotypes, *Eur. J. Immunol.,* 8, 853, 1978.

131. **Woodland, R. and Cantor, H.,** Idiotype-specific T helper cells are required to induce idiotype-positive B memory cells to secrete antibody, *Eur. J. Immunol.,* 8, 600, 1978.

132. **Julius, M. H., Cosenza, H., and Augustin, A. A.,** Enrichment of hapten-specific helper T cells using anti-immunoglobulin combining site antibodies, *Eur. J. Immunol.,* 10, 112, 1980.

133. **Janeway, C. A.,** Idiotypes, T cell receptors, and T-B cooperation, *Contemp. Top. Immunobiol.,* 9, 171, 1981.

134. **Janeway, C. A., Murgita, R. A., Weinbaum, F. I., Asofsky, R., and Wigzell, H.,** Evidence for an immunoglobulin-dependent antigen-specific helper T cell, *Proc. Natl. Acad. Sci. U.S.A.,* 74, 4582, 1977.

135. **Bottomly, K., Mathieson, B. J., Cosenza, H., and Mosieri, D. E.,** Idiotype specific regulation of the response to phosphorylcholine by T cells from mice with high and low levels of circulating idiotype, in *B Lymphocytes in the Immune Response,* Cooper, M., Mosier, D. E., Scher, I., and Vitetta, E., Eds., Elsevier/North-Holland, Amsterdam, 323, 1980.

136. **Shiozawa, C., Singh, B., Rubenstein, S., and Diener, E.,** Molecular control of B cell briggering by antigen specific T cell derived helper factor, *J. Immunol.,* 188, 2199, 1977.

137. **Geha, R. S.,** Regulation of human B cell activation, *Immunol. Rev.,* 45, 275, 1979.

138. **Ballieux, R. E., Heijnen, C. J., Uytdehaag, F., and Zegers, B. J. M.,** Regulation of B cell activity in man: role of T cells, *Immunol. Rev.,* 45, 3, 1979.

139. **Kontiainen, S. and Feldmann, M.,** Suppressor-cell induction *in vitro.* IV. Target of antigen-specific suppressor factor and its genetic relationships, *J. Exp. Med.,* 147, 110, 1978.

140. **Ju, S. T., Benacerraf, B., and Dorf, M. E.,** Idiotypic analysis of anti-GAT antibodies; interstrain and interspecies idiotypic cross-reaction, *Proc. Natl. Acad. Sci. U.S.A.,* 75, 6192, 1978.

141. **McDougal, J. S. and Gordon, D. S.,** Generation of T-helper cells *in vitro.* II. Analysis of supernates derived from T-helper cell cultures, *J. Exp. Med.,* 145, 693, 1977.

142. **Howie, S. and Feldmann, M.,** Immune response (Ir) genes expressed at macrophages-B-lymphocyte interactions, *Nature (London),* 273, 664, 1978.

143. **Feldmann, M., Howie, S., Erb., P., Maurer, P., Mozes, E., and Hämmerling, U.,** *In vitro* responses under I region control, in *Ir Genes and Ia Antigens,* McDevitt, H. O., Ed., Academic Press, New York, 1978, 315.

144. **Munro, A. J. and Taussig, M. J.,** Two genes in the major histocompatibility complex control immune response, *Nature (London),* 256, 103, 1975.

145. **Feldmann, M., Beverly, P. C. L., Woady, J., and McKenzie, I. F. C.,** T-T- interactions in the induction of suppressor and helper T cells: analysis of membrane phenotype of precursor and amplifier cells, *J. Exp. Med.,* 145, 793, 1977.

146. **Taussig, M. J. and Finch, A. P.,** Detection of acceptor site on human lymphocytes for antigen-specific T cell factors, *Nature (London),* 270, 151, 1977.

147. **Jerne, N. K.,** Toward a network theory of the immune system, *Ann. Immunol. (Paris),* 125C, 373, 1979.

148. **Bernabe, R. R., Martinez-Allonso, C., and Coutinho, A.,** The specificity of nonspecific concanavalin A induced helper factors, *Eur. J. Immunol.,* 9, 546, 1979.

149. **Asherson, G. L., Zembala, M., Thomas, W. R., and Perera, M. A. C. C.,** Suppressor cells and the handling of antigen, *Immunol. Rev.,* 50, 3, 1980.

150. **Ptak, W., Zembala, M., and Gershon, R. K.,** Intermediary role of macrophages in the passage of suppressor signals between T cell subsets, *J. Exp. Med.,* 148, 424, 1978.

151. **Taniguchi, M. and Tokuhisa, T.,** Cellular consequences in the suppression of antibody response by the antigen-specific T-cell factor, *J. Exp. Med.,* 151, 517, 1980.

152. **Tada, T. and Hayakawa, K.,** Antigen-specific helper and suppressor factors, *Progress in Immunology,* Vol. 4, Fougereau, M. and Dausset, J., Eds., Academic Press, New York, 1980, 389.

153. **Ben-Neriah, Y.,** Personal communication.

INDEX

A

Acetylcholine receptor (AChR), 8—9, 96
AChR, see Acetylcholine receptor
Acquired hypogammaglobulinemia, 82
Activated T lymphocyte enrichment, 135—137
Activating mAbs, 7, 8
Activation of cells, 10
Adenylate cyclase, 104
AEF, see Allogeneic effect factor
AFP, see α-Fetoprotein
Agglutinins, 92, 93
AKV2, see Endogenous ecotropic virus of AKR
    mice
Allogeneic effect factor (AEF), 115—118
    biological effects of, 115—116
    secretion of by T cell hybridomas, 116—118
Allosteric blocking, 46
AMLR, see Autologous mixed lymphocyte
    reaction
Analysis
    biochemical, 121—122, 125—127
    idiotypic, 104—105
Anaphylaxis, 2
Anemia, 97
Anti-AChR antibodies, 96, 97
    pathogenicity of, 9
Antibody-dependent cytolysis of target cells, 5
Antibody response, 138—139
Anti-2,4-dinitrophenyl, 2
Anti-DNA antibodies, 98
Anti-DNP, 4
Antierythrocyte antibodies, 97—98
Antigens
    carcinoembryonic, 14
    differentiation, 24
    GBS, 15
    Ia, 78
    parasite surface, 15
    protein, 144—146
    Sm, 102
    streptococcal, 15
    synthetic polypeptide, 147—148
    T cell, 72—78
Antigen-specific functional hybridomas, 137—138
Antigen-specific helper factor, see T cell antigen-
    specific helper factor
Antigen-specific Ia-bearing T cell factors,
    155—157
Antigen-specific suppressor factors, 160
Anti-Ia antibody inhibition, 116—118
Anti-V_H antibodies, 140
Anti-V_L antibodies, 140
Antinuclear antibodies, 94
Antinucleic acid antibodies, 98—102
Antireceptor antibodies, 104
Anti-Sm antibodies, 102—104
Anti-T cell mAbs, 83
Antithymocyte antibodies, 97—98

A (continued)

Assays, see also specific assays and tests,
    124—125
    binding, 27—28
    conditions and procedures for, 26—27
    ELISA, 4, 5
    ELMIA, 15
    enzyme, 4, 5, 15, 16
    fluorescence, 28
    immuno-, 15
    surface fluorescence, 11—12, 28, 46
Autoantibodies, 92—96
Autoimmune diseases, 95—104
Autoimmune thyroiditis, 105
Autoimmunity, 91—111
Autologous mixed lymphocyte reaction (AMLR),
    54—58
Avidity of antibodies, 25

B

Backbone, 98
Bacterial infections, 14—16
Basophil degranulation, 5
Benzoquinonium chloride, 8
Binding assays, 27—28
Binding site, 151—152
    distribution of, 41—42
    linear map of, 29—41
Biochemical analysis, 121—122
    of T cell hybridoma MAF, 125—127
Biological activity inhibition by anti-Ia
    antibodies, 116—118
Biological effects of AEF, 115—116
Biological receptors, 8—11
Biology, developmental, 12
Blocking, 46
Bone marrow transplantation, 84
Breakdown fragments
    natural, 29
Breast cancer, 14
α-Bungarotoxin, 8, 96

C

Cancer, 14
Carbamylcholine, 8
Carcinoembryonic antigens, 14
Carcinoma of colon, 14
Cardiolipin, 94
Cell hybridization, 114, 115, 134
Cells
    activation of, 10
    differentiation of, 11
    heterogeneity among, 55—58
    Langerhans', 77
    mast, 5

red blood, 97
responder, 58—60
T, see T cells
target, 5
Cell surface components, 72
Cell surface marker identification, 11—12
CGG-specific ThF, 143
Characterization, 27—29
Cholinergic ligands, 8
α-Chymotrypsin, 33
Chymotrypsin PEC-MAP, 33
Clostripain, 35
Cold agglutinins, 92, 93
Collagenase PEC-MAP, 36
Colon carcinoma, 14
Complement components, 8
Components
    cell surface, 72
    complement, 8
Conformation restraints, 35
Construction of somatic cell hybrid, 115
Cross-reactive idiotypes, 95
Cytolysis, 5
Cytomegalovirus infection, 82

D

Deglycosylated gp70, 28—29, 35
Degranulation, 5
Denatured (single-stranded) DNA, 98
Determinants
    idiotypic, 95
    V_H surface, 139—143
Developmental biology, 12
Development of embryo, 12
Diabetes, 10
Diagnostic uses of mAbs, 12—16, 83
Differentiation
    antigen, 24, 72
    cell, 11, 135
    lymphocyte, 80—81
    of T cells, 135
2,4-Dinitrophenyl (DNP), 2, 93
Diseases, see also specific diseases
    experimental autoimmune, 95—104
    graft-vs.-host, 84
    Graves', 104
    infectious, see Infections
Distribution
    of antibody-binding sites, 41—42
    of enzyme-cleavage sites, 41—42
Diversity of molecules, 24
DNA, 93
    denatured (single-stranded), 98
    messenger, 12
    native (double-stranded), 98
    recombinant, 12
DNA-histone, 94
DNP, see 2,4-Dinitrophenyl
Domains, 38
    localization of, 38—41
Double-stranded DNA, see Native DNA

Drosophila melanogaster, 11

E

Ecotropic viruses, 28, 46
Eels, 8, 96
Elastase, 34
ELISA, see Enzyme-linked immunosorbent assay
ELMIA, see Enzyme-linked monoclonal antibody
        inhibition assay
Embryo development, 12
Endogenous ecotropic virus of AKR mice
        (AKV2), 28
Endogenous gp70 expression, 25
Enrichment of activated T lymphocytes, 135—137
Enzyme assays, 4, 5, 15, 16
Enzyme-cleavage site distribution, 41—42
Enzyme-linked immunosorbent assay (ELISA), 4,
        linked monoclonal antibody inhibition
        assay (ELMIA), 15
Epitopes, 95
ER, see Estrogen receptor
E rosette receptor, 74
Erythroleukemias, 46
Escherichia coli, 8, 11
Estrogen receptor (ER), 14
Experimental autoimmune diseases, 95—104
Experimental models of SLE, 97—103
Experimental myasthenia gravis, 96—97
Expression of endogenous gp70, 25

F

Fauscher retrovirus, 46
FcR, see Fc receptors
Fc receptors (FcR), 4, 5
    Ig, 9—10
α-Fetoprotein (AFP), 13
Fluorescence assays, 28
F-MuLV, see Friend virus
Fragment breakdown, 29
Friend retrovirus, 46
Friend virus (F-MuLV), 28
Functional hybridomas, 113—132, 137—138
Fusion and immunization, 25—26

G

β-Galactosidase, 7—8
GBS, see Group B streptococcus
Gene products of MHC, 152
Generation
    of mAbs, 72—73
    of T cell hybridomas, 135—138
Genetic restriction of T cell factor activity,
        158—159
G_{IX}^-, 25, 26
Glycoproteins, 13
    gp70, see gp70

Glycosidic residues, 42
Glycosylation, 28—29, 42—44
gp70
    breakdown products of, 29
    deglycosylated, 28—29, 35
    endogenous expression of, 25
    heterogeneity of, 48
    retroviral, 24
    tertiary structure of, 41—49
Graffi, 48
Graft-vs.-host disease, 84
Graves' disease, 104
Group B streptococcal (GBS) antigen, 15
Growth hormone, 13

H

HA_1, 44
HA_2, 44
Haptenic groups, 148—150
HAT, see Hypoxanthine-aminopterin-thymidine
HB, see Hepatitis B
V_H determinants, 139—143
Heavy chains of Ig, 48
Helper factor, 160
    T cell antigen-specific, see T cell antigen-
    specific helper factor
(T,G)-A--L-specific, 138—139
Helper/inducer T cell subset, 75—76
Hemolytic anemia, 97
Hepatitis B (HB), 82
    immunodiagnosis of, 14—15
Heterogeneity
    among cells, 55—60
    among responder cells, 58—60
    of gp70, 48
HGG, see Human gamma globulin
HGH, see Human growth hormone
Homologies, 48
Hormones, human growth, 13
HRS, 48
Human gamma globulin (HGG), 144
Human growth hormone (HGH), 13
Hybridization of somatic cells, 114, 115, 134
Hypersensitivity reactions, 2
Hypogammaglobulinemia, 82
Hypoxanthine-aminopterin-thymidine (HAT), 26

I

Ia antigens, 78
Ia-bearing T cell factors, 155—157
Identification of cell surface markers, 11—12
Idiotypes
    analysis of, 104—105
    cross-reactive, 95
    determinant of, 95
IF, see Interferon
IgE, 2—5
IgE protein, 4

Ig FcR, 9—10
Ig heavy chains, 48
Immune precipitation, 28—29
Immunization and fusion, 25—26
Immunoassay for streptococcal antigen, 15
Immunodeficiencies, 81
Immunodiagnosis, 14—16
Immunofluorescence, 46
Immunogens, 25
Immunological responses, 134
Immunology, 11
Immunoregulatory factors, 113—132
Immunosuppressive agents, 83
Immunotherapeutic agents, 105—106
Inactivating mAbs, 7
Infections, see also specific infections, 82
    bacterial, 14—16
    cytomegalovirus, 82
    hepatitis B, 82
    parasitic, 14—16
    viral, 14—16
Infectious mononucleosis, 82
Influenza, 44
Inhibition of biological activity by anti-Ia
    antibodies, 116—118
Initial characterization, 27—29
Insulin, 10
Insulinomimetic mAbs, 10
Insulin-resistant diabetes, 10
Interactions
    regulatory, 78—80
    sites of for T cell factor, 159—162
Interferon (IF), 6, 7, 73
Isoelectric points, 99

K

Kidney transplants, 84

L

Langerhans' cells, 77
Leukemia, 81, 82
Leukemogenic retroviruses, 24
Ligands, 8, 93
Linear map of binding sites, 29—41
Listeria monocytogenes, 122, 124
Localization of domains, 38—41
Lupus, 97—103
Lymphocytes, 5
    activated T, 135—137
    differentiation of, 80—81
    T, see T cells
Lymphokines, 114
Lymphomas, 135
    T cell, 46

M

Macrophages, 5

Mφ activating factor (MAF), 122—127
  production of by T cell hybridoma, 124—127
  T cell hybridoma, 125—127
MAF, see Mφ activating factor
Malaria parasites, 15
Mast cell degranulation, 5
Maturation of T cells, 80
MCF, see Mink cell foci
Mechanisms of T cell factor activity, 158—162
Melanoma, 14
Membrane proteins, 13
Mesocestoides corti, 16
Messenger DNA, 12
Metastatic breast cancer, 14
Mice, 28, 48, 97—99
  tumors in, 46
Mink cell foci (MCF), 46
Mitogenic activity, 73
Mixed lymphocyte reaction (MLR), 54—58
MLR, see Mixed lymphocyte reaction
M-MuLV, see Moloney virus
Molecular diversity of multigene families of
    proteins, 24
Molecular structure
  of retroviral glycoprotein gp70, 24
  of T cell factors, 152—155
Moloney (MP2) peptide maps, 48
Moloney retrovirus, 46
Moloney tumors, 46
Moloney virus (M-MuLV), 28
Monoclonal autoantibodies
  in experimental autoimmune disease, 95—96
  spontaneously occurring, 92—95
Monocytes, 5
Mononucleosis, 82
Monospecificity, 8
Multigene families of proteins, 24
Multiple recombinational events, 48
Multiprotein complexes, 11
Murine IgE, 2—5
Murine retroviruses, 28
Myasthenia gravis, 9
  experimental, 96—97
Myoblasts, 12

N

Native (double-stranded) DNA, 98
Natural breakdown fragments, 29
Neurobiology, 12
Neuroblastoma, 14
Nonlineage specific antibodies, 77—78
Nonspecific immunoregulatory factors, 113—132
Nuclear medicine, 14
Nucleic acids, 98
Null mAbs, 7

O

OA, see Ovalbumin

Oligonucleotides, 98
Ovalbumin (OA), 2
Ovalbumin-specific murine IgE antibody, 2

P

p15e-binding sites, 44—46
Pan T cell antibodies, 73—75
Parasites, 15
Parasitic infections, 14—16
Passive cutaneous anaphylaxis (PCA) test, 2
Pathogenicity of antiAChR antibodies, 9
Patient-imaging technique, 14
PCA, see Passive cutaneous anaphylaxis
PEC-MAP, 32, 35
  chymotrypsin, 33
  collagenase, 36
  trypsin, 35
  V8 protease, 37
Penicillinase, 34
Peptides, 13
  mapping of, 29—30
Phagocytosis by macrophages, 5
Phospholipids, 99
Polynucleotides, 98
Polypeptide antigens, 147—148
Polyprotein, 46
Precipitation, 28—29
Precursor protein, 46
Preleukemic thymocytes, 46
Protease PEC-MAP, 37
Protecting mAbs, 7
Protein antigens, 144—146
Proteins, 13
  IgE, 4
  membrane, 13
  multigene families of, 24
  precursor, 46
  purification of, 6—7
  ribosomal, 11
  soluble, 5—11
  structure of, 24
Proteolytic attack, 41
Purification, 24
  ease of, 12
  of proteins, 6—7

R

R-9-derived ThF, 140—141
Radioallergosorbent test (RAST), 16
Radioimmunoassay (RIA) 4—6, 13, 14
RAST, see Radioallergosorbent test
Rauscher-derived recombinant (R-MCF), 28
Rauscher MCF retrovirus, 46
Rauscher (R319) peptide maps, 48
Rauscher virus, 27—28
Reactivities, 30
  against retroviruses, 46—49
Receptors, 5—11

acetylcholine, 8—9, 96
biological, 8—11
E rosette, 74
estrogen, 14
Fc, see Fc receptors
T cell factors and, 157—158
transferrin, 78
TSH, 104
Recombination, 12, 24
multiple, 48
Rauscher-derived, 28
Red blood cell antibodies, 97
Regulatory interactions between T cell subsets,
78—80
Renal transplants, 84
Residues of glycosides, 42
Responder cell heterogeneity, 58—60
Restraints in conformation, 35
Retroviral glycoprotein gp70, 24
Retroviruses, see also Viruses
AKV2, 46
Fauscher, 46
Friend, 46
leukemogenic, 24
Moloney, 46
murine, 28
Rauscher MCF, 46
reactivity against, 46—49
Rheumatoid factors, 92
RIA, see Radioimmunoassay
Ribosomal proteins, 11
R-MCF, see Rauscher-derived recombinant
RNA, 98

S

Schistosome, 16
Secretion of AEF, 116—118
Self-gene products, 54
Self-recognition, 66
Single-stranded DNA, 98
Sites
antibody-binding, 41—42, 151—152
enzyme-cleavage, 41—42
of interaction of T cell factor, 159—162
p15e-binding, 44—46
SLE, see Systemic lupus erythematosus
Sm antigen, 102
Soluble proteins, 5—11
structure-function relationship of, 7—8
Somatic cell hybridization, 114, 115, 134
Specific antibodies to parasites, 15
Specificity, 6, 12, 15, 24, 25
Specific T-helper cell function, 138—144
Spermatogenesis, 12
Spontaneously occurring monoclonal
autoantibodies, 92—95
SRBC, 144—146
Steric blocking, 46
Streptococcal antigens, 15
Streptococcus group B, 15

Structure-function relationships
among lymphokines, 114
biological receptors, 8—11
soluble proteins, 7—8
Structures
gp70, 41—49
molecular, 24
protein, 24
Subsets of T cells, 72, 76—80
Sugar-phosphate backbone, 98
Suppressor/cytotoxic T cell subset, 76—77
Suppressor factors, 144—150
antigen-specific, 160
T cell, see T cell suppressor factor
Surface antigens, 15
Surface components of cells, 72
Surface markers of cells, 11—12, 28, 46
Surface V_H determinants, 139—143
Synthetic polypeptide antigens, 147—148
Systemic lupus erythematosus (SLE), 97—103

T

Taenia hydatigena, 16
Target cells, 5
T cell antigen defined by mAbs, 73—78
T cell antigen-specific helper factor (ThF), 138,
144
CGG-specific, 143
R-9-derived, 140—141
T cell differentiation antigens, 72
T cell factors, 151—162
receptors and, 157—158
T cell growth factor (TCGF), 118—122
production of, 119—122
properties of, 118—119
T cell hybridomas, 113—132, 135—138
T cell leukemias, 82
T cell lymphomas, 46
T cell replacing factor (TRF), 138
T cells, 12, 46, 72, 73—80, 82, 83, 135, 144—162
activated, 135—137
differentiation stage of, 135
function of, 60—65, 138—144
helper type, 138—144
maturation of, 80
pan antibodies of, 73—75
subsets of, 72, 75—80
T cell suppressor factor (TsF), 138, 148—150
specificity of to protein antigens, 144—146
TCGF, see T cell growth factor
Tertiary structure of gp70, 41—49
Tests, see specific tests; Assays
(T,G)-A--L-specific helper factor, 138—139
Theileria, 16
Therapeutic applications, 83—84
ThF, see T cell antigen-specific helper factor
Thrombasthenia, 13
Thryoglobulin, 105
Thymocytes, 46
Thymocyte specific antibodies, 77

Thymus, 80
Thyroiditis, 105
Thyrotropin (TSH), 104
  receptors of, 104
Torpedo eel (*Torpedo californica*), 8, 96
Toxoplasma gondii, 16, 122
Transferrin receptor, 78
Transformation, 49
  viral, 134
Transplantation, 83
  bone marrow, 84
  renal, 84
TRF, see T cell replacing factor
Trypanosoma cruzi, 122
Trypanosoma sp., 16
Trypsin PEC-MAP, 35
TsF, see T cell suppressor factor
TSH, see Thyrotropin
Tumors
  AKR, 46
  immunodiagnosis of, 14

Moloney, 46

V

V8 protease PEC-MAP, 37
V_H determinants, 139—143
Viruses, see also Retroviruses
  ecotropic, 46
  endogenous ecotropic, 28
  Friend, 28
  immunodiagnosis of, 14—16
  Moloney, 28
  Rauscher, 27—28
  transformation of, 134

X

Xenotropic sequences, 46